ERG, VER and Psychophysics

Documenta Ophthalmologica
Proceedings Series volume 13

Editor H. E. Henkes

Dr. W. Junk bv Publishers The Hague 1977

ERG, VER and Psychophysics
14th I. S. C. E. R. G. Symposium
Louisville, Kentucky, USA,
May 10-14, 1976

Edited by Theodore Lawwill

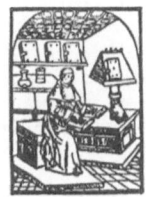

Dr. W. Junk bv Publishers The Hague 1977

Cover design: Max Velthuijs

© Dr W. Junk b.v. Publishers 1977

Softcover reprint of the hardcover 1st edition 1977

ISBN 978-94-010-1314-7   e-ISBN-13: 978-94-010-1312-3
DOI: 10.1007978-94-010-1312-3

CONTENTS

Electroretinography and Psychophysics

Electroretinography-Clinical Correlations

INTRODUCTION

In Dedication to Hermann Burian (1906-1974)

T. LAWWILL

(Louisville)

This 14th Symposium of the International Society for Clinical Electroretinography is dedicated to the memory of a great ophthalmologist, great physiologist, former officer of this Society, and my professor, Hermann Martin Burian.

Dr. Burian was a visual physiologist and an ophthalmologist. His physiology heritage was the finest. His father, Richard, was an eminent European physiologist who at the time of Dr. Burian's birth was director of the Stazione Zoologica in Naples.

The family later moved to Leipzig and Belgrade, where Dr. Burian's father held professorships.

Hermann Burian's ophthalmological academic heritage was also outstanding. After graduating from medical school in 1930 in Belgrade, he became a student of Tschermak and along the way worked with such famous men as Siegrist, Goldmann and Weigert.

In 1936, Dr. Burian came to the USA to join the Dartmouth Eye Institute. Here he worked in ocular motility under Professor Bielschowsky and in physiological optics under Professor Ames. He was chief ophthalmologist of the Darmouth Eye Institute from 1942-45. He was in the private practice of ophthalmology in Boston for six years before moving to Iowa City, Iowa where, for twenty years, he practiced and taught ophthalmology and carried out research on many problems in ophthalmology and visual physiology.

Dr. Burian's two main interests were strabismus and electrophysiology, but this did not keep him from publishing outstanding work on glaucoma, congenital anomalies, and color vision.

Of his over 200 publications, at least 30 had to do with electrophysiology. In 1952, he published on 'The Cerebral Electrical Response to Intermittent Photopic Stimulation in Amblyopia Ex Anopsia'. The initial reason for his electrophysiological studies was to have a tool to study visual processing in the amblyopia of strabismus. By 1953, his interest in ERG was much wider, as shown by his publication 'Electroretinography and Its Clinical Applications'.

Dr. Burian was always able to apply his broad knowledge to clinical problems. He did not gather knowledge for knowledge's sake, but for the good of mankind.

From his first publication, together with his sister, a Serbo-Croatian-Ger-

1

man dictionary commonly referred to locally as a 'Burian', and his third publication 'The Treatment of Tuberculosis with Fatty Substances' to his book published posthumously with von Noorden, the common theme of clinical applicability can be seen.

To leave out the remembrance of Dr. Burian's personality would be to leave out a most important part of his effectiveness. Dr. Burian was a culturally educated man who loved people. It was often that he could be located in a gathering at ISCERG by his convivial laughter ringing out above the noise of the crowd. When he was located he would be conversing simultaneously in three of his five languages and simultaneously translating for each member of the group.

Dr. Burian's enthusiasm was unending and infectious. In the six months he spent in my laboratory in 1973, he completely won everyone's heart and added an interest which accelerated our work manyfold.

Dr. Burian's often stated hope for ISCERG was that it would be truly international and truly clinical. This reflects Dr. Burian: he was truly international, truly clinical, and truly an energetic and productive scientist.

I am happy that Dr. Burian's Widow, Mrs. Gladys Burian Else, can be with us today to see her many old friends among the group and to share this remembrance of Dr. Burian who meant so much to many of us.

THE CORRELATION OF ELECTROPHYSIOLOGICAL AND PSYCHOPHYSICAL MEASURES: VECP

LORRIN A. RIGGS

(Providence, Rhode Island)

ABSTRACT

Electrical responses to visual stimulation are conveniently recorded without risk to human subjects: from the eye, by the use of a contact lens electrode; and from the brain, by electrodes appropriately located on the scalp.

The VECP originates from the massed activity of large numbers of cortical neurons. Individual impulse (spike) potentials do not appear on scalp electrodes because of the severe attenuation of any such signals by the intervening dura, bone and skin tissues that have a high electrical impedance. It is thus the pre- and post-synaptic graded potentials of brain cells, perhaps with the participation of glial cells, that are most likely to generate the complex series of waves that appear in the typical VECP record.

Single flash procedures, once used almost exclusively in visual electrophysiology, are now yielding to more complex methods of stimulus presentation.

No simple comparison can be made between a subject's report of what he sees and the VECP waves that arise from the same visual stimuli. The subjective report can describe, for example, the appearance of such complex stimuli as letters of the alphabet, people's faces, or a landscape extending off into the distance. There is no way in which gross electrodes can differentiate among the effects of such detailed visual scenes. Nor is there any likelihood that the VECP can rival psychophysical methods for detecting stimuli that are so small that they activate only a few receptors and neural conducting units.

Despite the limitations just mentioned, the VECP has often been shown to provide reliable measurements of certain parameters of visual performance.

In summary, the VECP can be used to supplement or replace subjective methods of experimental and clinical evaluations of certain visual functions. Some limitations on the sensitivity of VECP methods have been overcome, but not those due to indirectness and diffuseness of conduction from active cortical sites to the electrodes on the surface of the scalp. Psychophysical procedures are therefore still needed, but their validity is enhanced by the adoption of forced-choice or other relatively bias-free methods of observation. The correlation between VECP and psychophysical measures is highest where the signal-to-noise ratio of each can be enhanced by application of the new advances in signal detection theory.

Electrical responses to visual stimulation are conveniently recorded without risk to human subjects: from the eye, by the use of a contact lens electrode; and from the brain, by electrodes appropriately located on the scalp. Fig. 1 summarizes these connections and the resulting electroretinogram (ERG) and visually evoked cortical potential (VECP) waves. Armington (see below) will describe the relation of the ERG to human psychophysical data, and the present paper is concerned with the VECP.

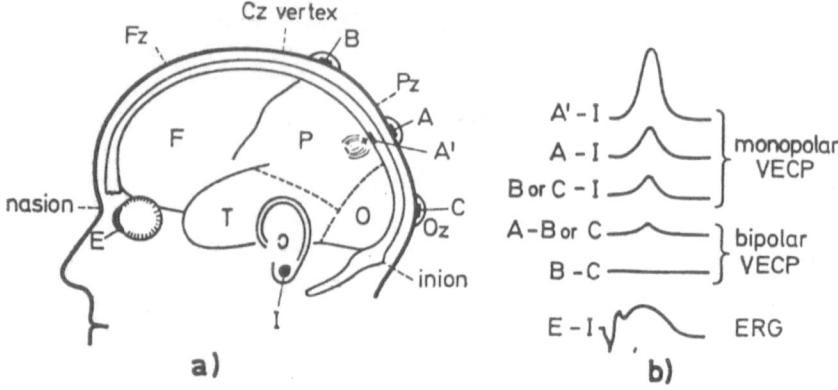

Fig. 1. a) Placement of electrodes for recording the ERG and VECP from from a human subject.

b) Hypothetical VECP to a simple source-sink transient at A', as it would appear if recorded from the designated electrode pairs; and ERG recorded with contact lens electrode at E. (Adapted from Riggs & Wooten, 1972).

ORIGIN OF THE VECP

No brief account of the VECP can give an adequate description of the relationships between the underlying brain cell responses and the response potential waves that are actually recorded between electrodes at particular locations on the scalp. The following are generalizations that have some support on evidence reviewed at greater length in recent summaries of the literature (Riggs & Wooten, 1972; Regan, 1972; Mackay & Jeffreys, 1973).

The VECP originates from the massed activity of large numbers of cortical neurons. Individual impulse (spike) potnetials do not appear on scalp electrodes because of the severe attenuation of any such signals by the intervening dura, bone and skin tissues that have a high electrical impedance. It is thus the pre- and post-synaptic graded potentials of brain cells, perhaps with the participation of glial cells, that are most likely to generate the complex series of waves that appear in the typical VECP record.

Problems of recording the VECP

The diffuseness of the conductance path from the cortex to the scalp electrodes is such that localization of the source is rather imprecise. Thus, in Fig. 1, a source of potential at point A' or at any other neighboring point on the cortex may equally well impress a voltage change upon a scalp electrode shown at C with reference to an indifferent electrode on the earlobe at I. Still another difficulty is that 'unwanted' activity is always present with the use of such gross, remote electrodes. Muscle and skin tissue, for example, may produce electrical 'noise' that is relatively well conducted to the electrodes, as are the spontaneous EEG waves from the brain itself. Each of

4

these extraneous sources may contribute potential waves in the same frequency band as the VECP signals; and the amplitudes of these waves may reach 50 to 100 μv. Thus, the 'raw' VECP record shows no possibility of isolating the stimulus-generated responses, the most interesting of which seldom exceed 15 μv. This seemingly hopeless situation, which prevailed until about 15 years ago, has yielded to the following technical advances.

1. Signal-averaging computers: A large number of VECP responses are cumulated, and the computer is time-locked to the onset of each visual stimulus. It then cumulates, stores and displays the algebraic average of potentials existing between the input electrodes at successive times following the stimulus onset. The noise components tend to manifest randomly occurring positive and negative deviations from the baseline as the averaging process continues; while the stimulus-generated VECP tends to built up consistently positive and negative waves at characteristic latent times after the stimulus onset. Thus the 'noise' averages out, and the shape of the VECP signal emerges more and more clearly throughout the process of cumulation. From 64 to 256 cumulations are typically needed for adequate display of the VECP waveform. Additional circuits can be used to display the variability or other statistical parameters, in addition to the average response potential wave.

2. Electronic filters: Low-pass and high-pass filters are typically used in the input to the amplifier. Thus the extremely low-frequency potentials such as the slow drift of electrode contact potentials and the electrodermal changes are excluded, as are also the irrelevant high-frequency effects such as voltage line transients and switching artifacts.

3. Lock-in amplifiers: These devices are particularly successful when used with stimuli at medium to high repetition rates. They give rapid indications of the amplitude of a response potential wave when the device is tuned to the fundamental frequency (or a harmonic of the frequency) of the stimulus. They are thus a viable alternative or adjunct to the average response computer when the complete waveform information is not needed. Furthermore, they can also indicate, by a vector analysis principle, the phase lag of the response waves with respect to the stimulus cycle.

Topological factors

'Monopolar' recording (see Fig. 1) involves a single electrode near the site of generation of the signals of interest. Potentials between this 'active' electrode and a remote 'indifferent' electrode then reflect to the greatest degree those voltages originating near the active one. The indifferent one is often placed on a site, such as the ear lobe, in which little muscular or other biological noise is present. In 'bipolar' recording, two electrodes are placed within the active zone in order to maximize the amplification of signals generated in the region lying immediately between them. The bipolar electrodes may, for example, be placed over the right hemisphere in an attempt to exclude responses generated in the left. However, this attempt is only partially successful because of the diffuse electrical conduction paths as mentioned above. Multipolar arrays of electrodes have been used, together

5

with computer processing, to permit an estimate of the lateral and longitudinal locations of points in the brain from which various VECP waves originate. In the most elaborate studies of this kind isopotential maps have been developed for a two-dimensional display of this information, and in some cases the temporal sequence has been indicated by the use of time-lapse computer-generated plots.

Potential maps obtained from multipolar arrays confirm the fact that particularly strong VECP signals are generated in each hemisphere near the occipital pole at the O_z location (see Fig. 1). This is consistent with the fact that, in man, this represents the primary visual projection area, on striate cortex, of pathways originating in the macular region of the retina. A small test stimulus typically produces VECP waves of maximum amplitude when delivered to the central fovea (Potts & Nagaya, 1965). Larger and larger responses are produced as the size of the centrally fixated spot is increased up to about 5° to 10° in diameter. Further increases in size produce little additional amplitude of VECP. However, these generalizations have numerous exceptions because (a) there are individual differences of brain anatomy between subjects (b) upper and lower fields may evoke responses that differ in phase or polarity, thus partially cancelling one another (c) light scatters widely beyond the focal region with high-intensity spots of small area (d) patterned and chromatic stimuli may evoke VECP waves that differ in origin and waveform from white flash stimuli; in particular, it may be that complex stimuli activate particular classes of responding units in striate and extrastriate regions of the occipital and parietal cortex. A further generalization is that the VECP, in contrast to the ERG, is much better correlated with photopic than with scotopic visual activity and exhibits much more selective responding to the contour, motion and color aspects of the stimulus field. Only with specially chosen experimental conditions it is possible to obtain VECP records originating from the scoptic visual system (Wooten, 1972).

METHODS OF STIMULATING THE VECP

Single flash procedures, once used almost exclusively in visual electrophysiology, are now yielding to more complex methods of stimulus presentation. The advantage of this is that separate visual functions can thereby be isolated. Among these are photopic vs. scotopic activity, chromatic vs. luminance responses, contrast sensitivity functions, binocular interactions, and spatial and temporal resolution. These require correspondingly complex systems of optical stimulation and data processing; hence they have not yet been widely adapted for clinical electrophysiology.

Stimulus alternation procedures

Of greatest importance is the principle of phase alternation. This was first introduced as a means of minimizing stray light effects in ERG recording (Riggs, Johnson & Schick, 1964) but has since become widely adopted in VECP experiments (Riggs, 1974).

6

Fig. 2 illustrates some of the principal stimulus patterns: In each case the observer fixates near the center of the pattern, and the stripes or checks of the pattern undergo periodic alternation. Thus each point in the retinal field is alternately exposed to each element of the pattern. Checkerboard targets produce large VECP waves, and hence are used for clinical investigation of localized field defects, errors of refraction, and circulatory disorders.

Transient stimulation of the VECP

Fig. 3 illustrates s series of records from an unpublished VECP study by Robert Moore. (Moore, 1976) The stimulus is a sinusoidal grating pattern. The pattern is generated on the face of a cathode ray oscilloscope, momentarily replacing a homogeneous field of equal liminance. Note that the amplitude goes down and the implicit time rises as the stimulus contrast is diminished. Figs. 4 & 5 contain measurements of these two functions. They confirm the fact that implicit time measures yield more reliable data than do amplitude measures with the method of transient stimuli (Vaughan, Costa & Gilden, 1966).

Periodic stimulation of the VECP

This method is most efficient for research in which lock-in amplifiers or response-averaging computers are employed to process the data.

Typically, one of the stimulus configurations in Fig. 2 is used with phase alternation at a frequency from 2 to 25 hz. Waveform information is lost, but large-sample mean amplitudes are reliably obtained. The usefulness of this method has been shown in studies of contrast sensitivity as a function of spatial frequency, blurring of vision due to refractive error, comparative studies of human and animal vision, and evidences of binocular rivalry and suppression.

CORRELATIONS BETWEEN THE VECP AND PSYCHOPHYSICS

No simple comparison can be made between a subject's report of what he sees and the VECP waves that arise from the same visual stimuli. The subjective report can describe, for example, the appearance of such complex stim-

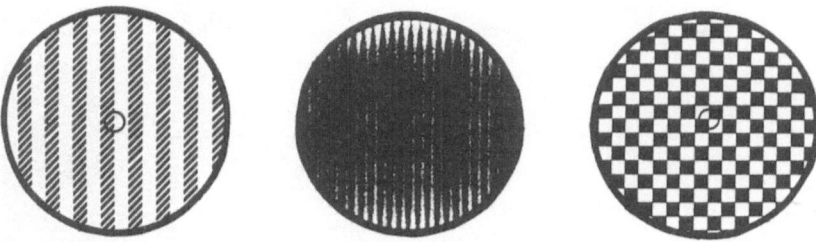

Fig. 2. Three types of pattern used in stimulating the eye with phase-alternation: Square-wave grating, sine-wave grating and checkerboard (Adapted from Riggs, 1974).

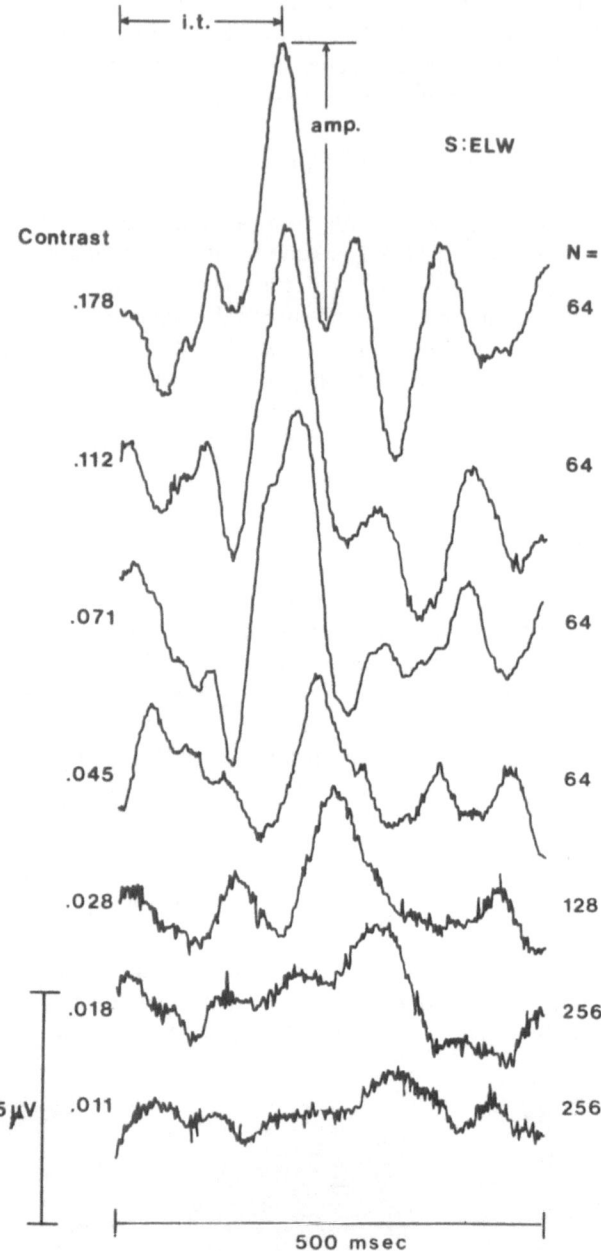

Fig. 3. Series of VECP records in response to transient presentations of sinusoidal grating at the various contrast levels indicated at left. Note the increase of implicit time (i.t.) and decrease of amplitude as contrast is reduced (Moore, 1976).

8

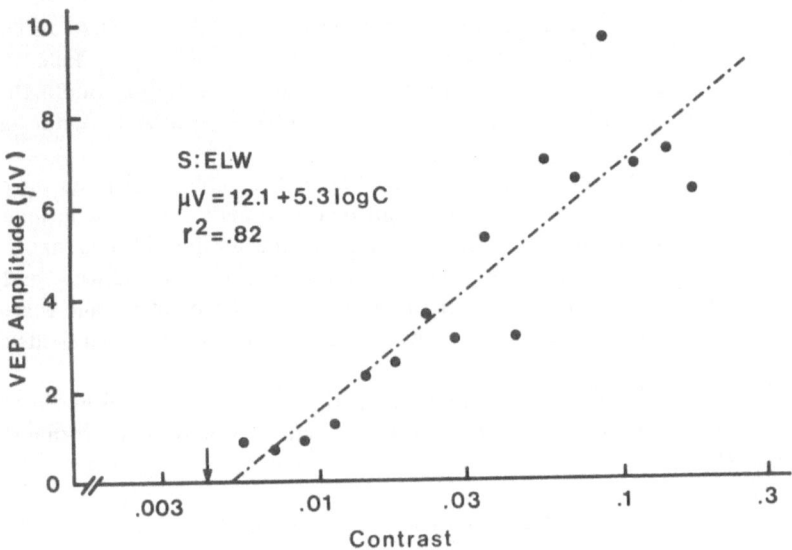

Fig. 4. Measured amplitudes of VECP as a function of contrast. Arrow denotes psychophysical contrast threshold for the same subject (Moore, 1976).

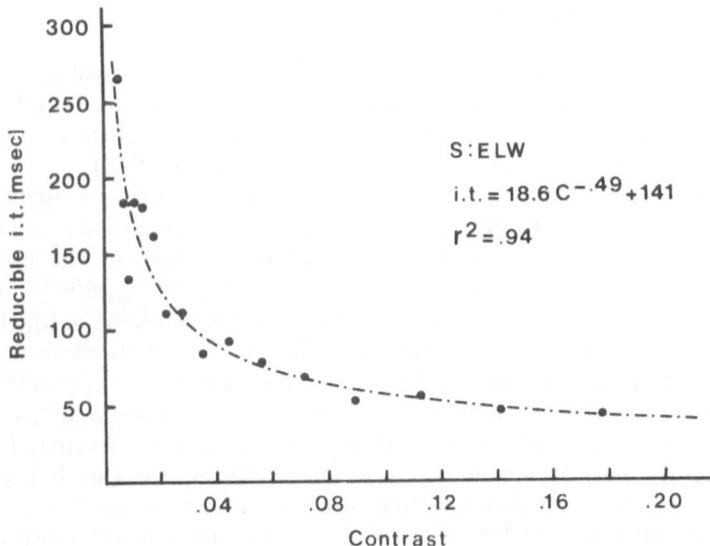

Fig. 5. A good fit ($r^2 = .94$) is provided by an equation in which an asymptote of 141 msec is taken to be the irreducible portion of i.t. for this subject (Moore, 1976).

uli as letters of the alphabet, people's faces, or a landscape extending off into the distance. There is no way in which gross electrodes can differentiate among the effects of such detailed visual scenes. Nor is there any likelihood that the VECP can rival psychophysical methods for detecting stimuli that are so small that they activate only a few receptors and neural conducting units.

Another limitation of the VECP is that it can only reveal transient or periodically changing responses; it cannot record directly the long-continued viewing of a steady pattern or afterimage. Still another limitation is that the VECP emphasizes cortical responses that take place at a relatively early stage of processing within the primary areas of visual projection, and that it also represents most heavily the activation of foveal and parafoveal fields of vision.

Despite the limitations just mentioned, the VECP has often been shown to provide reliable measurements of certain parameters of visual performance (Riggs, 1976).

Methodological comparisons

Finally, certain comparisons of methodology can be made between VECP recording and psychophysics. First, a raw measure of response amplitude in the VECP may conceivably be compared with psychophysical magnitude estimation. But both are nonlinear, and generally unreliable means of scaling the effects of visual stimulation. Thus, for example, one obtains only a qualitative and unreliable measure of spectral sensitivity by presenting the subject with equal-energy stimuli at all wavelengths and measuring the amplitude of VECP, meanwhile asking him to give estimates of the brightness. Much better, and more likely to yield comparable results, is to determine for each wavelength, the energy necessary to produce a criterion amplitude of VECP; or to reach a certain probability that the subject will detect the stimulus in a psychophysical judgment situation. Best of all are procedures arising out of the development, in electronic engineering, of the theory and practice of signal detection (Green & Swets, 1966; Egan, 1975).

Here, the basic concept is that a receiver operates to detect a stimulating 'signal' against a fluctuating background of 'noise'. Receiver operating characteristic (ROC) curves can be constructed on the basis of test trials in which noise alone, or signal plus noise, are present. The sensitivity of the receiver is computed on the basis of results from this procedure in which the percentages of correct and incorrect identifications are tabulated for various stimulus intensities. In the VECP case this typically involves cumulating a sufficient number of response potential waves so that a minimum signal is determined. The average amplitude is then reliably greater in response to the signal plus noise than in cumulations where no signal is present. In psychophysics, the analogous determination of a minimum signal is made by tabulating the percentage of 'yes' judgments that the subject makes when noise alone is present ('false alarms') and when various intensities of signal are present ('hits'). From these results ROC curves may be plotted and values of d' (discriminability index) computed. A simplified version is the well-known 'forced-choice' procedure of psychophysics. The great advantage of all these new psychophysical procedures is that they largely do away with the troublesome variations of threshold due to changes of observer criterion and bias. They should therefore replace the classical methods of psychophysics for research purposes and, ideally, for clinical evaluations as well.

The psychophysical procedure of reaction time measurement is analogous to the implicit time measurements that have been described for the VECP (Vaughan, Costa & Gilden, 1966). In each case, curves relating latent time of response to stimulus intensity are plotted. A criterion latency is then selected, and sensitivity is stated in terms of the reciprocal of stimulus energy necessary to meet the criterion in either the electrical (VECP) or psychophysical (threshold) situation.

CONCLUSION

In summary, the VECP can be used to supplement or replace subjective methods of experimental and clinical evaluations of certain visual functions. Some limitations on the sensitivity of VECP methods have been overcome, but not those due to indirectness and diffuseness of conduction from active cortical sites to the electrodes on the surface of the scalp. Psychophysical procedures are therefore still needed, but their validity is enhanced by the adoption of forced-choice or other relatively bias-free methods of observation. The correlation between VECP and psychophysical measures is highest where the signal-to-noise ratio of each can be enhanced by application of the new advances in signal detection theory.

REFERENCES

Egan, J.P. Signal detection theory and ROC-analysis. New York: Academic Press, 1975.

Green, D.M. & Swets, J.A. Signal detection theory and psychophysics. New York: Wiley, 1966.

MacKay, D.M. & Jeffreys, D.A. Visually evoked potentials and visual perception in man. In Jung, R. [Ed.]. Central Visual Information B. Volume VII/3, Handbook of sensory physiology. Berlin: Springer, 1973.

Moore, R.K. Unpublished study of the VECP at the Hunter Laboratory of Psychology, Brown University, 1976.

Potts, A.M. & Nagaya, T. Studies on the visual evoked response. 1. The use of the 0.06 degree red target for evaluation of foveal function. *Invest. Ophth.*, 4, *303-309* (1965).

Regan, D. Evoked potentials in psychology, sensory physiology and clinical medicine. New York: Wiley, 1972.

Rietveld, W.J., Tordoir, W.E.M. & Duyff, J.W. Contribution of fovea and parafovea to the visual evoked response. *Acta physiol. pharm. Neerl.*, 13, *330-339* (1965).

Riggs, L.A., Johnson, E.P. & Schick, A.M.L. Electrical responses of the eye to moving stimulus patterns. *Science*, 144, *567* (1964).

Riggs, L.A. & Wooten, B.R. Electrical measures and psychophysical data of human vision. In Jameson, D. & Hurvich, L.M. [Eds]. Visual Psychophysics. Volume VII/4, Handbook of sensory physiology. Berlin: Springer, 1972.

Riggs, L.A. Responses of the visual system to fluctuating patterns. *Amer. J. Optom. & Physiol. Optics,* 51, *725-735* (1974).

Riggs, L.A. Human vision: some objective explorations. *Amer. Psychologist,* 31, *125-134* (1976).

Vaughan, H.G., Jr., Costa, L.D. & Gilden, L. The functional relation of visual evoked response and reaction time to stimulus intensity. *Vision Res.,* 6. *645-656* (1966).

Wooten, B.R. Photopic and scotopic contributions to the human visually evoked cortical potential. *Vision Research,* 12, *1647-1660,* (1972).

Author's address:
Walter S. Hunter Laboratory of Psychology
Brown University
Providence, Rhode Island 02912
USA

VISUAL ACUITY AND CHECKERBOARD POTENTIALS WITH DEFOCUSING LENSES

G. VAN LITH, W. VAN MARLE
G. BARTL & S. VIJFWINKEL-BRUININGA

(Rotterdam/Leyden/Graz)

INTRODUCTION

Mainly because of the topography of the visual cortex, the VECPs reflect to a large extent the function of the posterior pole (Van Lith & Henkes, 1970). This is not only the case for pattern evoked potentials, but also for luminance evoked potentials. Despite this, the latter give hardly any information about one of the main foveal functions, viz. the visual acuity. One of the reasons is that the evoked potentials are highly variable; another reason is that luminance evoked potentials and visual acuity represent two totally different functions, the former being a measure of light sensitivity whereas the latter also includes a contrast function. Cortical potentials evoked by a pattern stimulus represent both functions, luminance and contrast, in a variable relation depending on checksize and contrast between the checks.

From literature (Spekreijse, 1966; Rietveld et al., 1967; Harter, 1970) it is known that the smaller the checksize is and the less the contrast between the checks, the more the evoked potentials will be dominated by the contrast component and the more they will represent foveal function.

Conversely, the luminance component and perifoveal function will dominate the response, when large checks and high contrasts are used. This difference in representation of the pattern evoked potentials is very important when their measurement is applied for clinical purposes. It means that the smaller the checksize and the less the contrast, the more the response will correlate with, but will also be dependent on, visual acuity — whether its cause is a refractive error, media opacity, retinal abnormality or disturbance in the visual pathway.

This dependence can be investigated in patients with cataract or macular degenerations. Apart from this method, which would take several years to investigate, contour sharpness of the pattern can also be diminished with defocusing lenses. This influence of defocusing lenses has already been described in a number of papers (Spehlmann, 1965; Harter & White, 1968; Harter & White, 1970; Millodot & Riggs, 1970; Dawson, Perry & Childers, 1972; Arden & Lewis, 1973; Regan, 1973). Of these Harter & White (1970) use various checksizes. We wanted to know the influence of both the checksize and the contrast.

METHOD

Since optico-mechanical equipment or equipment using polaroid plates do not allow checksize and contrast to be easily altered, we built an electronic pattern generator, which controls a monochrome TV-monitor (van Marle & van Lith, in press). Such a system has already been demonstrated by Arden at the XIIIth Symposium of the ISCERG (Arden, 1977).

A pattern-reversal stimulus of 4.9 Hz and a flashed-pattern stimulus of 1.9 Hz and 40 msec duration were applied. For both stimuli the mean luminance was 120 asb. From a pilot study, we learned that with checksizes of 10′ subtense visual angle and a contrast of 10% or less the responses were much smaller than those obtained with larger checks and higher contrasts. Therefore, checksizes of 20′, 40′ and 80′ visual angle with 20%, 40% and 80% contrast respectively were used for further study. They will be labelled as 20′-20%, 40′-40% and 80′-80%.

After amplification, 128 responses were averaged. For the pattern reversal stimulation a bandpass filter tuned at 9.8 Hz (quality 3.5) was used; for the flashed pattern stimulation the bandwidth was 0.1-75 Hz (3db points). The electrode position in the midline which gave the highest response with reference to the ear was always used. Usually this was at the 5% or 15% position above the inion (10%-20% EEG system).

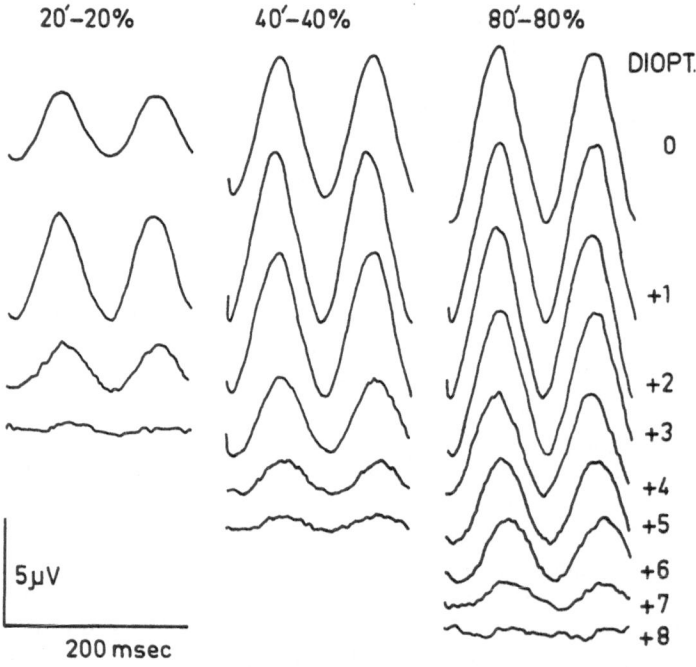

Fig. 1. Actual recordings of the visually evoked cortical potentials (VECPs) obtained with a pattern-reversal stimulus of various checksize (20′-40′-80′) and various contrast (20%-40%-80%) without (o) and with defocusing lenses (+1 till +8 Diopters) in front of the eye.

14

RESULTS

Figure 1 and 2 show the actual recordings of the VECPs obtained with pattern-reversal stimuli and flashed-pattern stimuli, respectively. The influence of the defocusing positive lenses is obvious in these recordings as well as in the graphs of figures 3 and 4. In figure 3 the amplitude of the sinusoidal evoked potentials is plotted versus the dioptric power of the defocusing lenses, in figure 4 at the left side the amplitude of the first positive peak of the flashed pattern evoked potentials and at the right side that of the negative peak. The positive peaks have been measured from the baseline, the negative peaks from the top of the positive peaks.

Using the pattern reversal stimulus (fig. 3) the 20'-20% response becomes nearly zero with +2.5 Diopters, the 40'-40% response with +5 Diopters and the 80'-80% response with +8 Diopters. It means that the larger the checks and the contrast are, the less the influence of defocusing and hence of refraction anomalies and perhaps also of media opacities, on the height of

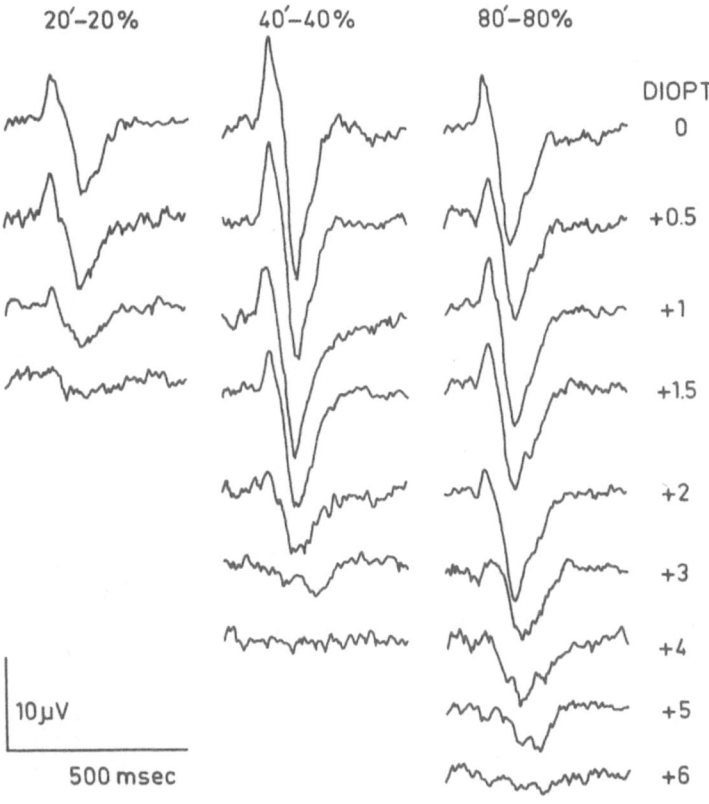

Fig. 2. Actual recording of the VECPs obtained with a flashed pattern stimulus. See also figure 1.

15

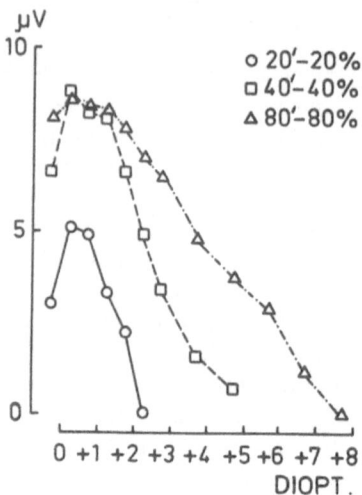

Fig. 3. Height of the pattern-reversal responses plotted against the dioptic power of defocusing lenses.

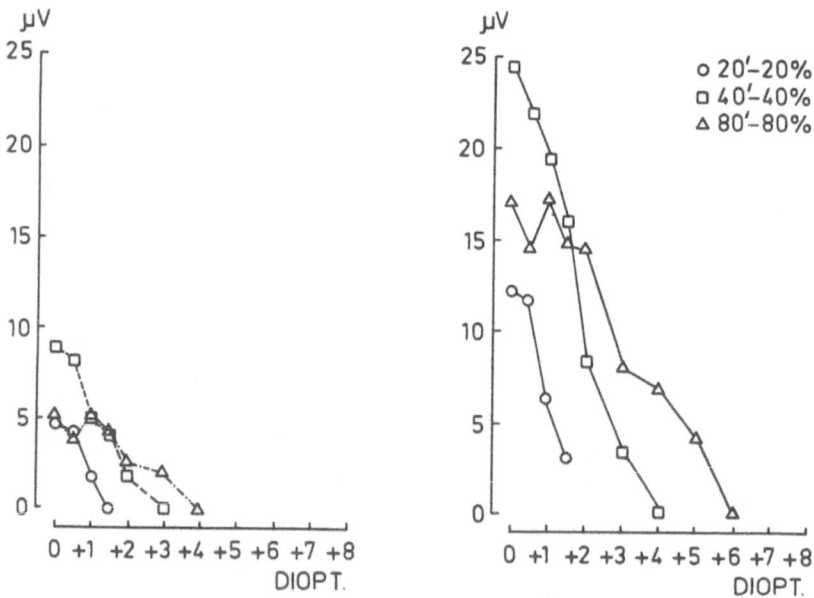

Fig. 4. Height of the positive peak (left) and negative peak (right) of a flashed-pattern response plotted against the dioptric power of defocusing lenses.

the response will be. This difference can possibly be used to differentiate between a group of abnormalities which diminish contour sharpness and other diseases. In neuritis, for example, we often see that the large check responses are equally lowered as compared with small check responses. Conversely, it is found that in amblyopia large check responses become even higher than those of the normal eye (Sokol & Bloom, 1973).

The difference in influence of the defocusing lenses is less for the negative peak of the flashed pattern response (fig. 4, right) and almost absent for the first positive peak (fig. 4, left). The latter has already become zero with +4 Diopters when evoked with the 80'-80% stimulus. This would mean that these responses are less suitable for a differential diagnosis as mentioned above.

From the experiments in this subject, two conclusions may be drawn, the first being that the influence of the defocusing lenses is less the larger the checksize and the greater the contrast. This was confirmed in 9 other subjects. The second conclusion is that the decrease of this influence with increasing checksize and contrast seems to be less in the negative peak of the flashed pattern response and is surely less in its positive peak. In the other subjects this second conclusion could only be confirmed as far as the positive peak is concerned and not for the negative peak. The results of the latter appeared to be the same as those of the pattern reversal stimulation.

Variability was rather high in our group of normal subjects and approximately the same for all stimulus parameters. With a 40'-40% reversal stimulus, the amplitudes of the responses without defocusing lenses ranged from $3\,\mu V$ to $10\,\mu V$, with a mean of $6.6\,\mu V$. Even when these values were put on a 100% basis, the variability with the lenses is rather high and much higher than those of the visual acuity. This is shown for the 20'-20% pattern reversal responses in figure 5. These responses, were chosen for comparison since they corresponded best with the decrease in the visual acuity.

The results of only 7 subjects are drawn in figure 5, the variability of the other three being even greater.

DISCUSSION

With our TV system the largest responses are found with 20' or 40' checks; with 10' checks the responses are always obviously lower. Spekreijse (1966) and Regan (Regan & Richards, 1971) found maximum responses with only 10' checks. The explanation for this difference may be that with a TV set as used by us the contour sharpness is less than that with the sophisticated mirror system of Spekreijse. In contradistinction to luminance evoked electroretinograms and cortical potentials, the pattern evoked cortical potentials obtained with small checksizes and contrast demonstrate a rather good correlation with visual acuity when defocusing lenses are used. Corresponding with visual acuity, however, they can contribute less to differential diagnosis if it is lowered. The use of checks of various sizes and contrasts may provide the solution, since diseases lowering the contour sharpness will influence small checksize responses much more than large checksize responses. This is very probably not the case in optic neuritis and in amblyopia. What happens

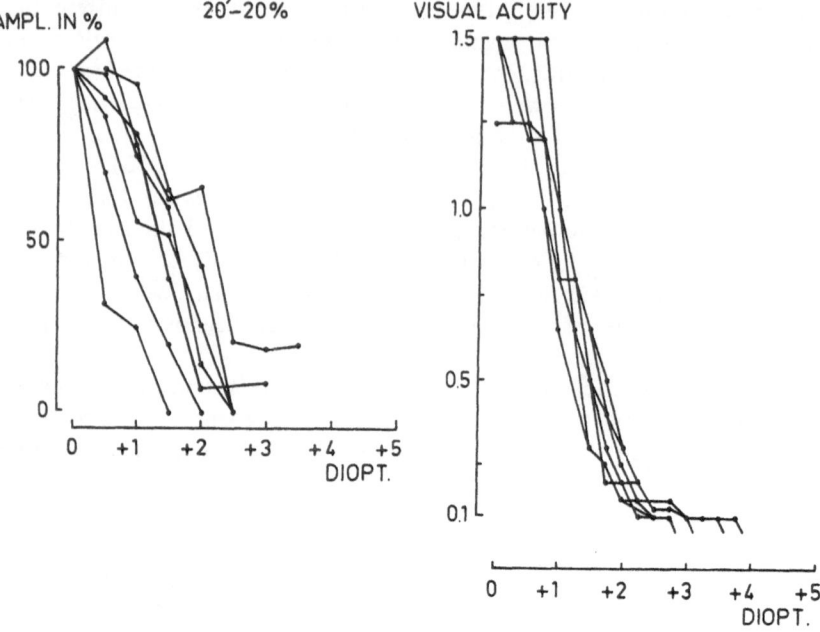

Fig. 5. Decrease of the visual acuity (right) and a 20'-20% pattern-reversal response with defocusing lenses obtained in 7 subjects.

in other diseases of the optic nerve and in macular diseases is still to be explored.

Since variability per individual was very small, comparison between a normal and a pathological eye in one person is feasible. Interindividual variability, on the other hand, is rather high. This, however, is only a problem when a lowered response is found and can be solved by investigating a large group of normal subjects. Then it must become possible to predict how large the chance is that a lowered response is found.

SUMMARY

Pattern evoked cortical potentials are influenced by defocusing lenses. This influence is less the larger the checksize is and the greater the contrast. It might be that this difference can be used for differential diagnosis of various causes of a lowered visual acuity.

REFERENCES

Arden, G.B. & Lewis, D.R.H.: The pattern visual evoked response in the assessment of visual acuity. *Trans. Ophthal. Soc. U.K.* 93, *39-48* (1973).

Arden, G.B.: Communication. Proc. XIII ISCERG Symposium, Israël April 1975; ed. by E. Auerbach. *Doc. Ophthal. Proc. Series* 11, *31-38* (1977).

Dawson, W.W., Perry, N.W. & Childers, D.G.: Variations in human cortical response to patterns and image quality. *Invest. Ophthal.* 11, *789-799* (1972).

Harter, M.R. & White, C.T.: Effects of contour sharpness and check-size on visually evoked cortical potentials. *Vision Res.* 8, *701-711* (1968).

Harter, M.R.: Evoked cortical responses to checkerboard patterns: effect of check-size as a function of retinal eccentricity. *Vision Res.* 10, *1365-1376* (1970).

Harter, M.R. & White, C.T.: Evoked cortical responses to checkerboard patterns: effect of check-size as a function of visual acuity. *Electroenceph. clin. Neurophysiol.* 28, *48-54* (1970).

Lith, G.H.M. van & Henkes, H.E.: The relationship between ERG and VER. *Ophtal. Res.* 1, *40-47* (1970).

Marle, G.W. van & Lith, G.H.M. van: A TV-stimulator for visually evoked potentials. *Electronic Engin.* (to be published).

Millodot, M. & Riggs, L.A.: Refraction determined electrophysiologically. *Arch. Ophthal.* 84, *272-278* (1970).

Regan, D. & Richards, W.: Independence of evoked potentials and apparent size. *Vision Res.* 11, *679-684* (1971).

Regan, D.: Rapid objective refraction using evoked brain potentials. *Ivest. Ophthal.* 12, *669-679* (1973).

Rietveld, W.J., Tordoir, W.E.M., Hagenouw, J.R.B. et al.: Visual evoked responses to blank and to checkerboard patterned flashes. *Acta. Physiol. Pharmacol. Neerl.* 14, *259-285* (1967).

Sokol, S. & Bloom, B: Visually evoked cortical responses of amblyopes to a spatially alternating stimulus. *Invest. Ophthal.* 12, *936-939* (1973).

Spehlman, R.: The averaged electrical responses to diffuse and to patterned light in the human. *Electroenceph. clin. Neurophysiol.* 19, *560-569* (1965).

Spekreijse, H.: Analysis of EEG responses in man. Thesis. The Hague, Junk, 1966.

Author's addresses:
G. van Lith
Eye Hospital
Erasmus University
Rotterdam, The Netherlands
(partly: Eye Dept, University of Leyden)

W. van Marle & S. Vijfwinkel-Bruininga
Eye Hospital
Erasmus University
Rotterdam, The Netherlands

G. Bartl
Researchfellow
Universitäts-Augenklinik
Graz, Austria

INFLUENCE OF STIMULUS DURATION AND AREA ON THE SPECTRAL LUMINOSITY FUNCTION AS DETERMINED BY SENSORY AND VECP MEASUREMENTS

E. ZRENNER

(Bad Nauheim/Frankfurt a.M.)

ABSTRACT

Spectral luminosity functions were determined by measuring the radiation power of monochromatic test lights of 2° and 10° in diameter during exposure to white light of 30,000 td. Criterion was (a) the achromatic threshold, (b) the chromatic threshold, (c) a small constant amplitude in the visually evoked cortical potential (VECP).

With a test light duration of 10 ms the achromatic threshold exhibited a spectral luminosity function similar in shape to the CIE V_λ-curve, except for a slightly increased sensitivity in the shortwave region of the spectrum. Using the chromatic threshold as index, a general loss of sensitivity was found, i.e. a small (0.1 log unit) photochromatic interval in the longwave and a large (0.5 log unit) photochromatic interval in the middle and shortwave region of the spectrum relative to the achromatic threshold sensitivity. The spectral luminosity function obtained, using the VECP threshold amplitude criterion as index, was different from that using sensory criteria and exhibited an increased sensitivity near 600 nm and a loss in the green part of the spectrum.

With a test light duration of 400 ms no photochromatic interval was observed; both the sensory and the VECP luminosity function exhibited an increased sensitivity in the longwave part of the spectrum, resulting in a three-peak function. With stimulus diameter of 2°, spatial summation was found only in the function determined by the VECP with 10 ms stimulus duration.

The double sensitivity peak in the longwave region obtained with 400 ms stimulus duration or with suprathreshold stimulus intensity could be described by a linear subtraction of the predominant red and green sensitive fundamental function (R and G resp., defined in VECP experiments). The curve obtained by sensory threshold measurements with 10 ms stimulus duration, however, could be described only by linear addition of R and G functions. This indicates that under strong white adaptation the establishing of color opponency processes as determined by threshold measurements is evidently influenced by stimulus duration.

If we assume that just visible flashes of duration longer than the maximum integration time are a special kind of suprathreshold stimulation, the color opponent system would be activated if a certain number of quanta above the threshold is exceeded, whether the suprathreshold condition is defined by the critical stimulus duration or stimulus intensity.

Measurements by some authors of the spectral sensitivity functions by means of the visually evoked cortical potential (VECP) indicated some dissimilarities to the functions determined psychophysically (Armington, 1964; Cavonius, 1965; Cigánek & Ingvar, 1969; Siegfried, 1971), while other investigators found a close resemblance between sensory and electrical measurements (Regan, 1970; Adachi-Usami *et al.*, 1974; Zrenner *et al.* 1975). The differences may be based upon the different response criteria chosen or upon different conditions of stimulation. Since the experiments of Svaetichin & MacNichol (1958) on lower vertebrates and of De Valois *et al.* (1966) and Wiesel & Hubel (1966) on mammals, the existence of two types of neural units associated with cone vision has been well established: (a) color opponent cells which show inhibitory effects in response to one wavelength region but excitatory effects to another, and (b) non-opponent cells which indicate some degree of summation. Recently, Padmos & Norren (1975) found indications for color opponency also by recording graded potentials in the visual cortex of monkeys. Using microelectrodes in monkey cortex, Gouras (1974) found some cells which showed color opponency at threshold, while others required suprathreshold stimuli for its manifestation.

The present study demonstrates that experiments using intense white adaptation exhibit color opponency also in the gross potential of the visual cortex of man. The measurement of spectral sensitivity functions by sensory thresholds compared with those using a VECP amplitude criterion reveals the important role of stimulus duration and suprathreshold stimulation for establishing the interaction of color opponent mechanisms. This interaction can be described mathematically by a simple procedure using linear subtraction resp. addition of VECP fundamental spectral sensitivity functions obtained under conditions of strong chromatic adaptation (Zrenner & Kojima, 1977).

METHODS

The experiments were performed on the normal trichromatic observer J.H. (age 24) during exposure to white light of 30,000 td, 5.500° K, and on 4 normal trichromatic observers (age 19 to 26) during exposure to monochromatic light. The color vision of the subjects was determined with Ishihara plates, Nagel anomaloscope, Farnsworth Panel D-15, and Farnsworth-Munsell 100-Hue test. The subject fixated in Maxwellian view (pupil dilated) on the center of a circular adaption field 15° in diameter on which test stimuli of 10° or 2° in diameter were concentrically superimposed, both originating from a xenon arc lamp and controlled by electromagnetic shutters. The pupillary radiant intensity I_p (CIE, 1970) at 10 wavelengths in the range of 451 nm to 650 nm was determined as follows: The irradiance E was measured with a radiant flux meter (Model 8330 A, Hewlett-Packard) at different distances (d) from the plane where the subject's pupil would be. The value of $E \cdot d^2$ yields I_p, the pupillary radiant intensity expressed in $nW \cdot sr^{-1}$. For each interference filter in the test beam (Schott, type AL, bandwidth 20 nm) an equivalent density was calculated and interposed to equalize irradiance. The VECP was recorded by a gold disk electrode placed 3 cm above the inion; the indifferent electrode was attached to the earlobe. The potentials were amplified (WP-Instruments, DAM 6A), led through a bandpass filter of 0.8-250 Hz and averaged by a Nicolet 1070 computer. The reciprocal of the absolute pupillary radiant intensity I_p necessary for a criterion amplitude of 4 μV, 4.5 μV or 6 μV (not varied intraindividually), interpolated from 4-5 VECP recordings and plotted against the wavelength, was used as a measure of the sensitivity of the observer.

In the experiments with white adaption light, stimuli of 10 ms and 400 ms duration were presented with a repetition rate of 1.1 per sec. Before and after each averaging cycle, the achromatic (colorless sensation) and chromatic (colored sensation) thresholds were determined by an up-and-down method for small samples (Dixon, 1965) in the VECP measurement test light intensities were presented in random order, beginning slightly (0.3 log unit) above the visual threshold; the observer had to report his color sensation before and after each averaging procedure.

In the experiments with chromatic adaptation three monochromatic lights were used for background illumination: (a) blue-green (μ = 489 nm) to depress selectively the assumed predominant blue and green sensitive mechanisms, (b) purple (422 nm + 630 nm) to depress the blue and red mechanisms, and (c) yellow (574 nm) to depress the red and green mechanisms. The retinal illumination of the adaption field was compared and adjusted to the white adapting source as used in the above experiments by means of sensory threshold measurements in order to obtain photopic equivalence under all conditions. In the chromatic adaptation experiments, stimuli of 20 ms duration and 10° subtense were presented.

The linear subtractive procedure (see text) was calculated with a DECLAB 11/40 computer (Digital Equipment) by the method of least squares.

RESULTS

VECPs in response to a series of light pulses of increasing intensity I_p are shown in fig. 1A. Under the conditions chosen (602 nm test stimulus of 10 ms duration, superimposed on a white background of 30,000 td) the first distinctly marked positive component P_1 (peak latency 95-125 ms) became visible at about a 0.3 log unit stimulus intensity above the subjective achromatic threshold. The negative component N_1 (peak latency 55-85 ms) appeared at about 0.9 log unit. The amplitude of the main feature (N_1-P_1) of the response increased with stimulus intensity (fig. 1B). The dynamic range of the response was small, about 1.1-1.9 log unit. The wave's shape did not vary systematically with stimulus wavelength. However, at very short and very long wavelengths, the slope of amplitude vs. log I_p was seen to be slightly lowered; therefore, a low amplitude criterion was chosen.

Averaged spectral sensitivity curves of 4 normal trichromatic observers as determined by a VECP amplitude criterion of 4.5 μV are depicted in fig. 2. The functions R, G and B were obtained during exposure to strong colored light of 30,000 td in order to diminish the sensitivity of two of the assumed three color mechanisms; this method of selective chromatic adaptation permits isolation of the third color mechanism in psychophysical (Wald, 1964) and VECP measurements (Kellermann & Adachi-Usami, 1972/1973; Zrenner & Kojima, 1977). Thus, the remaining functions represent the long-, middle- and shortwave color vision mechanisms as detected at the cortical

23

level. The sensitivity loss of the R function was about 0.2-0.4 log unit lower than Stiles' (1959) π_5 mechanism between 470 nm and 560 nm. The G function showed a similar loss between 570 nm and 630 nm in comparison with Stiles' π_4 mechanism. This indicates a possible subtractive interaction of R and G resulting in a narrower function. In addition, compared to Stiles' π_1 mechanism, the B function in the VECP is shifted about 10 nm towards longer wavelengths. The lines drawn in fig. 2 approximate the experimental data by smooth functions, later used for the linear subtraction of R and G functions in order to indicate the relative weight of both mechanisms during white adaption.

As opposed to the above experiment using strong colored light for selective adaptation fig. 3 shows the increment spectral sensitivity functions during steady exposure to a white background of 30,000 td.

With the large stimulus field (10°) and test flashes of long duration (400 ms) the threshold sensation (half-filled and open squares) is never colorless. The sensitivity curve determined by means of the VECP (filled squares) as well as the sensory measurements exhibit broad functions with sensitivity peaks near 610 nm and 525 nm, but a trough near 575 nm. The shape of the curve can be described roughly by a linear subtraction similar to the model of Sperling & Harwerth (1971): The solid line in fig. 3A represents the values obtained by linear subtraction of the functions R and

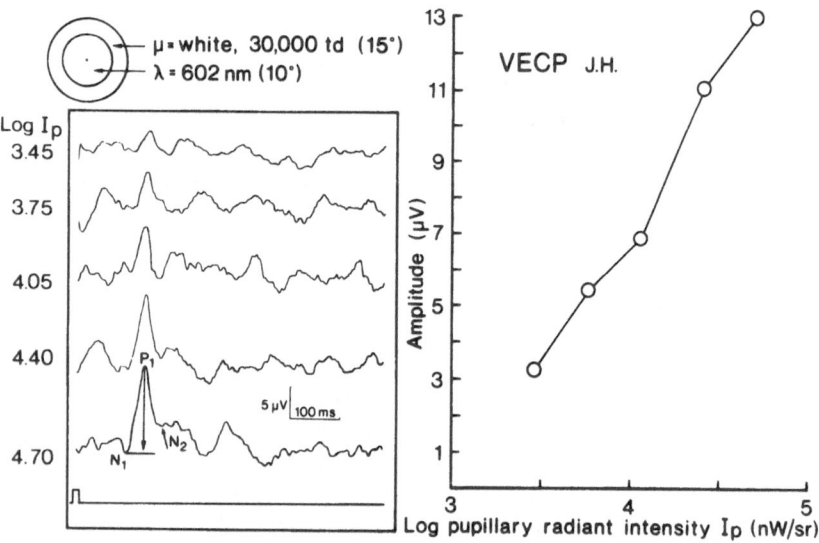

Fig. 1. *A:* Averaged VECPs (n = 128) of a normal trichromatic observer in response to circular test stimuli of 10° subtense radiant intensity I_p superimposed on a steady background of 15°. Spectral composition of test pulse (λ) and adaptation light (μ) as indicated. The incidence of the light pulse is shown by upward deflection of the lowermost record.

B: Plot of amplitudes N_1-P_1 in the VECP vs. pupillary radiant intensity I_p. From this the sensitivity was calculated by interpolating the inverted I_p needed for a 4.5 μV amplitude criterion.

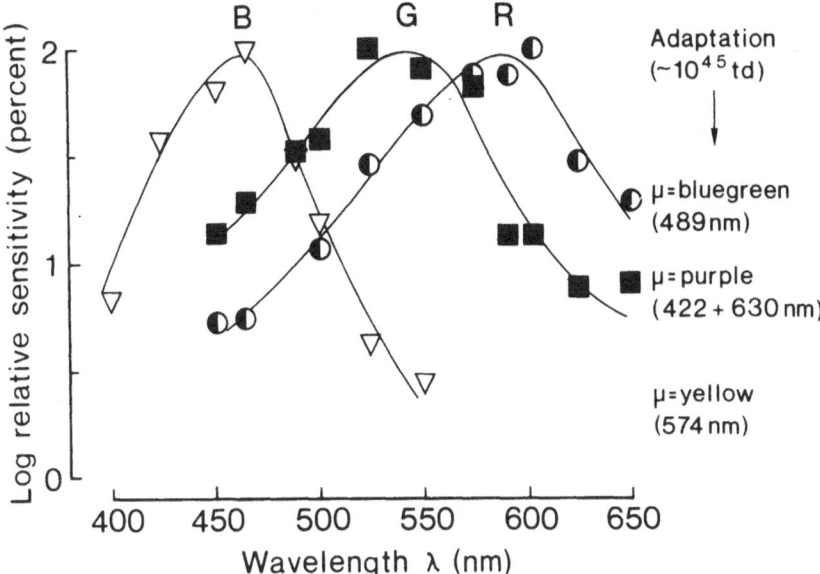

Fig. 2. Spectral sensitivity curves of 4 normal trichromatic observers averaged as determined by the reciprocal pupillary radiant intensity necessary for a 4 μV amplitude criterion N_1-P_1 in the VECP. Sensitivity functions are arbitrarily displaced along the ordinate and plotted in log percent of the maximum. The functions R,G, and B were obtained during exposure to a steady background of blue-green (R), purple (G) and yellow (B), of 30,000 td of 15° subtense, centered on the fovea. Thin lines were drawn by hand to fit the data.

G shown in fig. 2. The sensitivity peak in the green range of the spectrum near 525 nm is described by the expression $M = G - k_1 \cdot R$ (left part), the peak in the longwave part by $L = R - k_2 \cdot G$ (right part). The values of k_1 and k_2 were computed (DECLAB 11/40) to give the best fit between the experimental data and the resulting function using a least mean square error criterion. Being relative values, k_1 and k_2 represent the relation between R and G for a given stimulus condition. The B mechanism is not considered here. In both the sensory and the VECP measurements in fig. 3A, k_1 is smaller than k_2, indicating that the participation of G in the subtractive process is greater than that of R.

Shortening of the stimulus duration to 10 ms (fig. 3B) causes a loss of the trough at 574 nm and approaches the spectral sensitivity function determined by achromatic thresholds (half-filled circles) to the CIE photopic spectral luminosity curve (dotted line). The photochromatic interval between the achromatic threshold (half-filled circles) and the chromatic threshold (open circles) is small in the red part of the spectrum and becomes larger towards the green and the blue-green range. The VECP sensitivity function (filled circles) on the other hand retains the trough evidenced at

25

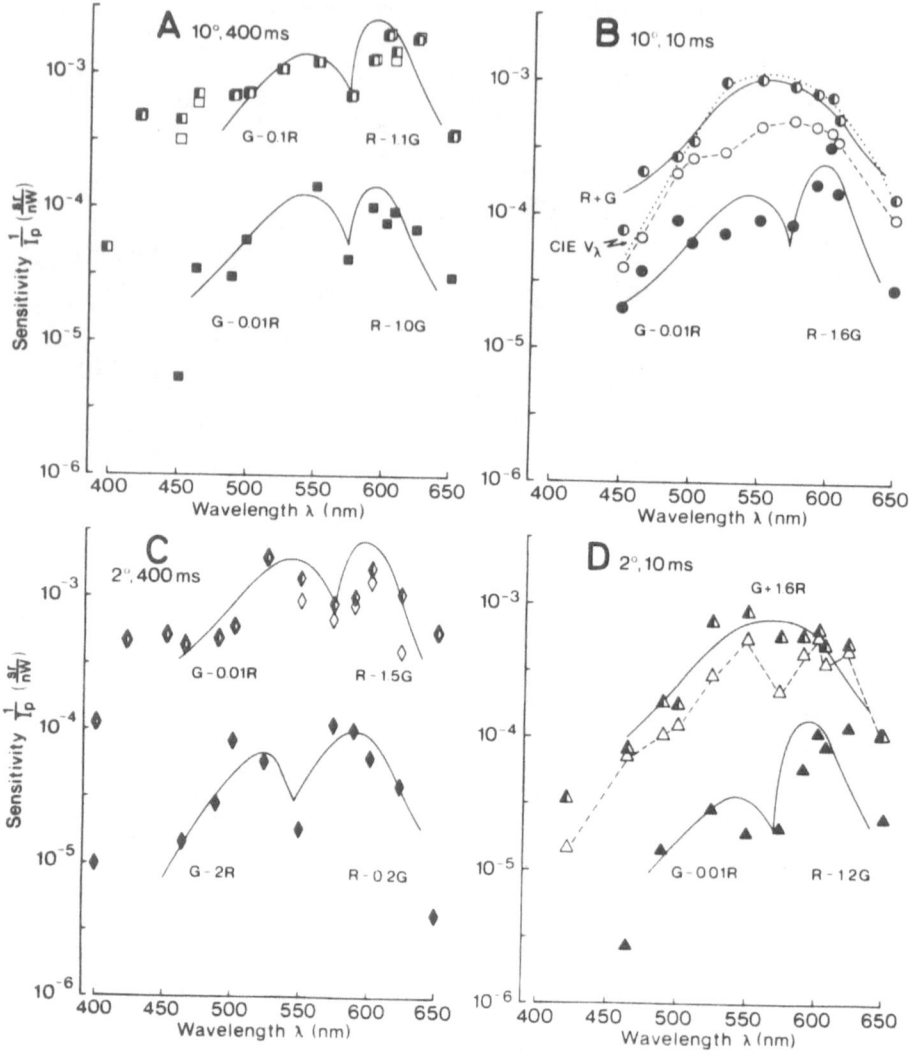

Fig. 3. Spectral sensitivity functions as obtained by determination of sensory achromatic thresholds (half-filled symbols), chromatic thresholds (open symbols, in B and D connected by dashed lines) and VECP criterion thresholds N_1-P_1 amplitude of 4.5 μV (filled symbols) between 400 and 650 nm. Each value represents the average of three experiments with observer J.H. during exposure to a white background of 15° subtense (30,000 td, 5500 °K). The solid lines represent the logarithm of the absolute values as obtained by linear subtraction of functions $k_1 \cdot R$ and $k_2 \cdot G$ (from fig. 2) as indicated near the resulting functions (see text). The dotted line is the CIE photopic spectral luminosity curve. Area centered on the fovea and duration of monochromatic test pulses: A: 10° subtense, 400 ms (squares); B: 10° subtense, 10 ms (circles); C: 2° subtense, 400 ms (rhombs); D: 2° subtense, 10 ms (triangles).

26

longer stimulus times. The peak in the red is increased and comes close to the sensitivity of the subjective threshold in this region; this fits the experiments of Krüger and Gouras (1976), who found a predominance of red sensitive cells in the monkey. Whereas the psychophysically determined sensitivity curves can be described only by an addition of R and G function ($k_1 = k_2 = 1$, upper solid line), the VECP sensitivity function requires subtraction of R and G (lower solid line, $k_1 < k_2$).

Experiments with a test light diameter of 2° and stimuli of 400 ms duration (fig. 3C) result in spectral sensitivity functions similar to those obtained with a 10° field as shown in fig. 3A. Despite the smaller area stimulated, the absolute sensitivity is not decreased. Apparently the temporal summation renders the spatial summation ineffective (Barlow, 1958). Compared with the sensory measurements (half-filled and open rhombs) the longwave peak and trough in the VECP sensitivity function (fig. 3C, filled rhombs) are shifted towards shorter wavelengths. This indicates the dominance of the R mechanism at higher radiant intensities as traced by the linear substraction of R and G ($k_1 > k_2$).

With a stimulus duration of 10 ms (fig. 3D) the achromatic threshold of the 2° test field (half-filled triangles) does not resemble a double peak curve, but comes closer to the CIE V_λ curve (as shown in fig. 3B, dotted line). The photochromatic interval is small and restricted to medium wavelengths, similar to that described in the experiment with a 10° test field but exhibiting a deep trough near 580 nm. The VECP sensitivity function (filled triangles) again shows a peak near 615 nm and a trough near 560 nm. Comparison with the 10° field, however, shows the absolute sensitivity to be decreased. This indicates that the upper limit of spatial summation provided by stimulus duration and background intensity was not fully achieved with the 2° condition.

DISCUSSION

Padmos & Graf (1974) and Padmos & Van Norren (1975) described local VECP spectral sensitivity functions in rhesus monkeys as exhibiting submaxima narrower than the primary functions of the color vision mechanisms. The present results are of similar nature and stress the conclusion of Gouras & Padmos (1974) that the graded response of the foveal striate cortex reflects color antagonistic interactions. The description of these interactions by a simplified linear subtractive procedure (with reference to the linear subtractive interaction model developed by Sperling & Harwerth (1971) in psychophysical measurement) was done merely to differentiate between subtractive and non-subtractive processes, rather than to define the parameters of the color opponent mechanism.

The effect of stimulus duration upon the spectral sensitivity in the sensory measurements was explained by Ikeda & Boynton (1962) in terms of shifts in the threshold vs. stimulus duration. Regan & Tyler (1971) found that the critical duration for the detection of wavelength change at the subjective threshold is longer than that for detection of luminance change. Recently, King-Smith (1975) described stimulus duration dependent differences in spectral sensitivity functions by sensory threshold measurements. He suggested that these differences could be caused by differences in the temporal and spatial integration properties of the luminance and opponent color systems.

In contrast to the reports discussed above, the VECP thresholds utilized in the present work permitted the determination of spectral sensitivity functions at light levels above the sensory threshold. With such suprathreshold measurements color opponent interactions are seen under all conditions of stimulus duration or intensity used. In the sensory threshold measurement, however, the color opponent interactions are seen only for long stimulus durations. These results can be explained if we assume that the maximum integration time also represents a type of threshold and that just visible flashes of longer duration than the maximal integration time are a special kind of suprathreshold stimulation. Thus, the color opponent system would be activated if a certain critical number of quanta above the threshold is exceeded, whether the suprathreshold condition is defined by the critical stimulus duration or stimulus intensity.

Sperling & Harwerth (1971) state that the interaction between the red and the green receptor responses increases as the fovea is adapted to higher levels of white light. We may add that this also occurs as the degree of suprathreshold stimulation is increased. On the other hand, the influence of adaptation may be different for the individual color vision mechanisms (Zrenner et al., 1977). Taking into consideration all these factors, the CIE photopic spectral luminosity function, very well fitted by Regan's (1970) sensitivity measurements by means of the second harmonic of the VECP, does not completely describe human photopic spectral sensitivity.

In agreement with the psychophysical experiments of Monroe (1924), Graham & Hsia (1969), Bouman & Walraven (1972), Eichengreen (1976), the maximum of the photochromatic interval was found in the green range. The general increase of the photochromatic interval with stimulus field confirms the finding of Bouman & Walraven (1957); at wavelengths near 575 nm, however, the photochromatic interval decreases with the increasing of test field, as previously shown by Tittarelli (1967).

The small contribution of the blue mechanism to color opponency described by Gouras (1974) in the foveal striate cortex of the monkey is also seen in the present VECP measurement in man: In the shortwave part of the spectrum, sensitivity is lower in the VECP than in the sensory measurements indicating that the contribution of the short wave mechanism to the N_1-P_1 VECP criterion is small, as reported by Zrenner & Kojima (1976) for the P_1-N_2 criterion. Also, the variation in topographical structure of the visual cortex between individuals may effect the spectral sensitivity functions, especially during white adaptation which involves all mechanisms.

Being a gross potential, the VECP provides a somewhat coarse tool for describing such compound functions as the photopic spectral sensitivity. Moreover, in our experimental set-up, we are limited to 14 test wavelengths separated by intervals of about 20 nm. Nevertheless, the results obtained with this method of investigation point to general patterns in the processing of visual information by color opponent mechanisms.

ACKNOWLEDGMENTS

I am grateful to Prof. E. Dodt for helpful discussion, to Miss Brita Maschen and Monika Baier for technical assistance and to Dr. O. Ludwig and Mr. K. Rockenfeller for their helpful advice on statistical problems.

REFERENCES

Adachi-Usami, E., J. Heck, V. Gavriysky & F.-J. Kellermann: Spectral sensitivity function determined by the visually evoked cortical potential in several classes of colour deficiency (cone monochromatism, rod monochromatism, protanopia, deuteranopia). *Ophthal, Res.* 6, *273-290* (1974).

Armington, J.C.: Relations between electroretinograms and occipital potentials elicited by flickering stimuli. Proc. 2nd ISCERG Symp. Amsterdam 1963, *Doc. Ophthal.* 18, *194-206* (1964).

Barlow, H.B.: Temporal and spatial summation in human vision at different background intensities. *J. Physiol.* 141, *337-350* (1958).

Bouman, M.A. & P.L. Walraven: Some color naming experiments for red and green monochromatic lights. *J. opt. Soc. Am.* 47, *834-839* (1957).

Bouman, M.A. & P.L. Walraven: On threshold mechanisms for achromatic and chromatic vision. *Acta Physiol.* 36, *178-189* (1972).

Cavonius, C.R.: Evoked response of the human visual cortex: Spectral sensitivity. *Psychon. Sci.* 2, *185-186* (1965).

CIE: International Lighting Vocabulary, 3rd Ed., CIE Publication No. 17, Paris 1970.

Cigánek, L. & D.H. Ingvar: Colour specific features of visual cortical responses in man evoked by monochromatic flashes. *Acta physiol. scand.* 76, *82-92* (1969).

De Valois, R.L., I. Abramov & G.H. Jacobs: Analysis of response patterns of LGN cells. *J. opt. Soc. Am.* 56, *966-977* (1966).

Dixon, W.J.: The up-and-down methode for small samples. *J. Am. Statist. Ass.* 60, *967-978* (1965).

Eichengreen, J.M.: Separate chromatic thresholds for binary hue stimuli. *Vision Res.* 16, *321-322* (1976).

Gouras, P.: Opponent colour cells in different layers of foveal striate cortex. *J. Physiol.* 238, *583-602* (1974).

Gouras, P. & P. Padmos: Identification of cone mechanisms in graded responses of foveal striate cortex. *J. Physiol.* 238, *569-581* (1974).

Graham, C.H. & Y. Hsia: Saturation and the foveal achromatic interval. *J. opt. Soc. Am.* 59, *993-997* (1969).

Ikeda, M. & R.M. Boynton: Effect of test-flash duration upon the spectral sensitivity of the eye. *J. opt. Soc. Am.* 52, *697-699* (1962).

Kellermann, F.-J. & E. Adachi-Usami: Spectral sensitivities of colour mechanisms isolated by the human visual evoked response. *Ophthal. Res.* 4, *199-210* (1972/73).

King-Smith, P.E.: Visual detection analysed in terms of luminance and chromatic signals. *Nature* 255, *69-70* (1975).

Krüger, J. & P. Gouras: Many cells in visual cortex use wavelength to detect borders and convey information about colour. Exp. Brain Res. (in press, personal communication).

Monroe, M.M.: The energy value of the minimum visible chromatic and achromatic for different wave-lengths of the spectrum. Psychol. Rev. Publ. 34, Psychol. Monographs No. 158 (1924).

Padmos, P. & V. Graf: Colour vision in rhesus monkey, studied with subdurally implanted cortical electrodes. 11th ISCERG Symp. Bad Nauheim 1973, *Doc. Ophthal. Proc. Series* 4, *307-314* (1974).

Padmos, P. & D.V. Norren: Increment spectral sensitivity and colour discrimination in the primate, studied by means of graded potentials from the striate cortex. *Vision Res.* 15, *1103-1113* (1975).

Regan, D: Objective method of measuring the relative spectral luminosity curve in man. *J. opt. Soc. Am.* 60, *856-859* (1970).

Regan, D. & C.W. Tyler: Temporal summation and its limit for wavelength changes: An analog of Bloch's law of color vision. *J. opt. Soc. Am.* 61, *1414-1421* (1971).

Siegfried, J.B.: Spectral sensitivity of human visual evoked cortical potentials: A new method and a comparison with psychophysical data. *Vision Res.* 11, *405-417* (1971).

Sperling, H.G. & R.S. Harwerth: Red-green cone interactions in the increment-threshold spectral sensitivity of primates. *Science* 172, *180-184* (1971).

Stiles, W. S.: Colour vision: The approach through increment threshold sensitivity. *Proc. Nat. Acad. Sci. USA* 45, *100-114* (1959).

Svaetichin, G. & E.F. MacNichol, Jr.: Retinal mechanisms for chromatic and achromatic vision. *Ann. N.Y. Acad. Sci.* 74, *385-404* (1958).

Tittarelli, R.: Photochromatic interval as a function of spot size: A controversy. Atti Fondazione G. Ronchi 22, No. 3 (1967).

Wald, G.: The receptors of human color vision. *Science* 145, *1007-1017* (1964).

Wiesel, T.N. & D.H. Hubel: Spatial and chromatic interactions in the lateral geniculate body of the rhesus monkey. *J. Neurophysiol.* 29, *1115-1156* (1966).

Zrenner, E. & M. Kojima: Colour vision mechanisms isolated by chromatic adaptation in normals and dichromats as detected by the visually evoked cortical potential (VECP). 13th ISCERG Symp. Israel, 1975. *Doc. Ophthal. Proc. Series* 11, *115-121* (1977).

Zrenner, E. & M. Kojima: The visually evoked cortical potential (VECP) in dichromats. Colour Vision Deficiences III. Int. Symp., Amsterdam 1975. *Mod. Probl. Ophthal.* 17, *241-246* (1976).

Zrenner, E., V. Gavriysky & F.-J. Kellermann: Further studies on the colour mechanisms in the human visually evoked cortical potential (VECP) isolated by selective chromatic adaptation. Proc. 2nd ERG Conf. Wroclaw, Vol. 1, 7-16 (1975).

Zrenner, E., M. Kojima & E. Jankov: Untersuchung ders Farbsinns mit der Methode der visuell evozierten corticalen Potentiale (VECP). *Ber. Dtsch. Ophthal. Ges.* 74, *717-722* (1977).

Author's address:
Max-Planck Institut für Physiologische und klinische Forschung
W.G. Kerckhoff-Institut
Parkstrasse 1
D-6350 Bad Nauheim
FRG

LOCAL AND SPATIAL DISTRIBUTION OF PHOTOPIC AND SCOTOPIC RESPONSES IN THE VISUAL FIELD AS REFLECTED IN THE VISUALLY EVOKED CORTICAL POTENTIAL (VECP)

M. KOJIMA & E. ZRENNER

(Bad Nauheim/Frankfurt a.M.)

ABSTRACT

Visually evoked cortical potentials (VECP) were elicited by test fields between 5° and 110° in diameter under scotopic and photopic conditions. Photopic and scotopic responses in the VECP were identified by implicit time measurements (70-200 ms for the photopic, 180-400 ms for the scotopic response).

The slope of the implicit time vs. luminance curves was steeper under scotopic than under photopic conditions. The change of slope was identified by the spectral luminosity functions as the transition from rod to cone activity.

With a test stimulus of 30 times absolute threshold the scotopic response was obtained not before 10 minutes in darkness. The maximum height of response was reached after 35 minutes of dark adaptation.

Spatial summation of the scotopic response was seen for test flashes between 5° and 110° in diameter (central fixation).

Moving a test field of 5° in the visual field, the sensitivity of the scotopic response (based on the implicit time) increased from the center towards the nasal periphery with a maximum at about 20°. Further move to 40° eccentricity decreased the scotopic sensitivity gradually. The photopic sensitivity decreased strongly as the stimulus field moved from center to nasal periphery.

Sensitivity measurements based on an implicit time criterion of the VECP closely agree with the known distribution of rod and cone cells and the sensory threshold measurements of the scotopic and photopic system.

Due to the magnification properties of the visual cortex, the visually evoked cortical potential (VECP) in man reflects mainly the activity of the foveal and parafoveal parts of the retina (Potts *et al.*, 1965; De Voe *et al.*, 1968). However, under appropriate conditions of stimulation it has been possible to record cortical signals of scotopic origin, predominantly in VECP components marked by long implicit time (van Balen & Henkes, 1960).

Vaughan (1964) identified the break in the implicit time vs. intensity plots as the transition of rod to cone VECP. Using the scotopic VECP as a clinical test of peripheral retinal function, Adams *et al.* (1969) found abnormal responses in patients with night blindness, while the photopic VECP was normal; the reverse was seen in patients suffering from macular degeneration. In 16 patients with hemianopsia Kojima *et al.* (1972) observed asymmetries between the responses from the two hemispheres by means of the scotopic VECP. Using an implicit time criterion Huber & Adachi-Usami (1972) found the spectral sensitivity of the scotopic VECP to agree well with the scotopic CIE luminosity function.

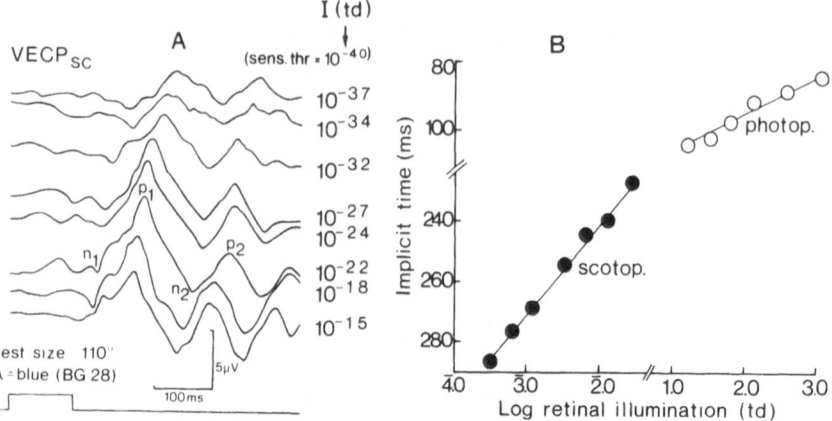

Fig. 1. A: Scotopic VECPs of observer A.R. (N = 64) in response to a blue light (BG 28, Schott) after 40 min of dark adaptation. Upward deflection indicates positivity of the scalp electrode (p_1, p_2). Size of test fields 110°, central fixation. Duration of test light 110 ms as indicated by lowermost record. The numbers beside records denote the retinal illumination in troland (td).
B: Implicit time of the first positive peak p_1 in the VECPs vs. log test light intensity (as illustrated in A) and of the photopic VECP (not illustrated in A) recorded in response to an orange light (OG 5, Schott) during exposure to blue light (BG 28, Schott) of 50 td. Observer O.A.

The present study was conducted to investigate the spatial distribution of retinal sensitivity by means of scotopic and photopic VECP. Moreover, spatial summation of the scotopic response was determined for test flashes up to 110° in diameter.

METHODS

The optical stimulator provides two beams originating from a xenon arc source (XBO 150 W, Osram). After being focussed at electro-magnetic shutters, both beams illuminated a diffusing acrylic screen 10 cm in diameter positioned between 3 and 15 cm in front of the eye. Size and retinal location of the test flash were controlled by appropriate diaphragms attached to the screen. The subject lay in a dark room and fixated on a dim red lamp through a hole 1 mm in diameter. The active scalp electrode was fixed with collodion 4% (Merck) at Oz (according to the international 10-20 EEG system). The signals were amplified, filtered (bandpass 1-40 Hz), displayed and averaged (N = 32 or 64) by a Nicolet 1070 computer. To avoid contamination with the background activity, the light stimulus was manually triggered. In order to prevent adaptation effects by the stimulus light, the minimum stimulus interval used was 1.5 s. Four normal students served as subjects; before the beginning of the experiment, they were dark adapted for 40 min.

RESULTS

Typical recordings of the scotopic VECP in response to a blue test light of 110° are demonstrated in fig. 1A. The major components are indicated by lower case letters; they show implicit time (interval between stimulus onset and peak of individual wave) between 200 and 400 ms; the interval between major peaks remained constant, the implicit time decreased as retinal illumination was increased (fig. 1B, filled circles). Under photopic conditions (orange light stimuli presented on a blue background of 50 td) the slope of the function relating implicit time of p_1 vs. retinal illumination was much less (fig. 1B, open circles) than under scotopic conditions. The slopes were about 25 ms/log change in retinal illumination for the scotopic and about 10 ms/log change in retinal illumination for the photopic responses. Similar findings in VECP measurements were made previously by Vaughan (1964) who demonstrated a break in the implicit time vs. luminance curve. He concluded, and we agree, that the steeper slope of the curve was due to stimulation of the retinal rods.

As previously described by Huber & Adachi-Usami (1972), the scotopic origin of the potentials recorded can be shown also by measurements of the VECP amplitude during dark adaptation. Moreover, as fig. 2 shows, also the implicit time of p_1 increases with the time course of dark adaptation: After a 5 min exposure to white light of 10,000 td, test flashes of constant intensity (30 times absolute threshold) evoked no response before 10 min in darkness (fig. 2). Then the amplitude of p_1 increased to a constant value of 5 μV during 35 min in the dark. During the same time, the implicit time decreased monotonically from 277 ms after the 10th minute to 250 ms after 40 min. Being response curves, not threshold measurements, different curves are expected with higher or lower test light intensities.

Further proof of the scotopic nature of the electrocortical component recorded above was obtained by measurement of the spectral sensitivity function in the dark adapted eye. For this purpose, implicit time vs. intensity curves of the scotopic VECP were produced for six different stimulus wavelengths (fig. 3). The slope of these functions stayed parallel with test lights between 425 and 601 nm, which indicates that only one mechanism is responsible for its generation. With test lights of 651 nm a steeper function is seen in the upper part of the curve, which is not consistent with the results shown in fig. 1B because of the different condition used. Scotopic vision is characterized by an achromatic sensation and by a central scotoma. However, with test lights beyond 650 nm there is no photochromatic interval and the test light — even at threshold intensity — appears red. Therefore, the break in the implicit time vs. intensity with 651 nm stimulus indicates at least participation of more than one mechanism.

The VECP spectral sensitivity curve derived from measurement of the implicit time of p_1 under scotopic conditions agrees both with the curve determined by measurement of the sensory thresholds and with the scotopic CIE luminosity function (fig. 4, upper part). Under photopic conditions, the VECP sensitivity in the shortwave range of the spectrum is higher than the CIE curve (fig. 4, lower part). It best matches preferably Wald's (1945)

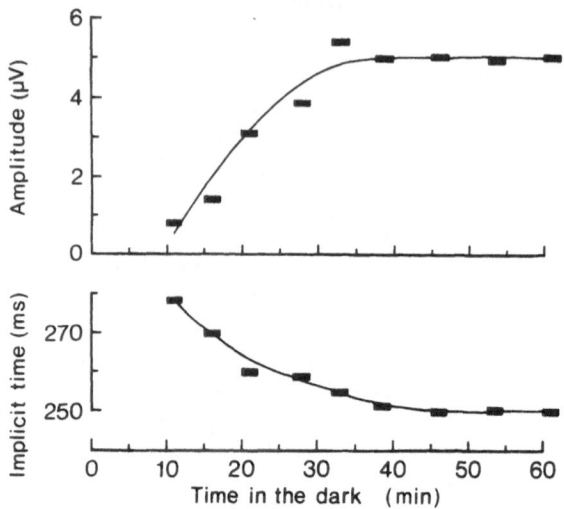

Fig. 2. Graphs relating p_1 amplitude (above) and implicit time (below) of the scotopic component of the VECP during dark adaptation in response to a blue test light of 110 ms duration of $10^{-2.4}$td (about 30 times absolute threshold) following 5 min pre-adaptation to white light of 10,000 td. Interstimulus interval 2 s. Time necessary for averaging (N = 64) indicated by the horizontal length of symbols. Observer A.R.

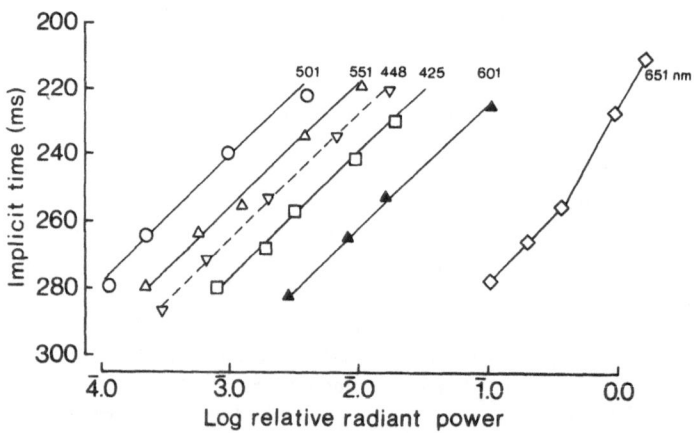

Fig. 3. Implicit time vs. intensity plots of the scotopic VECP after 40 min of dark adaptation for six stimulus wavelengths as indicated. Size of test field 110°. Data were obtained by measurement of the implicit time of component p_1. Values at 448 nm (indicated by broken line) are displaced to higher intensities by 0.25 log units to prevent overlap. Observer O.A.

curve of extrafoveal cones showing increased sensitivity in the blue caused by the lack of the macular pigment and the higher portion of blue cones, conditions produced by the large size of the stimulus presently used.

Spatial summation as reflected by the scotopic VECP was first shown by Adachi-Usami & Kellermann (1973) at least up to a stimulus diameter of 18°. From the present measurements using different diameters of test field up to 110°, we concluded that spatial summation occurred within the whole retinal area investigated (fig. 5). Using a double logarithmic scale, a linear relationship between stimulus area and threshold responses was found up to 25° in the sensory and up to 50° in the measurements of the scotopic VECP. With larger fields, i.e. including peripheral parts of the retina, the slope decreases. The curve based on the criteria of the implicit time exhibits

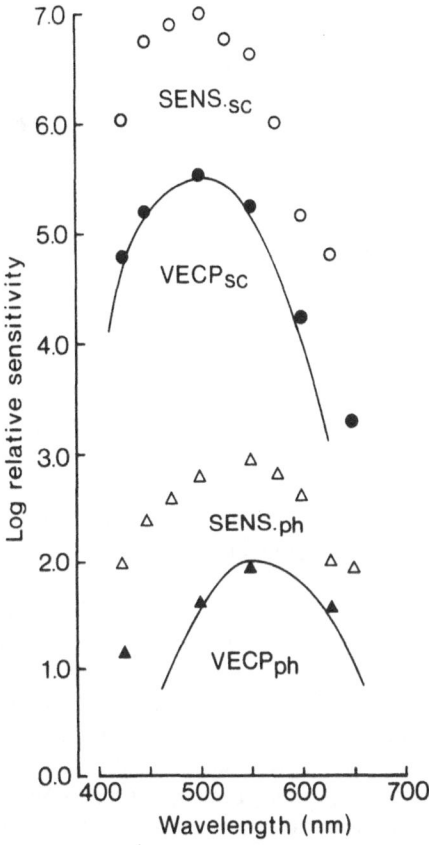

Fig. 4. Spectral sensitivity functions derived from sensory thresholds (open symbols) and from VECP measurements (filled symbols) under scotopic (circles, above) and photopic conditions (triangles, below). The photopic curve was obtained during exposure to white light of 100 td. The VECP data were obtained from measurements of radiant intensity necessary for an implicit time criterion of 250 ms in the dark adapted state and 180 ms during light adaptation. The solid lines are the CIE scotopic (above) and the CIE photopic luminosity function (below). Size of test field 110°. Observer O.A.

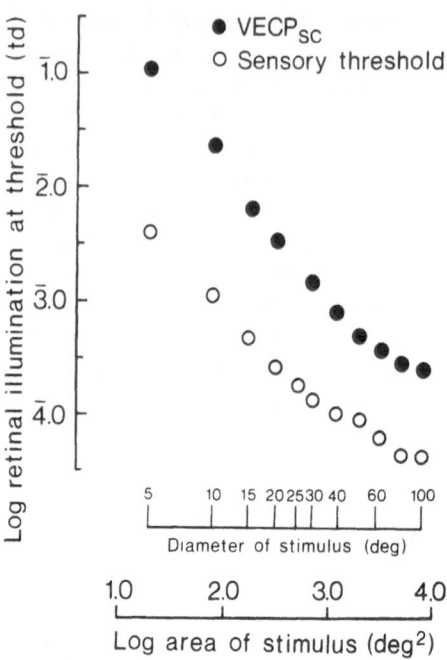

Fig. 5. Graph relating diameter (5° to 110°) of scotopic stimulus (blue light BG 28 of 110 ms) and log retinal illumination at sensory threshold (open circles) and at VECP implicit time criterion of 250 ms (filled circles). Dark adapted observer O.A.

a slightly steeper slope than that obtained by the sensory threshold (cf. Adachi-Usami & Kellermann, 1973). Retinal inhomogeneity i.e. the increasing number of rods up to about 20° eccentricity may be responsible for the changing slope of the area-threshold curve.

In another experiment an attempt was made to investigate retinal inhomogeneity by measuring regional differences in sensitivity within the peripheral retina. In this experiment the sensitivity of the temporal retina was determined by measuring the retinal illumination necessary for a constant p_1 implicit time of the scotopic VECP in response to a blue test stimulus of 5° in diameter, eccentrically presented in different places of the visual field up to 40° from the fovea. The data obtained after 40 min dark adaptation indicate that the sensitivity of the peripheral retina first increases up to a maximum near 20°, then it decreases gradually to the periphery (fig. 6A, filled symbols). The corresponding sensory data exhibited the same distribution at a somewhat (about 10 times) lower level of test light illumination (fig. 6A, open symbols). The same experiment performed under photopic conditions (steady exposure to blue light of 50 td, orange test flashes) revealed a reverse function (fig. 6B), which is in agreement with similar findings of van Lith & Henkes (1968). The photopic VECP data based on the implicit time criterion of 190 ms indicates a steep decrease of sensitivity towards the peripheral retina, particularly up to 10° (filled triangles). The decrease of sensitivity by the sensory threshold was smaller (open triangles) in the periphery as compared with the VECP measurement.

DISCUSSION

Previous authors (Wooten, 1972; Huber & Adachi-Usami, 1972) have shown, and we agree, that careful selection of adaptive and test light conditions provides differentiation between scotopic and photopic responses in the VECP. Comparing the criteria chosen (amplitude or implicit time) in the peripheral retina beyond 20°, the amplitude of the scotopic VECP decreases strongly as a function of increasing eccentricity of stimulation. This counterfeits a loss of sensitivity. However, the measurement of the implicit time criterion by means of the scotopic VECP confirms the well known increase of sensitivity from 0° up to 20° eccentricity; it shows only a slight decrease of sensitivity between 20° and 40° eccentricity. Therefore, only the use of the implicit time as the criterion permits reliable measurement of the local peripheral retinal sensitivity.

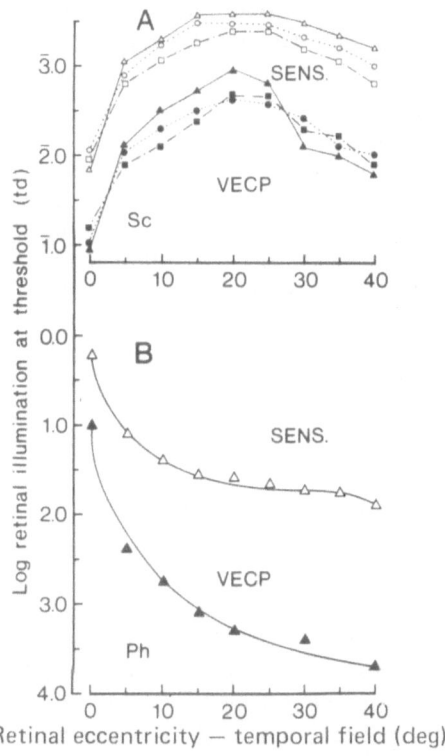

Fig. 6. Local distribution in the temporal retinal field as determined by measurement of retinal illumination necessary for sensory threshold (open symbols) and constant implicit time criterion in the VECP (filled symbols) for test lights of 5° subtense.
A: Data obtained under scotopic conditions (40 min of dark adaptation, blue test light, BG 28 Schott). Implicit time criterion 260 ms. Three observers.
B: Data obtained under photopic conditions (steady exposure to blue light of 50 td, orange test light, OG 5 Schott). Implicit time criterion 190 ms. Observer O.A.

The scotopic origin of the components recorded was identified by measurements of the spectral sensitivity function and by recording the implicit time changes in darkness (dark adaptation curve). Spatial summation determined by scotopic VECP was seen up to test light diameters of 110°, a result not described previously in VECP literature.

Despite the well known predominance of cone activity in the VECP (for review, see Potts & Marriot, 1965), the contribution of rods can be utilized in the VECP to such an extent that the sensitivity of peripheral retinal fields to stimuli 5° in diameter can be determined up to a 40° eccentricity. Along the horizontal meridian the photopic and scotopic VECP threshold generally agrees with the number of cones and rods respectively, as reported by Østerberg (1935) as well as with the thresholds based on sensory (Stiles & Crawford, 1937; Sloan, 1947) and pupillary measurements (Dodt & Alexandridis, 1968).

In the comparison of foveal and peripheral thresholds, notable differences are seen under photopic conditions between sensory and electro-cortical determinations. Since the VECP is strongly affected by the position of the recording electrode (Gastaut & Régis, 1965), these differences may be caused or modified by the magnified projection of the foveal field onto the visual cortex (Holmes, 1918).

In the determination of regional retinal sensitivity, careful attention has to be payed to the state of adaptation. VECP measurement of peripheral retinal thresholds requires a dark adaptation time of at least 40 min, stimulus intensities of 1 to 1.5 log units above the sensory threshold, and stimulus intervals of at least 1.5 s. At 40° eccentricity, only under these conditions could VECP amplitudes large enough to permit clear determination of implicit time (1.5-2.0 μV) be obtained. This may explain why previous investigators missed the scotopic VECP with stimuli applied to the peripheral retina (van Lith, personal communication).

COMMENT

In the evaluation of the electrical measurement of threshold in the retinal field, the contribution of stray light to the electrical response is of major importance. Depending on the size of the area stimulated, the electroretinogram threshold as measured with single test flashes is between 10^1 and $10^{5.5}$ units above the sensory threshold (reviewed by van Lith, 1966). In the present determination of scotopic VECP thresholds, the test flashes at the criterion level were about 1 log unit above the sensory threshold. According to Le Grand (1937) and De Mott & Boynton (1958) the amount of stray light decreases by 2 log units at 10° eccentricity from the retinal field illuminated and by 1 log unit at 3°. Therefore, in the above measurements stray light is effective only within 3° from the border of the stimulus field.

ACKNOWLEDGEMENT

We are grateful to Prof. E. Dodt for helpful discussions.

REFERENCES

Adachi-Usami, E. & F.-J. Kellermann: Spatial summation of retinal excitation as obtained by the scotopic VECP and sensory threshold. *Ophthal. Res.* 5, *308-316* (1973).

Adams, W.L., G.B. Arden & J. Behrman: Responses of human visual cortex following excitation of peripheral rods. *Brit. J. Ophthal.* 53, *439-452* (1969).

Balen, A.T.M., Van & H.E. Henkes: Recording of the occipital lobe response in man after light stimulation. *Brit. J. Ophthal.* 44, *449-460* (1960).

CIE: International Lighting Vocabulary, 3rd Edition, Paris 1970, Publication No. 17.

De Mott, D.W. & R.M. Boynton: Retinal distribution of entopic stray light. *J. opt. Soc. Am.* 48, *13-22* (1958).

De Voe, R.G., H. Ripps & H.G. Vaughan, Jr.: Cortical responses to stimulation of the human fovea. *Vision Res.* 8, *135-147* (1968).

Dodt, E. & E. Alexandridis: Electroretinography and pupillography as supplementary tools in the evaluation of retinal function in man. 6th ISCERG Symp. Erfurt 1967; VEB Georg Thieme, Leipzig 1968, pp. 459-466.

Gastaut, H. & H. Régis: Visually evoked potentials recorded transcranically in man. In: L.D. Proctor & W.R. Adey (eds.): The Analysis of Central Nervous System and Cardiovascular Data using Computer Methods (1964 Symposium), Washington, NASA 1965, pp. 7-34.

Holmes, G.: Disturbances of vision by cerebral lesions. *Brit. J. Ophthal.* 2, *253-384* (1918).

Huber, C. & E. Adachi-Usami: Scotopic visibility curve in man obtained by the VER. In: G.B. Arden (ed.) The Visual System: Neurophysiology, Biophysics, and Their Clinical Application. Proc. 9th ISCERG Symp. Brighton 1971, Adv. exp. med. Biol. 24, 189-198, Academic Press New York 1972.

Kojima, M., H. Abe & K. Iwata: The VER in patients with hemianopsia. Folia Ophthal. Jap. 23, 962-968 (1972).

Le Grand, Y.: Recherches sur la diffusion de la lumière dans l'oeil humain. *Rev. Opt.* 16, *241* (1937).

Lith, G.H.M., Van: Simultane Bestimmung der elektroretinographischen und sensorischen Reizschwelle. *Vision Res.* 6, *185-197* (1966).

Lith, G.H.M., Van & E. Henkes: The local electric response of the central retinal area. 6th ISCERG Symp. Erfurt 1967, VEB Georg Thieme, Leipzig 1968, pp. 163-170.

Østerberg, G.: Topography of the layer of rods and cones in the human retina. *Acta Opthal. Kbh. Suppl.* 6, *1-102* (1935).

Potts, A.M. & F.H.C. Marriot: Studies on the visual evoked response. I. The use of a 0.06 degree red target for evaluation of foveal function. *Invest. Ophthal.* 4, *303-309* (1965).

Sloan, L.L.: Rate of dark adaptation and regional threshold gradient of the dark adapted eye. Pnysiologic and Clinical Studies. *Am. J. Ophthal.* 30, *705-720* (1947).

Stiles, W.S. & B.H. Crawford: The effect of a glaring light source on extrafoveal vision. *Proc. Roy. Soc (London)* 122 B, *255* (1937).

Vaughan, H.G., Jr.: The perceptual and physiologic significance of visual evoked responses recorded from the scalp in man. In: Burian and Jacobson (eds.) Clinical Electroretinography. *Vision Res. Suppl. 203-223* (1964).

Wald, G.: Human vision and the spectrum. *Science* 101, *653-658* (1945).

Wooten, B.R.: Photopic and scotopic contribution to the human visually evoked cortical potential. *Vision Res.* 12, *1647-1660* (1972).

Author's address:
Max-Planck-Institut für Physiologische und
Klinische Forschung, W.G. Kerckhoff-Institut
Parkstr. 1
D-6350 Bad Nauheim FRG

GRATING ACUITY IN TWO SISTERS
WITH TAPETORETINAL DEGENERATION*

MURRAY WOLKSTEIN, ADAM ATKIN & IVAN BODIS-WOLLNER

(New York, N.Y.)

ABSTRACT

Grating detection was studied in two sisters with tapetoretinal degeneration. Both had normal Snellen acuity scores, but the older complained of blurred vision, while the younger had no visual complaints. In the older, a high spatial frequency deficit was found by both psychophysical and evoked potential methods, and a generalized foveal sensitivity loss was demonstrated by static perimetry. In contrast, the younger sister had normal grating detection and static perimetry results.

INTRODUCTION

Visual acuity can be measured by determining the finest detectable grating (Mayer, 1754). In subjects with normal vision, or with cataract or refractive error, acuity scores determined by this grating method are in agreement with Snellen measurements (Green, 1970). When the visual pathways are involved, the agreement is less perfect (Bodis-Wollner, 1972; Bodis-Wollner & Diamond, 1973).

The number of pairs of black and white bars per degree of visual angle is termed the 'spatial frequency' of the grating. The 'cut-off frequency' is the highest detectable spatial frequency at 100% contrast. For lower spatial frequencies, contrast provides a measure of grating detectability (Schade, 1956). The minimum contrast required to detect a given grating is the contrast threshold, and its inverse value is the contrast sensitivity. The plot of the latter as a function of the spatial frequency is a 'contrast sensitivity curve'. Abnormalities of a given patient's contrast sensitivity are best demonstrated by a normalized plot called a 'visuogram' (Bodis-Wollner, 1972; Bodis-Wollner & Diamond, 1973). This is a plot of the ratio of the patient's contrast sensitivity to that of the average normal at corresponding spatial frequencies.

The contrast sensitivity curves of normals with 20/20 Snellen acuity show little intersubject variability (Campbell & Green, 1965), and change predictably with visual blurring due to refractive error. In patients with cerebral lesions involving the visual pathways, the curve is no longer predictable from the visual acuity measurement (Bodis-Wollner, 1975).

* Supported in part by NIH Grant No. EY-00340, and by the Clinical Center for Research in Parkinson's and Allied Disorders, NIH Grant No. NS 11631-03.

41

Looking now at a more peripheral level of the visual pathways, we have been investigating spatial contrast sensitivity functions in retinal disease. Findings in two sisters with tapetoretinal degeneration are reported.

METHODS

Gratings with a sinusoidal luminance profile were generated on an oscilloscope screen by standard methods (Bodis-Wollner, 1972). The screen subtended four degrees of arc at a distance of 144 cm.

For psychophysical measurements, the grating was turned on and off at the rate of 0.4 Hz. The luminance of the homogenous screen during the 'off' phase was equal to the mean luminance of the pattern (40 foot-lamberts). At each spatial frequency tested, the contrast of the grating was varied, and at each contrast level, the patient was asked if he detected the grating. As in previous work, fifty percent detectability was taken as contrast threshold (Bodis-Wollner, Hendley & Atkin, 1976). The extrapolated cut-off frequency for the average normal subject with 20/20 Snellen acuity is 42 cycles/degree under our test conditions (Bodis-Wollner, 1972; Bodis-Wollner & Diamond, 1973).

For evoked potential (EP) measurements, silver disc electrodes were placed occipitally and temporally, with a forehead ground (Bodis-Wollner, Hendley & Atkin, 1976). The stimulus grating (0.7 contrast) was phase-alternated at a rate of 8 Hz ('counterphase flicker': Kelly, 1971). Scalp potentials were fed to a differential amplifier, filtered with corner frequencies of 1.5and 60 Hz, and averaged with a Nicolet 1072 computer.

Opthalmological evaluation included: Snellen acuity with chart luminance of 40 foot-lamberts; AO HRR pseudo-isochromatic plates and Farnsworth D-15 panel; Goldmann dynamic and static perimetry (the latter with a 0.1 deg target on standard background brightness of 93 foot-lamberts); and Goldmann-Weekers dark adaptometry. Electroretinography was performed under photopic conditions, and also after 10 minutes dark adaptation, using a modified Burian-Allen ERG electrode and a Grass PS-2 photic stimulator.

CASE HISTORIES

C.M.: A 19-year-old female complained of progressive 'blurry vision', difficulty reading, and decreased vision in the dark. Her visual acuity was 20/20-3 for each eye without correction. Her refractive error was +2.50 sphere, OU, but correction did not change acuity. Although C.M. could read the 20/20 line, she responded slowly. Her color vision was normal. Appreciation of Haidinger brushes was normal. Goldmann perimetry of each eye revealed a dense ring scotoma, field constriction for all isopters, and an 8-10° central field to the I/4 isopter (see Figures 1A and B).

Funduscopic examination showed normal discs and maculae, markedly attenuated vessels, and a whitish generalized mottling of the pigment epithelium, with occasional granules of pigment. The electroretinogram was extinguished. Dark adaptation, tested 11 degrees inferior to fixation, gave a monophasic curve. The early portion of the curve was elevated by about 1.5 log units. In five minutes C.M.'s threshold reached a plateau which corresponded to the dark adapted final cone threshold of normal observers. There was no evidence of a rod branch. After 40 minutes dark adaptation, the detectability of a foveally presented 3 degree red target was elevated about 0.3 log units.

M.M.: The 15-year-old sister had no visual complaints. M.M.'s Snellen acuity was 20/20-2 either without or with correction of +1.25 cylinder axis 90°. This was similar to C.M.'s acuity of 20/20-3, but M.M. promptly identified the letters of the chart. Funduscopic examination revealed retinal pathology, which was similar to C.M.'s, albeit somewhat less marked. Goldmann perimetry showed a marked constriction of central isopters and a relative scotoma which ringed fixation temporally, OU (Figures 1C and D). Color vision was normal. Dark adaptation showed a normal primary curve and rod-cone break, but the final rod threshold was elevated 1/2 log unit. The dark adapted threshold to a foveally presented 3 degree red target was normal. The photopic electroretinogram was subnormal, and neither the a-nor the b-wave amplitude increased with stimulus intensity or with dark

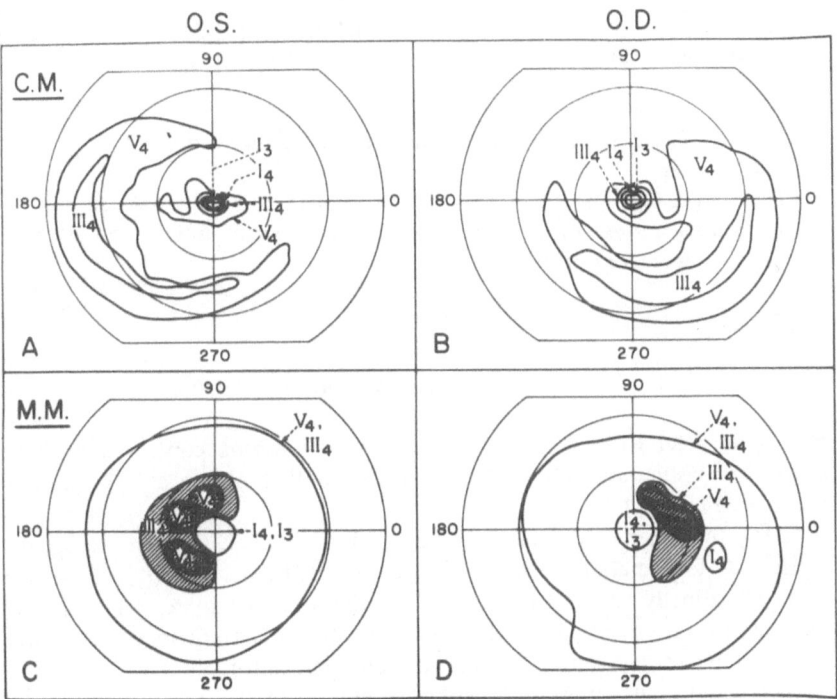

Fig. 1. Dynamic visual fields of C.M. (A and B) and M.M. (C and D). Both sisters had 20/20-Snellen acuity scores, annular scotomata, field constriction, and a central field larger than eight degrees. The concentric circles, from the outermost inward, indicate 90 deg, 60 deg, and 30 deg from fixation.

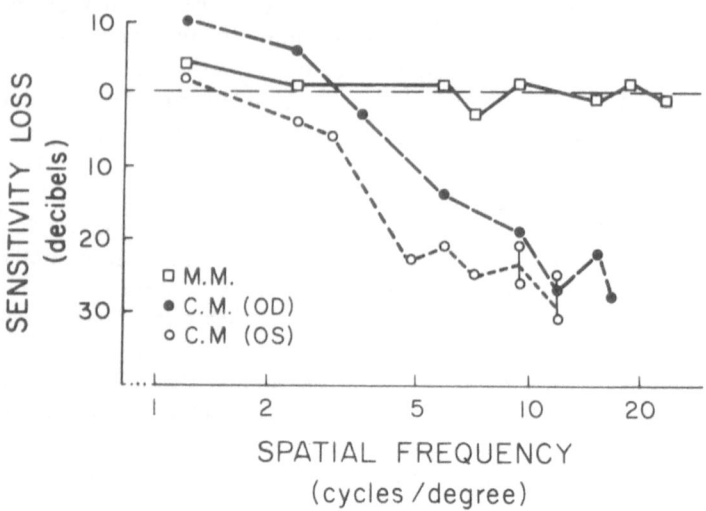

Fig. 2. Visuograms of C.M. and M.M. Plot of the ratio (ordinate) of patient's contrast sensitivity to that of the average normal at corresponding spatial frequencies (abscissa), expressed in decibels. (A 20-decibel loss corresponds to 1 log unit or tenfold threshold elevation; a 6 db loss corresponds to a twofold elevation). M.M. shows a perfectly normal visuogram. C.M. has high frequency loss for both OD and OS.

adaptation. The response to flicker at the rate of 30 flashes per second was also subnormal.

The two sisters' parents and five other sibling had no visual complaints: their visual acuities, fundus examination, Goldmann fields, and electro-retinograms were all normal.

RESULTS

A. Measurements of spatial contrast sensitivity

M.M. (the sister with no visual complaints) had a normal contrast sensitivity curve: her visuogram almost exactly matched that of the average normal observer (Figure 2).

C.M., the sister complaining of visual blurring, showed good grating detection at low spatial frequencies, but her contrast sensitivity started to drop abnormally from 4 cycles/degree, and the loss increased with frequency at a rate of about 12 db per octave. Her high frequency cut-off was about 17 cycles/degree for OD and 12 cycles/degree for OS.

The amplitudes of M.M.'s evoked potentials were within the normal range, but those of C.M. were well below normal at all spatial frequencies tested except the lowest (0.5 cycle/degree). For each sister, the EP results were generally consistent with the psycho-physical results. However, C.M.'s responses began to drop off at somewhat lower spatial frequencies in the evoked potential than in the psychophysical data.

B. Static perimetry

Static perimetry (Figure 3) showed a tenfold reduction in sensitivity to a 0.1 degree target over the central 4 degrees of C.M.s field. There was no reduction over the corresponding part of M.M.'s field.

DISCUSSION

The earliest pathology of tapetoretinal degenerations of the retinitis pigmentosa variety is a dystrophy of the rods and/or cones. Initially, these changes are most severe at the midperiphery of the retina and progress centripetally and centrifugally. In addition, a generalized narrowing of the retinal vessels occurs at an early stage. The condition is typically characterized by a progressive annular scotoma in the visual field, a markedly subnormal to extinguished electroretinogram, and an elevation of dark adapted thresholds. Both C.M. and M.M. had these classical clinical findings.

We were surprised to find a profound high frequency loss of contrast sensitivity in C.M., in view of 20/20 Snellen acuity and normal color vision. Her extrapolated grating acuity was 17 cycles/degree, OD, and 12 cycles/degree, OS. These cut-off frequencies are less than half the value which could be expected from her Snellen acuity. M.M., the younger sister, had completely normal contrast sensitivity and normal cut-off frequencies: i.e. normal grating acuity. The static perimetry results were consistent with these data; i.e. foveal sensitivity normal for M.M. and reduced for C.M.

The detection of high frequency gratings in humans is believed to be mediated by the central-most ganglion cells and their neural connections, as demonstrated in the primate and cat retina (Ikeda & Wright, 1972). Low spatial frequencies are thought to stimulate large ganglion cells with receptive fields extending beyond the foveal region. The ring scotoma of C.M. left a central island of about 8 degrees by 10 degrees intact to the I/3 isopter.

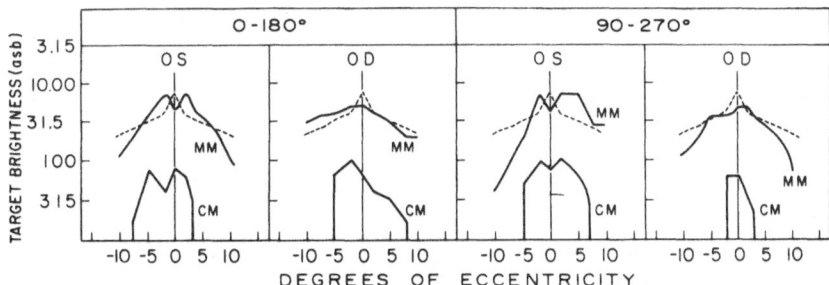

Fig. 3. Static perimetry of C.M. and M.M. obtained for the central fields on the Goldmann perimeter using the 'I' target subtending approximately 6' of arc at the eye. Background brightness was 93 foot-lamberts. Dotted lines represent the profile of a normal observer. Static profiles approximating the normal response were obtained from M.M. Depressed profiles represent C.M.'s responses. Results obtained in oblique meredians were similar.

Our grating target size is 4 degrees, and its detail is best detected by foveal vision. Consequently, one might expect that retinal photoreceptor pathology which gives rise to an annular rather than central scotoma would be associated with normal grating detection, or if anything, with low spatial frequency losses.

Whatever the pathophysiological explanation for the observed high-frequency loss, we are faced with the problem of dissociation between different measures of foveal vision. C.M., the sister with 'blurry vision', showed decreased grating acuity, high spatial frequency loss, and decreased foveal sensitivity measured by static perimetry and dark adaptometry. M.M., the sister without subjective complaints, had none of these abnormalities. But both patients had normal Snellen acuity scores. We wonder, therefore, about the limitations of current methods for measuring visual acuity.

REFERENCES

Bodis-Wollner, I. Visual acuity and contrast sensitivity in patients with cerebral lesions. *Science* 178, *769-771* (1972).

Bodis-Wollner, I. Visual acuity measurements with grating patterns. *The Lancet* I, *503-504* (1975).

Bodis-Wollner, I. & S.P. Diamond.. A method of testing and evaluating blurred vision in cerebral lesions. *Trans. Am. Neurol. Assoc.* 98, *9-12* (1973).

Bodis-Wollner, I., C.D. Hendley & A. Atkin. Evaluation by evoked potentials of dissociated visual functions in patients with cerebral lesions, in Desmedt, J. (ed): Visual Evoked Potentials in Man, Oxford, Clarendon Press, 1976.

Campbell, F.W. & D.C. Green.. Optical and retinal factors affecting visual resolution. *J. Physiol.* 181, *576-593* (1965).

Green. D.G. Testing the vision of cataract patients by means of laser generated interference fringes. *Science* 168, *1240-1242* (1970).

Ikeda, H. & M.J. Wright. Differential effects of refractive errors and receptive field organization of central and peripheral ganglion cells. *Vis. Res.* 12, *1465-1476* (1972).

Kelly, D.H. Theory of flicker and transient responses: II. Counterphase gratings. *J. Opt. Soc. Am.* 61, *632-640*, 1971.

Mayer, T. (1754) Comment. Gotting. IV, 97 and 135. In: 'Handbuch der Physiologischen Optik' by H.V. Helmholtz. Vol. I 3rd Edition with comments by Gullstrand, v. Kries, and Nagel (1911). Hamburg and Leipzig: L. Voss, pp. 31-32.

Schade, D.H. Optical and photoelectric analog of the eye. *J. Opt. Soc. Am.* 46, *721-739* (1956).

Author's address
Dept of Opthalmology
Mount Sinai School of Medicine
5th Ave & 100th Street
New York, N.Y. 10029
USA

PSYCHOPHYSICAL AND VECP EXAMINATIONS OF EMMETROPIA, MYOPIA, HYPERMETROPIA AND APHAKIA

Y. CHIBA, D. KANAIZUKA & E. ADACHI-USAMI

(Chiba/Hamamatsu)

ABSTRACT

The VECP to checkerboard pattern revearsal stimuli is studied in a number of situations where the area and the spatial distribution of the stimuli around the central retina are altered. As the results, the VECP threshold is proved to be strongly related to the central part of the retina.

In many cases of emmetropia, myopia, hypermetropia and aphakia, the corelation between the VECP and subjective measurements are studied. Summarized data prove that there are ± 0.5 dioptres differences between them.

Since Van der Tweel (1966) and Spekreijse (1966) reported checkerboard pattern reversal VECPs, a number of studies on this subject have been reported (Cambell & Maffei, 1970; Millodot & Riggs, 1970; Regan & Sperling, 1971; Behrman *et al.*, 1972; Huber *et al.*, 1972).

Because of the fact that this potential is simply sinusoidal in its waveform and no inter-individual difference is found, not only pure physiologists, but also clinicians have been trying to apply this method for diagnosing disease. We are also not an exception. A series of our studies (Chiba *et al.*, 1975; Chiba, 1976; Chiba, in press) on the VECP in several diseases of the visual pathway suggested that it is quite a useful tool to study diseases which impair central vision.

In the present paper, investigation of the changes of pattern reversal VECPs in subjects with refractive errors is performed and those results are compared with subjective measurements.

Prior to beginning clinical studies, some physiological properties of the checkerboard pattern reversal VECP related to the central portion of the retina were studied.

METHODS

Our device for producing the checkerboard pattern reversal is essentially the same as Behrman's, but greatly modified for practical purposes (Adachi *et al.*, 1975).

In order to get the visual angle of 15' for the individual checks of the polaroid checkerboard, the distance between the eye and the pattern sheet is set at 2.3 m.

The visual angle of the sheet and the luminance at the sheet are variable.

Frequencies of pattern reversal are around 12.0Hz.

Potentials are recorded from electrodes placed on the midline, 3 cm above the inion, and an indifferent electrode on the earlobe. Potentials are amplified with a bandpass of 1.5 Hz-300 Hz and fed into an averager. Two hundred responses are averaged. The averaged VECP is photographed by a polaroid camera or written by an inkwriting pen recorder or an X-Y recorder.

Cycloplegia is done with 1% atropine or 1% cyclopentolate.

The height between the peak and the trough of the sinusoidal output is measured as the amplitude of the VECP.

Thirty six subjects (43 eyes) are examined. They are 7 cases of emmetropia (9 eyes), 12 cases of myopia (12 eyes), 13 cases of hypermetropia (16 eyes) and 5 cases of aphakia (6 eyes).

RESULTS AND DISCUSSION

(A) Fundamental experiments in normal subjects

1. Effects of the luminance of the pattern sheet on the VECP

Changes of VECP amplitudes are studied at various pattern luminances. The visual angle of a piece of polaroid square is set at 15' and that of the entire pattern sheet is 2°30'. Frequency of pattern reversal is 12.0 Hz.

As shown in Figure 1, the maximum amplitude is obtained at a luminance of around 0.8 log ft-L, which is 3.5 log units above the sensory threshold.

The phase of the sinusoidal potential shifts to the left as the pattern luminance increases.

2. Area-intensity relationship and retinal location

1) Effects of area of the pattern sheet on the VECP

When the eye is centrally fixated, the areal effect of a pattern sheet on the VECP is studied.

Examined stimulus areas are 30', 1°00', 1°30', 2°00', 2°30', 3°00', 3°30' and 4°00'.

The pattern luminance required for the amplitude of 1.0 μV is measured at each stimulus field, and the values obtained are plotted against log area of stimulus field (Figure 2).

Up to an area of 2°30', VECP sensitivity increases linearly as the areal size increases.

At areal sizes greater than 2°30', no increase in VECP sensitivity is found.

2) Occlusion of the central stimulus area

Studies are done to determine the VECP sensitivity in different locations on the retina, excluding the areal effect.

The visual angle of the pattern sheet is set at 4° and the central area of it is occluded.

48

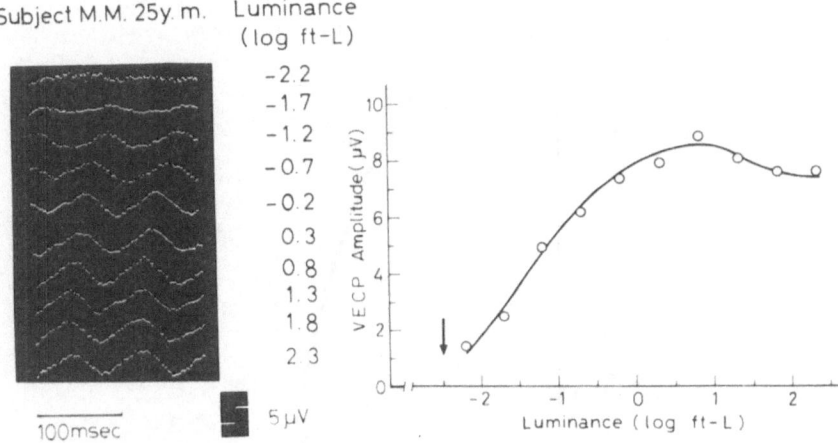

Fig. 1. The left half of the figure represents the actual VECPs at various pattern luminance. Pattern luminance is reduced by insertion of neutral density filters. On the right, VECP amplitudes are plotted against pattern luminance of the stimulus field. The arrow indicates sensory threshold. Frequency of pattern reversal, 12.0 Hz; Visual angle of an individual check, 15′.

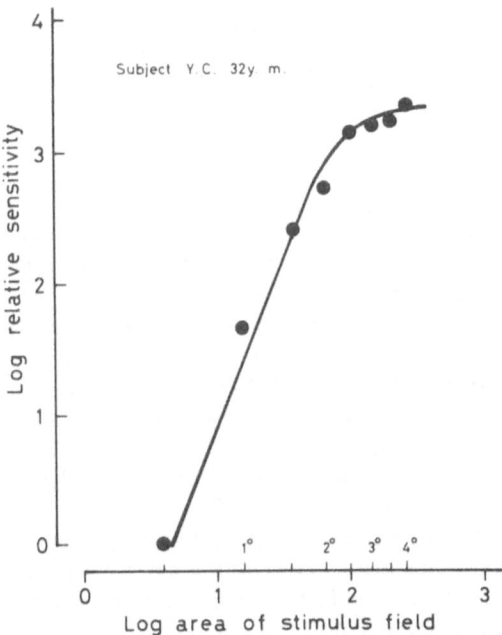

Fig. 2. Log relative sensitivity (criterion amplitude = 1.0 μV) of the VECP vs. log area of the stimulus field. Frequency of pattern reversal, 13.3 Hz; Visual angle of an individual check, 15′.

49

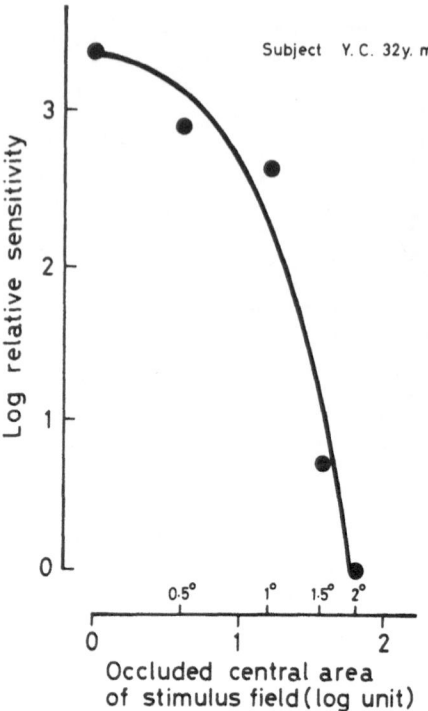

Fig. 3. Log relative sensitivity vs. the central area occluded. The entire stimulus field subtends 4° of visual angle. Frequency of pattern reversal, 13.3 Hz; Visual angle of a individual check, 15′.

As shown in Figure 3, no VECP is recorded when a central area of 2° is occluded. In this case, the remaining peripheral area is identical to the non-occluded central area of 3°30′.

This indicates that the decrease of VECP sensitivity depends not on the area itself, but on the retinal location.

To confirm these results, the VECPs to the central stimulus with visual angle of 1°30′ and the stimulus with the same area with the central area of 1°30′ occluded are compared (Figure 4). A remarkable reduction of the VECP sensitivity is seen when the central area is occluded.

3) Eccentricity from the fovea

The VECP changes when the stimulus falls at different distances from fixation are studied. The visual angle of the pattern sheet is set at 1° and the VECPs are recorded with the fixation point shifted nasally 1° and 2°.

As the fixation point is shifted peripherally from the foveal, the VECP sensitivity decreases and the VECP is not recordable when the fixation point is moved 3° from the fovea.

All the above mentioned results suggest that the pattern reversal VECP is strongly related to the central part of the retina up to 2° from the fovea.

The VECPs are recorded with various power lenses inserted in front of the eye.

For each power lens, the relationship between VECP amplitude and the pattern luminance is examined. The luminance where there is a linear relationship is found. This luminance is used for VECP examinations in patients.

VECP amplitudes are plotted against the lens diopters used. The lens for obtaining the maximum VECP amplitude is then compared with subjective visual acuity measurements. Both VECPs and sensory measurements of representative cases are shown in Figure 5 and 6.

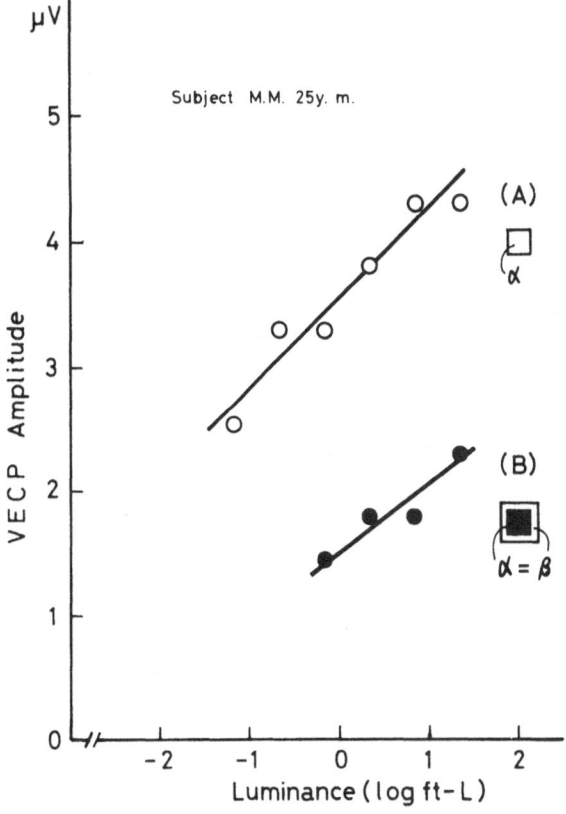

Fig. 4. VECP amplitude vs. pattern luminance of the stimulus field falling on the central retina. The stimulus (A) has a diameter of 1° 30′ in visual angle. And (B) has the same occluded with a peripherical band of equal area stimulated. The exposed area (α) is equal to the occluded area (β). Frequency of pattern reversal, 12.0 Hz: Visual angle of an individual check, 15′.

Comparisons between the lens diopters required for the subjective best visual acuity and for the maximum VECP amplitude are summarized in Table 1. The difference between the two measures (indicated as ΔD in Table) is extremely small.

In 1961, Van der Tweel introduced the application of sinusoidal modu-

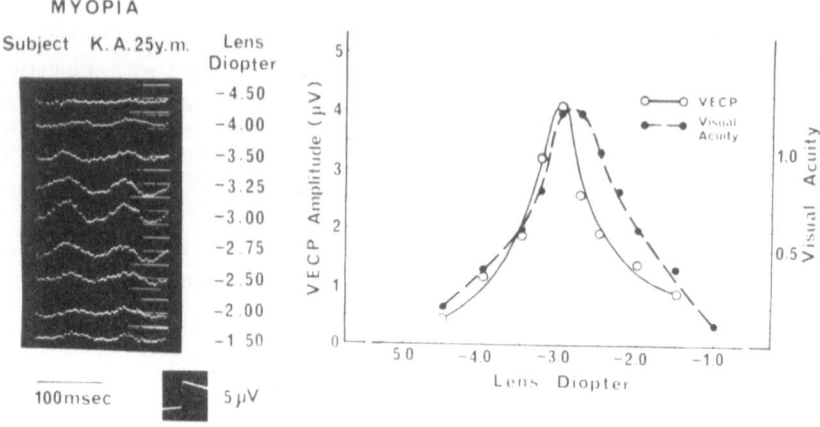

Fig. 5. The left half of the figure represents the actual VECPs of a myopic eye at various lens powers in diopters. On the right, VECP amplitudes (indicated with open circles) and visual acuity (indicated with dots) are plotted against lens power in diopters. Frequency of pattern reversal, 12.0 Hz; Visual angle of an individual check, 15'.

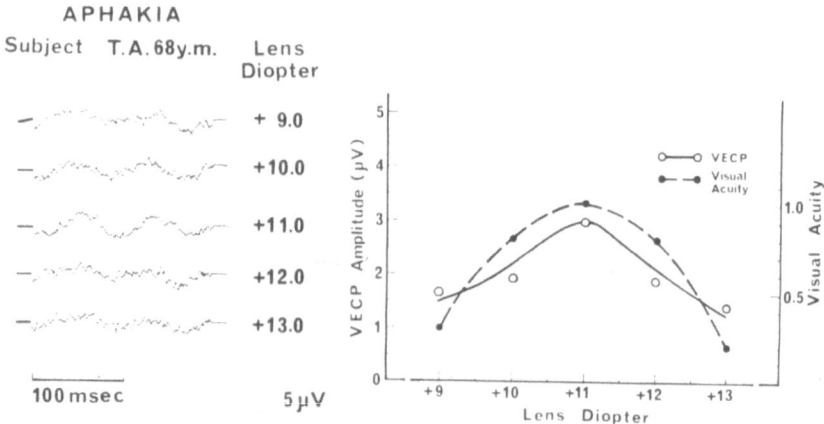

Fig. 6. The left half of the figure represents the actual VECPs of an aphakic eye at various lens powers in diopters. On the right, VECP amplitudes (indicated with open circles) and visual acuity (indicated with dots) are plotted against lens power in diopters. Frequency of pattern reversal, 12.0 Hz; Visual angle of an individual check, 15'.

52

Table 1. Summary of the results of refractive examination with VECP and subjective measurements.

	Name	Age	Sex	Side	Lens Diopter for maximum VECP Amplitude (A)	Lens Diopter for maximum Visual Acuity (B)	ΔD (A−B)
	T.I.	8	m	R	0.00	0.00	0.00
	S.S.	21	f	R	0.00	0.00	0.00
				L	0.00	0.00	0.00
	T.K.	23	f	R	0.00	0.00	0.00
Emmetropia	S.I.	25	m	R	0.00	0.00	0.00
				L	0.00	0.00	0.00
	M.M.	25	m	L	0.25	0.00	+0.25
	S.A.	27	f	L	0.00	0.00	0.00
	D.K.	43	m	L	0.00	0.00	0.00
	S.B.	9	m	R	− 0.75	− 1.00	+0.25
	Y.K.	22	f	R	− 1.50	− 1.75	+0.25
	K.S.	24	m	R	− 3.50	− 3.00	−0.50
	Y.S.	25	f	L	− 1.25	− 1.50	+0.25
	K.N.	25	f	R	− 2.50	− 2.50	0.00
Myopia	K.A.	25	m	L	− 3.00	− 2.75	−0.25
	Y.W.	26	f	L	− 5.00	− 5.00	0.00
	K.S.	31	m	L	− 1.00	− 1.00	0.00
	M.K.	33	f	R	−14.00	−14.00	0.00
	N.N.	37	f	L	− 1.50	− 1.50	0.00
	Y.K.	39	f	L	− 2.00	− 1.75	−0.25
	I.S.	48	m	R	−10.00	−11.00	+1.00
	Y.K.	7	f	R	+ 1.50	+ 1.50	0.00
				L	+ 4.50	+ 5.00	−0.50
	K.O.	9	m	R	+ 8.00	+ 9.00	−1.00
				L	+10.00	+10.00	0.00
	T.I.	10	m	R	+ 2.00	+ 1.50	+0.50
	K.O.	13	f	L	+ 2.00	+ 2.00	0.00
	K.O.	18	f	L	+ 1.25	+ 1.25	0.00
Hypermetropia	J.O.	23	f	R	+ 0.50	+ 0.25	+0.25
	M.B.	27	f	L	+ 0.50	+ 0.75	−0.25
	Y.C.	31	m	L	+ 0.50	+ 0.25	+0.25
	N.K.	42	m	R	+ 0.50	+ 0.50	0.00
	Y.K.	47	f	L	+ 1.50	+ 1.50	0.00
	U.Y.	53	m	R	+ 0.50	+ 0.50	0.00
	T.A.	62	f	R	+ 1.00	+ 0.50	+0.50
				L	+ 1.00	+ 1.00	0.00
	A.S.	64	m	R	+ 1.25	+ 1.00	+0.25
	T.I.	60	f	L	+11.00	+11.00	0.00
	H.O.	64	m	R	+ 9.00	+ 9.00	0.00
Aphakia	T.A.	68	m	L	+11.00	+11.00	0.00
	S.M.	69	m	R	+12.00	+12.00	0.00
				L	+11.00	+12.00	−1.00
	Y.K.	78	m	R	+11.00	+11.00	0.00

lated light in human evoked potentials. Then, Van der Tweel (1965, 1966), Spekreijse (1966, 1973), Regan (1971, 1973) have described a number of studies on potentials evoked by pattern reversal.

Other approaches to obtain pattern reversal stimuli have been tried by several authors (Millodot & Riggs, 1970; Behrman et al., 1972; Huber et al., 1972; Bornstein, 1975).

Spekreijse was the first who found that the amplitude of the VECP to pattern reversal stimuli was greatly reduced when the retinal image was defocused.

Then, possibilities of measuring refraction by means of this kind of VECP were reported by Millodot & Riggs (1970), Behrman et al. (1972), Huber et al. (1972), McCormack & Marg (1973), Regan (1973), Adachi et al. (1975) and Chiba et al. (1975).

The present study is similar, but includes a large number of clinical cases.

As seen in the summary table, slight differences between the VECP refraction measurements and the subjective visual acuity are found in cases of emmetropia, on the order of ± 0.25 D. In cases of myopia, the VECP results tend to shift more to + side of the sensory results. A good correspondence between the two is found in aphakic eyes.

The most important thing determined during these studies is the effect of accommodation on the VECP. If 0.5% tropicamide (usually used in the clinic for fundus examination) is used, the data are strongly affected by the insufficient cycloplegia. Therefore, in young subjects, cycloplegia should be done with Atropine in order to get reliable VECP refraction measurements.

REFERENCES

Adachi, E., Adachi, T., Kanaizuka, D. & Chiba, Y.: New stimulating devices for the checkerboard pattern reversal cortical evoked potentials. *Folia Ophthal. Jap.*, 26, *516-518*, 1975.

Behrman, J., Nissim, S. & Arden, G. B.: A clinical method for obtaining pattern visual evoked responses. 'The Visual System Neurophysiology, Biophysics, and Their Clinical Applications' Proc. 9th ISCERG Symp. in Brighton 1971, 199-203, Plenum Press, N.Y./Lond., 1972.

Bornstein, Y.: The pattern evoked responses (VER) in optic neuritis. *Albrecht v. Graefes Arch. klin. exp. Ophthal.*, 197, *101-106*, 1975.

Cambell, F.W. & Maffei, L.: Electrophysiological evidence for the existence of orientation and size detectors in the human visual system. *J. Physiol.*, 270, *635-652*, 1970.

Chiba, Y., Kanaizuka, D. & Adachi, E.: Studies on the visual evoked cortical potentials to checkerboard pattern reversal stimuli. Report 1. It's applications in refraction. *Jap. J. Clin. Ophthal.*, 29, *17-26*, 1975.

Chiba, Y.: Studies on the visual evoked cortical potentials to checkerboard pattern reversal stimuli. Report 2. Central serous chorioretinopathy. *Folia Ophthal. Jap.*, 27, *339-347*, 1976.

Chiba, Y.: Checkerboard pattern reversal VECP in optic neuritis. *Jap. Rev. Clin. Ophthal.* (in press)

Huber, C., Adachi-Usami, E. & Kellermann, F.-J.: Bestimmung von Refraktionsfehlern mittels der visuell evozierten Antworten im EEG. Bericht über die 71. Zusammenkunft der Deutschen Ophthalm. Gesellschaft in Heidelberg 1971. J.F. Bergmann, München, 548-551, 1972.

McCormack, G. & Marg, E.: Computer-assisted eye examination. II. Visual evoked response meridional refractometry. *Am. J. Opt. and Arch. Am. Acad. Opt.*, 50, *889-903*, 1973.

Millodot, M. & Riggs, L.A.: Refraction determined electrophysiologically. Responses to alternation of visual contours. *Arch. Ophthal.*, 84, *272-278*, 1970.

Regan, D. & Sperling, H.G.: A method of evoking contour-specific scalp potentials by chromatic checkerboard patterns. *Vision Res.*, 11, *173-176*, 1971.

Regan, D.: Rapid objective refraction using evoked brain potentials. *Invest. Ophthal.*, 12, *669-679*, 1973.

Spekreijse, H.: Analysis of EEG responses in man, Junk Publishers, The Hague, The Netherlands, 1966.

Spekreijse, H., Tweel, L.H. van der & Zuidema, Th.: Contrast evoked responses in man. *Vision Res.*, 13, *1577-1601*, 1973.

Tweel, L.H. van der: Some problem in vision regarded with respect to linearity and frequency response. *Ann. N.Y. Acad. Sci.*, 89, art. 5, *829-856*, 1961.

Tweel, L.H. van der & Verduin Lunel, H.F.E.: Human visual responses to sinusoidally modulated light. *Electroenceph. Clin. Neurophysiol.*, 18, *587-598*, 1965.

Tweel, L.H. van der & Spekreijse, H.: Visual evoked responses. 'The clinical value of electroretinography' ISCERG symp. Ghent 1966, 83-94, Karger, Basel/N.Y., 1968.

Authors' address:
Y. Chiba & D. Kanaizuka
Dept of Ophthalmology
School of Medicine
Chiba University
Chiba
Japan

E. Adachi-Usami
First Dept of Physiology
School of Medicine
Hamamatsu University
Hamamatsu
Japan

LOCALIZATION OF VISUAL EVOKED CORTICAL POTENTIALS IN HOMONYMOUS HEMIANOPIA*

Z. NAKAMURA & W.R. BIERSDORF

(Kawasaki/Columbus, Ohio)

INTRODUCTION

The human retina is split vertically at the fovea, with optic fibers from the temporal retina projecting to the occipital lobe on the same side of the head, while nerve fibers from the nasal retina cross at the optic chiasm and project to the occipital lobe of the opposite side. This semidecussation of the optic nerve results in the clinical phenomenon of homonymous hemianopia in cases of optic tract or pathway damage. Semi-decussation might therefore be expected to produce differing visual evoked cortical potentials on the two sides of the scalp. A number of studies have explored this question, with some finding differing VECP's over the two brain hemispheres.

In our previous research (Biersdorf & Nakamura, 1971; Nakamura & Biersdorf, 1971), VECP's were monopolarly recorded from multiple electrodes by half-field blank flash stimulation of normal eyes in a light-adapted condition. Isopotential contour maps of each VECP component were drawn. It was shown that the maxima of the early three VECP components were located in the parieto-occipital area of the hemisphere which corresponded to the half retina stimulated.

VECP's of seven cases of homonymous hemianopia have been recorded. The results support the theory on the localization of VECP sources previously proposed (Biersdorf & Nakamura, 1971, 1973).

METHOD

The apparatus was the same as previously reported (Nakamura & Biersdorf, 1971; Nakamura, 1975). A hemisphere of 60 cm diameter was illuminated with white light at 330 nit (96ft-L) with direct current to light adapt the eye and suppress rod function. An aperture (13 degree visual angle) at the center of the hemisphere in front of the subject admitted light from a xenon flash lamp and reflector through a red filter (Kodak Wratten No. 25) and a diffusor (transmission 76%). The intensity of the xenon flash lamp was maintained at a constant moderate level (O.3 Joule). Standard EEG electrodes

* This research supported in part by USPHS Research Grant No. EY00454.

(5 mm in diameter) of the chlorided silver type were attached to the scalp with electrode jelly following the International 10-20 EEG system. Monopolar recording was used with linked earlobes as the common reference. Amplication was by differential AC amplifiers with time constant 0.3 sec and high cut of 30 Hz. Five channels were recorded simultaneously with a two-channel signal averager and an FM tape recorder. Responses were displayed on an X-Y recorder. For contour mapping from ten electrode positions, five positions were first recorded twice and then the other five positions were recorded twice.

The patient was positioned with the eye to be tested at the center of the hemisphere with a chin rest 30 cm from the stimulus light. He was asked to look at a small black dot at the center of the 13 degrees red stimulus area while the other eye was occluded. Responses (200) to the red stimulus light flashing at a rate of 3.3 Hz were averaged. Masking noise provided by a phonostimulator made the clicks inaudible. The patient's pupil was not dilated. VECP's were also recorded in the same manner to stimulation of the other eye.

RESULTS

Fig. 1 shows photopic macular ERG's and VECP's of normal eyes. Three responses were simultaneously recorded from lower lid (ERG), parietal (Pz) and occipital area (Inion). Twenty eight average responses from twenty eight normal eyes were superimposed to show intersubjective variation as a criterion for clinical application.

As shown in previous papers, VECP's were widely distributed on the scalp (Nakamura & Biersdorf, 1971; Nakamura 1975). VECP's recorded in the photopic condition, however, were classified into two basic waveforms: Parietal type (P_z-VECP) and occipital type (Inion-VECP). The former is recorded from C_z, P_z, P_3, P_4, T_5, and T_6, while the latter is obtained from O_1, O_2, O_z, and the Inion. Early components of P_z-VECP are labeled component I (negative, peaking at 50.9 ± 4.8 msec), II (positive-69.1 ± 5.2 msec) and III (negative-91.5 ± 5.2 msec) as in Fig. 1. Fig. 2 illustrates isopotential contour maps of component II in response to full disc and half-field stimulation in a normal subject. For the derivation of these maps, VECP's are measured at constant latencies derived from the P_z-VECP peaks at all electrode locations. In response to half-field stimulation there is a positive maximum in the parietal area of the contralateral hemisphere and negative maximum at the occipital pole. Components of Inion-VECP do not show this contrast between the two hemispheres. Stimulation of the full disc in normals produces a positive maximum near P_z (sometimes double maxima near P_3 and P_4) with negative maximum at the occipital pole. The zero line for half-field stimulation tends to be linear, either vertical or slanting obliquely across the scalp. In contrast, the zero line for full-disc stimulation tends to form a semicircle around the occipital pole.

Following are the hemianoptic data.

Case 1: T.K. 18 year old female, left homonymous hemianopia (Fig. 3, 4). She was bruised in the left frontal area by a traffic accident in Au-

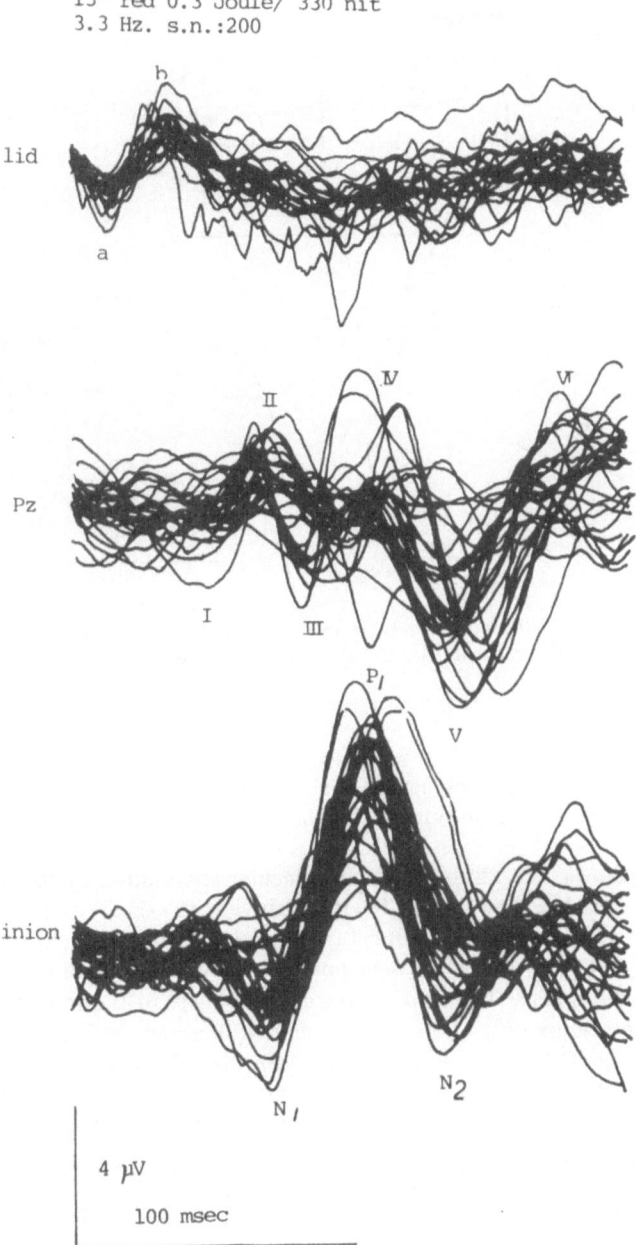

Fig. 1. Averaged ERG's and VECP's from 28 normal eyes from lower lid (ERG), parietal VECP (P_z) and inion VECP.

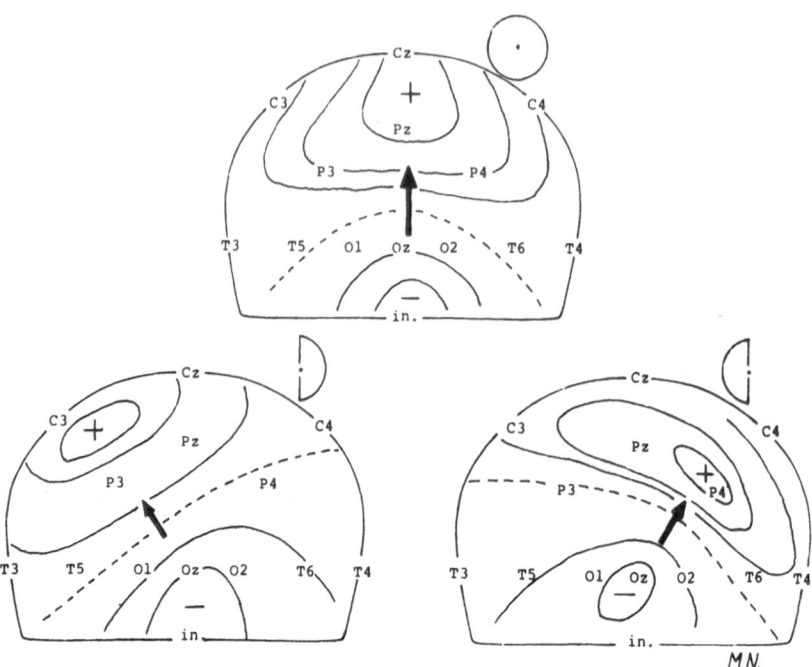

Fig. 2. Isopotential contour maps of the posterior scalp (component II) in response to full disc (top) and lateral half-disc stimulations. Dashed line is zero potential. Normal subject in photopic condition.

gust 1973, and lost consciousness for twenty days. Four months later she complained of left homonymous hemianopia (Fig. 3). V.D. = 1.5, V.S. = 1.0.

Fig. 3 shows VECP's to photopic macular stimulation of the right eye by the 13° red disc. The P_z-VECP with positive II (81 msec) and negative III (96 msec) were found at P_3 and T_5 in the left hemisphere, and reversed polarity P_z-VECPs (negative II and positive III) were found at P_4 and T_6 in the right hemisphere. The isopotential contour maps of II and III have been drawn as posterior projection views in Fig. 4. The zero-lines (broken lines) ran vertically (O.D.) or obliquely (O.S.) on the left hemisphere. Based on the theory of the previous papers (Biersdorf & Nakamura, 1971; 1973), the equivalent dipole source of components II and III is tangenital to the surface of the head and located near zero potential on a line connecting the negative and positive potential maxima. In this case, the source for components II and III is located in the left occipital area, on the intact side. The VECP maps from the stimulation of the left eye show essentially the same results. (Fig. 4)

Case 2: S.M. 43 year old male, left homonymous hemianopia. After a right occipital lobectomy was performed on September 10, 1973 because of a brain tumor of the right parieto-occipital region, he complained of left homonymous hemianopia (Fig. 5). V.D. = 1.2, V.S. = 1.2. The isopotential contour maps of components II and III were similar to case I and also indicate a VECP source in the left occipital region.

Case 3: T.H. 39 year old male, infarct of the left occipital lobe. On Nov. 4, 1964 he was suddenly attacked with severe headache in the left posterior region, vomiting, nosebleed and blurred vision. Later he complained of right homonymous hemianopia with incomplete macular splitting (Fig. 6) V.D. = 1.2, V.S. = 1.2. Potential contour maps showed that the maxima of components II (positive) and III (negative) were located in the right hemisphere on the intact side.

Five additional hemianopes were tested, of which two showed results similar to the above three. In one case, the right eye showed good contrast between the two side in component III, but did not in component II because of incomplete hemianopia. The left eye showed good contrast for both components. In one case of quadrantopia due to a brain infarct, component II showed some contrast while component III showed no differences. A final case of cerebral infarct showed a relative homonymous hemianopia to red and blue targets, and the VECP did not show good contrast between the two hemispheres.

The early components II and III, of the VECP to macular red light stimulation in light adaptation in cases of homonymous hemianopia showed a good contrast between both hemispheres. Components IV and later did not always show such contrast between the two hemispheres. The potential maps for full disc stimulation of a hemianopic patient are basically similar to the maps obtained from half-field stimulation of normal subjects (Biersdorf & Nakamura, 1971). For the hemianopes, the potential maxima of the

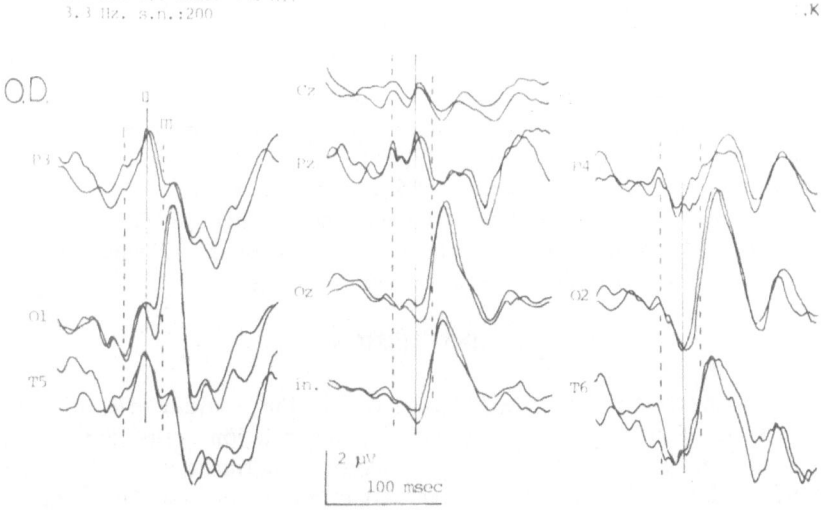

Fig. 3. Averaged VECP's from full disc stimulation of a left homonymous hemianope (Case 1). Two averages shown each position. Solid line-component II. Dashed lines-components I, III.

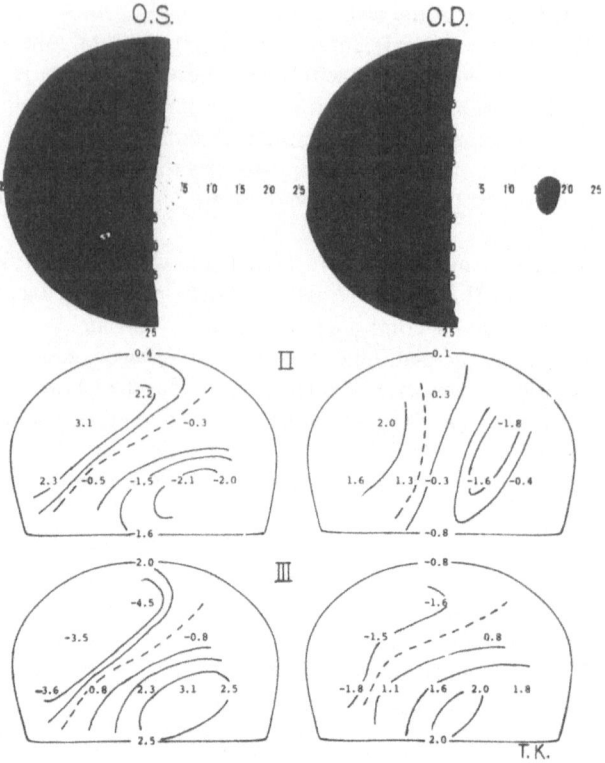

Fig. 4. Visual fields of same patient in Fig. 3 (Case 1). Isopotential contour maps of VECP components II and III shown for each eye.

early components occur over the parieto-occipital area of the healthy hemisphere, while for normals the maxima occur over the same area of the hemisphere corresponding to the half-field stimulated.

Preliminary data have been obtained using either ganzfeld or flashed checkerboard stimulation on some of these hemianopes. This data also showed polarity reversals between the two hemispheres.

DISCUSSION

The semidecussation of the optic nerve and the resulting effects on the VECP are of interest in two respects: for their relation to the clinical problem of hemianopia, and also for the analysis of normal optic pathway and brain organization. In analysing the VECP in homonymous hemianopia, a variety of approaches have been tried. One technique is the placing of electrodes over both cerebral hemispheres and recording VECP's to full field stimulation (Kojima *et al.*, 1972; Yonekura, 1973; Adachi *et al.*, 1971; Vaughan, Katzman & Taylor, 1963; Kooi, Güvener & Bagchi, 1965; Samson-Dollfus *et al.*, 1974; Faidherbe, Lennes & Joachim, 1974; Cohn, 1973). Variable results have been found. Sometimes VECP amplitudes have been reduced and latencies prolonged over the affected hemisphere, while in other cases amplitudes have been found reduced over the normal side. Other approaches that have been tried in a limited number of cases utilize the recording of VECP's to localized stimuli in the visual field (Regan & Heron, 1969; Müller *et al.*, 1974).

The lack of consensus on results points up several problems involved in VECP recording. One is the lack of knowledge on where in the brain the VECP is generated. Does it come from the primary visual area (area 17), or do parts of it come from association areas (18 and 19) Secondly, even for a constant site of origin the orientation of the source (e.g. radial or tangential to the scalp) can produce quite different VECP's at the same position on the scalp. Another question involves macular sparing and its effect on the VECP, when it is known that the VECP is primarily macular in origin. A related problem is that of stray light. A localized stimulus in a dark periph-

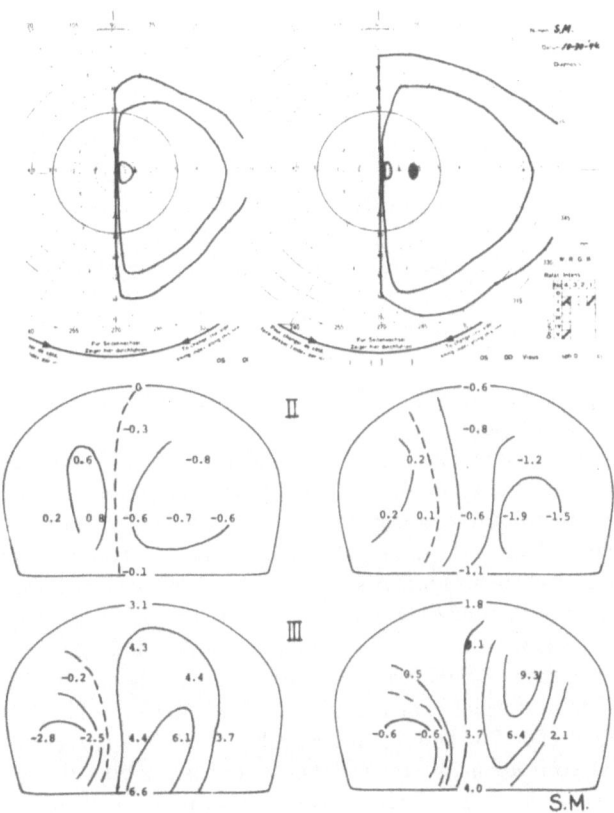

Fig. 5. Visual fields and isopotential contour maps (components II and III) for a left homonymous hemianope (Case 2).

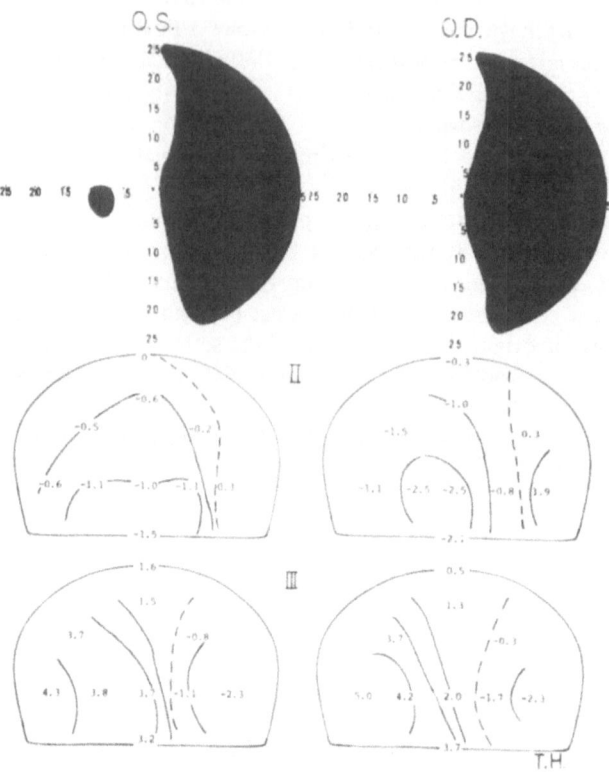

Fig. 6. Visual fields and isopotential contour maps (components II and III) for a right homonymous hemianope (Case 3).

eral field may stimulate the more sensitive macula by means of stray light, rather than the intended peripheral location.

The approach used here has developed out of research on normal subjects using partial field stimulation, and the results found on hemianopes are consistent with those previously found on normals. Two important aspects of the technique are (a) the use of a light-adapted surround with a moderately bright white light adaptation, and (b) the use of a red stimulus light. The reasons for selecting these conditions were to emphasize cone responses free of any possible rod interactions, and to eliminate any possible stimulation by stray light. Utilizing these conditions with lateral half field unpatterned flashes in normal subjects, it was found that three early components of the VECP (50, 70, and 95 msec peaks) were lateralized on the scalp. Isopotential contour maps showed a potential maximum in the parieto-occipital area of the hemisphere corresponding to the half-field stimulated with an opposite polarity potential maximum over the other hemisphere. Later VECP components were not lateralized on the scalp, although this is changed by the use of patterned flashes (Biersdorf & Nakamura, 1973).

Fig. 2 illustrates isopotential contour maps of component II in response to three different stimuli in a normal subject. When the right half field is stimulated, a positive maximum occurs in the left parietal area with a negative maximum near 0_z or on the right occipital area. The theoretical model for this potential distribution assumes an equivalent dipole tangential with the scalp located approximately near zero potential on the line connecting the two potential maxima. This places the source in the left hemisphere which corresponds to the right half field stimulated. Analogous results are obtained with left half field stimulation.

Stimulation of homonymous hemianopic patients show the same results as half-field stimulation of normal subjects. In a left homonymous hemianopia for example, a positive potential maximum for component II occurs in the parieto-occipital area of the left hemisphere with a negative maximum in the occipital area midline and to the right side. This corresponds to stimulation of the seeing half-field, as in half-field stimulation of normals. The hemianopes tested here have two characteristics: (a) macular splitting, i.e. complete half-macular scotoma, and (b) normal visual acuity, i.e. normal function of the other half macula. The results obtained are probably dependent on these characteristics (Kojima et al., 1972; Yonekura, 1973), although it is difficult to compare results with those from other laboratories with differing stimulus conditions.

In both hemianopes and normals, even though only a single VECP source in one hemisphere is active, positive potentials are recorded on one side of the head at the same time negative potentials are recorded on the other side of the head. These potentials can be of reduced amplitude over the abnormal hemisphere, or they can be of equal or even larger amplitude over the abnormal hemisphere. Only when polarities of these potentials and the distribution of these potentials on the scalp are considered in addition that the differences between normal and hemianopic VECP's are shown. As indicated, the zero line between positive and negative VECP's in hemianopes shows considerable variability between vertical and obliquity approaching but not reaching the horizontal. In contrast, the zero line for full disc stimulation of normal tends to form an arc around the occipital pole. Thus a small number of electrodes will not necessarily reveal the difference between a normal and an abnormal distribution. A minimum of several electrode positions are required to show the course of the zero line.

The VECP analysis presented here is also supported by results obtained on bitemporal hemianopes (Lehmann, Kavanagh & Fender, 1969; Kooi, Yamada & Marshall, 1973). In these rare cases, the fibers crossing at the chiasm are inactivated, so that stimulation of one eye produces excitation in the hemisphere on the same side. In case of Lehmann et al. for example, this produced a positive VECP component at 52 msec over the active hemisphere, while a negative component at the same latency was recorded over the other hemisphere. Thus again a single VECP source in one hemisphere produced potentials of opposite polarities on the two sides of the scalp. Taking the difference in reference electrode location into account, their isopotential contour maps are similar to those of this research.

SUMMARY

In order to study the relationship between the semidecussation of the optic nerve and the visual evoked cortical potential, photopic VECP's were monopolarly recorded from multiple electrodes on the scalps of eight patients with homonymous hemianopia. The locations of the amplitude maxima of the three early components of the parietal type of VECP were obtained by means of a contour mapping technique. The macular area (13°) of the patients was stimulated with unpatterned red flashes in a white light-adapted condition (330 nit, 96ft-L). In patients with good acuity and without macular sparing the positive maximum of component II was located over the parieto-temporal area of the intact hemisphere while a negative maximum was found on the other side of the head or near the occipital pole. Components I (50 msec on the average in normal subjects), II (69 msec) and III (91 msec) were similarily localized (polarity reversals between successive peaks). Later components did not usually show this contrast between the hemispheres. The potential contour maps are similar to those obtained from lateral half-field stimulation of normal subjects. The results can be explained by the theory of an equivalent dipole source in a volume conductor previously applied to the results in normals.

REFERENCES

Adachi, E. *et al.* VER of the intracranial lesion and its clinical application. *Folia Ophth. Jap.* 22, *403* (1971).

Biersdorf, W.R., & Nakamura, Z. Electroencephalogram potentials evoked by hemi-retinal stimulation. *Experientia* 27: *402* (1971).

Biersdorf, W.R, & Nakamura, Z. Localization studies of the human visual evoked response. Xth ISCERG Symposium. Doc. Ophth. Proc. Ser. 2, 137 (1973).

Cohn, R. Summated evoked cortical activity in homonymous visual field defects. *Trans. Am. Neurol. Assoc.* 98, *258* (1973).

Faidherbe, J., Lennes, G. & Joachim, M. Mean visual evoked potentials in hemionopsia. XIth ISCERG Symposium. Doc. Ophth. Proc. Ser. 4, 369 (1974).

Kojima, M. et al. The VER in patients with hemianopia. *Folia Ophth. Jap.* 23, *962* (1972).

Kooi, K.A., Güvener, A.M. & Bagchi, B.K. Visual evoked responses in lesions of the higher optic pathways. *Neurology* 15, *841* (1965).

Kooi, K.A., Yamada, T. Marshall, R.E. Field studies of monocularly evoked cerebral potentials in bitemporal hemianopsia. *Neurology* 23, *1217* (1973).

Lehmann, D., Kavanagh, R.N. & Fender, D.H. Field studies of averaged visually evoked EEG potentials in a patient with a split chiasm. *Electroenceph. clin. Neurophysiol.* 26, *193* (1969).

Müller, W. et al. Contributions to objective perimetry by means of the VER. XIth ISCERG Symposium. Doc. Ophth. Proc. Ser. 4, 323 (1974).

Nakamura, Z., & Biersdorf, W.R. Localization of the human visual evoked response. Early components specific to visual stimulation. *Amer. J. Ophth.* 72, *988* (1971).

Nakamura, Z. Studies on the clinical application of the human visual evoked potentials. (2) Macular function and VEP. *Acta Soc. Ophthal. Jap.* 79, *1192* (1975).

Nakamura, Z. Studies on the clinical application of the human visual evoked potentials.

(1) Size of the stimulus fields and VEP on the longitudinal positions of the scalp. *Acta Soc. Ophthal. Jap.* 78, *867* (1974).

Regan, D. & Heron, J.R. Clinical investigation of lesions of the visual pathway: a new objective technique. *J. Neurol. Neurosurg. Psychiat.* 32, *479* (1969).

Samson-Dollfus, D. *et al.* Interest of monopolae leads in visual evoked responses of lateral homonymous hemianopsia. XIth ISCERG Symposium. Doc. Ophth. Proc. Ser. 4, 363 (1974).

Vaughan, H.G. Jr., Katzman, R. & Taylor, J. Alterations of visual evoked response in the presence of homonymous visual defects. *Electroenceph. clin. Neurophysiol.* 15, *737* (1963).

Yonekura, Y. The visual evoked response (VER) in a patient with hemianopia. *Folia Ophth. Jap.* 24, *569* (1973).

Authors' address:
Z. Nakamura
Dept of Ophthalmology
St. Marianna University
Kawasaki
Japan

W.R. Biersdorf
Dept of Ophthalmology
Ohio State University
Columbus, Ohio
USA

AMPLITUDE VERSUS FREQUENCY CHARACTERISTICS OF VISUAL EVOKED CORTICAL POTENTIALS TO SINE WAVE MODULATED LIGHT IN DISEASE OF THE OPTIC NERVE

CH. HUBER

(Zürich)

ABSTRACT

The frequency dependence of visual evoked cortical potentials under stimulation with a large field sine wave modulated light is investigated in patients with affections of the optic nerve. Neuritis and optic atrophy results in a strong reduction of high frequency responses (above 20 Hz). In neuritis the attenuation may be reversible. Amblyopia wether due to squint or occlusion does not affect the high frequency responses as compared to the normal eye in the same subject. V.E.C.P. are obtainable in patients with retinitis pigmentosa in whom the ERG is extinct. The more advanced cases however show a strong reduction of high frequency responses, the V.E.C.P. reduction is not dependent on the presence of cataract. The method can be applied to infant and small children without general anesthesia as fixation is not essential.

In the last few years the stimulation technology in visual evoked cortical potentials (V.E.C.P.) has been so far improved that cortical responses can be used even for refraction or color vision testing. Unfortunately for the many patients whose vision is reduced to the perception of shadows those sophisticated stimuli are but a tale told by a doctor, but nevertheless soundless and signifying nothing. We have been looking for a Stimulus to elicit V.E.C.P. sensitive to affections of the visual system but also insensitive to opacities of the ocular media or erratic fixation pattern. A homogenous blank field whose intensity is modulated in time with a strong modulation depth has been found to be very little affected by opacities of the ocular media and if the stimulus size is made large enough a lack of steady fixation is also unimportant. On the other hand a maximal V.E.C.P. amplitude to sine wave modulated light is usually obtained in a frequency range around the alpha rythm where a great amount of individual variability in response amplitude is due to an insufficient attenuation of the alpha rythm (Trimble & Potts 1975). With higher stimulus frequency the amplitude of the responses decreases but the individual and interindividual differences are much smaller. High frequency responses in normal subjects have been measured up to 80 Hz under very bright square-wave flicker whereas the responses to frequencies over 50 Hz are only obtained under very bright light stimulation (Gavrisky 1974, Abe Kojima & Iwata 1974).

The summation area for high frequency responses in the range of 45 to 55 Hz has been described as larger than for lower frequency stimulus with a loss of high frequency response when the stimulus field was reduced to less than 15° (Regan 1969).

We have measured the variation in V.E.C.P. amplitude as a function of stimulus frequency in patients with affection of the optic nerve and retina. We used a large stimulus field of 40°, modulated at 97%. In normal subjects V.E.C.P. of identical amplitude can be obtained with a field size of only 10° and a modulation depth of only 30% as with 40° and 97% modulation depth. In low vision patients however it is an advantage to saturate the response as the question asked is usually not whether any response is of normal amplitude or not but if it is present at all. The variable parameter used to obtain different responses, was the stimulus frequency.

MATERIALS AND METHODS

The stimulator used is the same we have shown in Nof Ginossar (Huber 1975) with the only alteration that the projector is focussed on a translucent screen placed 40 cm in front of the subject. The light stimulus is produced by an ordinary Kodak slide projector whose luminance is modulated with a stationary and a rotating polaroid. The mean luminance on the screen is 60 cd/m^2, the modulation depth 97% ($\frac{I\ max - I\ min}{I\ max + I\ min}$). The stimulus field size is 40°. The stimulus frequency can be varied from 3 to 50 Hz.

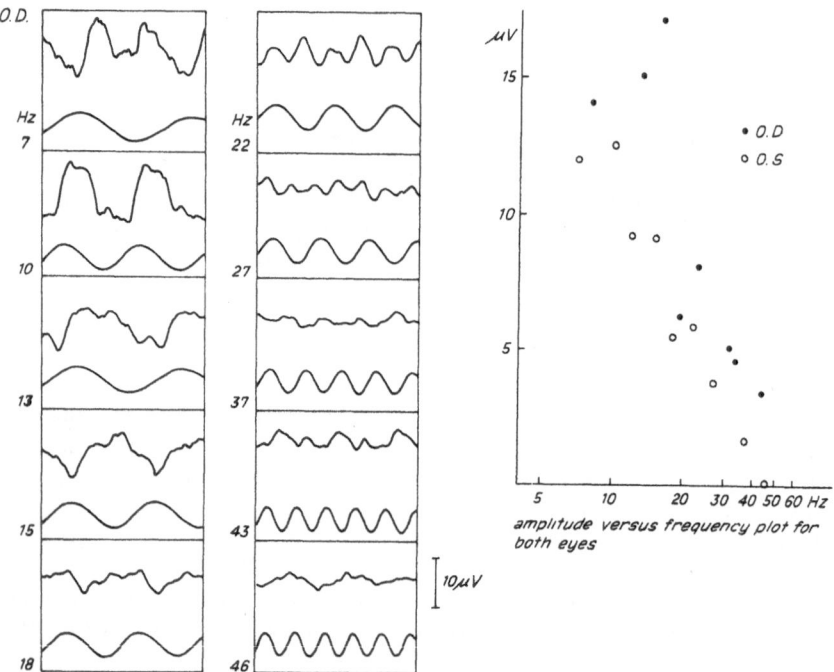

Fig. 1. left: V.E.C.P. to stimulation of the right eye with sine wave modulated light at different frequencies. Time base at 7 and 10 Hz = 200 msec. Time base at higher frequencies = 120 msec. right: Amplitude versus frequency plot of monocular V.E.C.P. for both eyes. The visual acuity in the left eye is reduced to finger counting after a traumatic cataract.

The EEG is recorded from a midline electrode 4 cm above the inion, one ear lobe is used as ground the other as reference. The band pass of the P.A.R. preamplifier is set from 3 to 100 Hz. The averager used is a Nicolet 1070 used in the Artifact rejection mode which allows rejecting any recorded sweep before the data is transferred to the memory, and so avoid reducing the amplitude of the recorded signal by contamination with any EEG segment without information content through overload of the preamplifier or Analog to digital converter of the averager. In a second channel of the averager the luminance change on the screen is recorded simultaneously with the V.E.C.P. to allow an exact measurement of frequency.

We record always more than one light-dark period as it is often possible only with an overview of two or more periods to decide whether a response is light induced or an artifact especially at the higher frequencies with small response amplitude.

At the start of the examination one eye is occluded and a first record is made at 12 Hz. If there is a sizable response, the stimulus frequency is slowly increased until no response can be elicited. If the response at 12 Hz is absent or minimal, the stimulus frequency is decreased until a response can be recorded. In most cases who are not absolutely blind, some slow frequency response can still be recorded. The choice of an amplitude instead of a latency measure is due to the fact that in cases with only very small potentials the choice of which peak to take for latency measurement is more a guess than a reliable decision (Van Lith 1973). When the frequency range where the response disappear has been determined, the same measurements are performed on the other eye and a plot of amplitude versus frequency for both eyes is drawn on a half logarithmic scale.

RESULTS

Subjects with intact retina or optic nerve show (fig. 1) a more or less regular reduction of V.E.C.P. amplitude in function of frequency. In our stimulus conditions the highest frequencies which can still elicit a response of more than 1 microvolt are in the range of 45-50 Hz. The frequency dependent amplitude reduction is very similar for both eyes, even if, as in the patient of fig. 1, there is a traumatic cataract in the left eye with a vision of finger counting O.S.

The waveform of the response is always very simple, consisting in the lower frequency range of a response at the stimulus frequency with often a sizable second harmonic component and at higher frequencies over 30 Hz only the stimulus frequency appears (van der Tweel & Verduijn Lunel 1965, Regan 1968) but surprisingly at frequencies between 40 and 50 Hz some patients show a response of only half the stimulus frequency. This is not an isolated artifact but may build up progressively at high frequency. In our curves those V.E.C.P. do not appear as we considered a cortical response present only if there were the same number of peaks in the V.E.C.P. and the light stimulus record. Although one wonders if in that situation what the patient percieves is or is not similar to a stimulus at half frequency with a much smaller modulation depth.

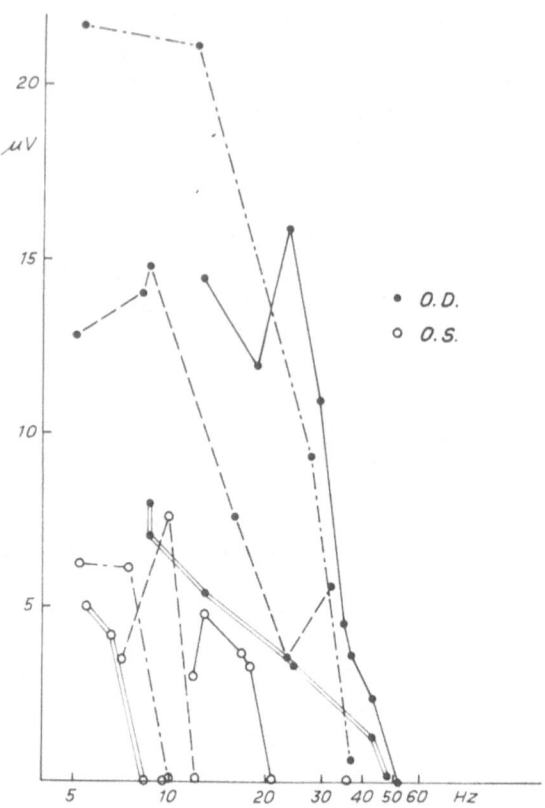

Fig. 2. Amplitude versus frequency plots of V.E.C.P. in 4 patients with atrophy of the left optic nerve. Strong reduction of high frequency responses in stimulation of the affected eyes. x———————x and x- - - - -x post traumatic atrophy. x-.-.-.x atrophy secondary to papillitis. x= = = = =x atrophy secondary to a pituitary adenoma.

AFFECTIONS OF THE OPTIC NERVE

The effect of an atrophy of the optic nerve is very impressive, not only are the responses at low frequency reduced but there is a consistent loss of responses over 20 Hz. The 4 patients in fig. 2 all have an atrophy of the left optic nerve with a reduction of vision to fingercounting or less and full vision in the right eye. There is a clear difference in the high frequency attenuation in the left eyes independently of the atrophy's origin (2 traumatic cases, 1 post neuritic, 1 pituitary adenoma).

In an other traumatic case the loss of high frequency response preceeds the atrophy and can be recorded immediately after an accident. The patient in fig. 3 suffered a stab with a wire below the right eye with a massive retrobulbar hematoma and an amaurotic pupil without any radiological lesion of the optic canal. The V.E.C.P. to stimulation of the right eye was strongly reduced and improved during a period of two months only at low frequency, the patient developed a classical optic atrophy in spite of a visual recovery to 0,4 with a field loss in the upper half field not quite reaching the macula. The left eye is normal.

RETROBULBAR NEURITIS

It is now well known that a retrobulbar neuritis (RBN) results in an increase of V.E.C.P. latency to pattern reversal stimulus (Halliday, McDonald & Mushin 1972, Milner, Regan & Heron 1974, Asselman Chadwick & Marsden 1975, Lehmann & Mir 1976) and in a reduction of amplitude as well as an increase in latency in V.E.C.P. to luminance change (Adachi, Kellerman & Makabe). We therefore also expected a reduction of high frequency responses in neuritis patients. We have followed electrophysiologically a young woman during an acute RBN and the following recovery in a manner similar to the case described by van der Tweel & Estevez (1974), who

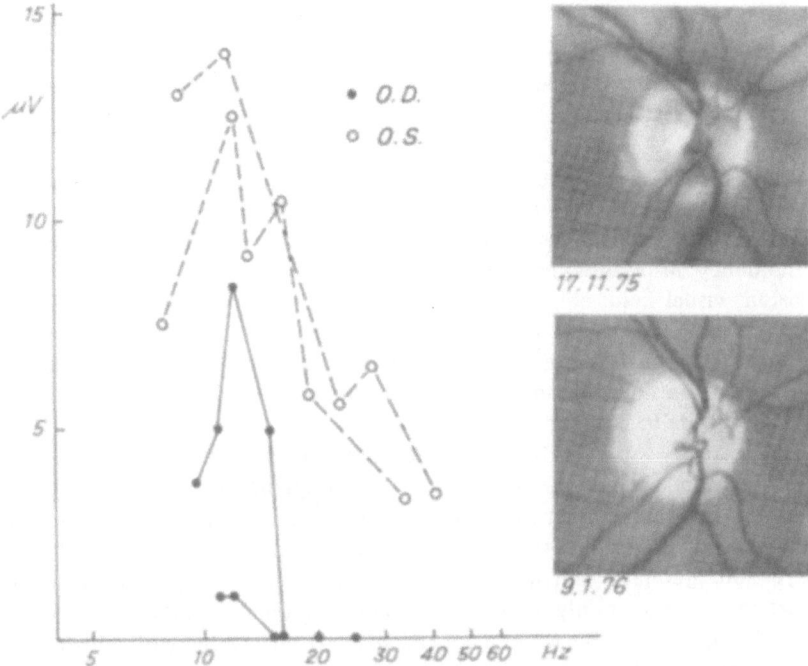

Fig. 3. Recovery of low frequency responses after a trauma of the right optic nerve in spite of the development or an atrophy of the right optic nerve. No recovery of high frequency responses. Lowest curve: V.E.C.P. to stimulation of the right optic nerve two days after the accident (17.11.75) Vision OD; finger counting, Upper filled curve: right eye after visible atrophy of the right optic nerve and improvement of visual acuity to 0,4 (9.1.76). Upper curves V.E.C.P. to stimulation of the left eye (17.11.75 and (9.1.76).

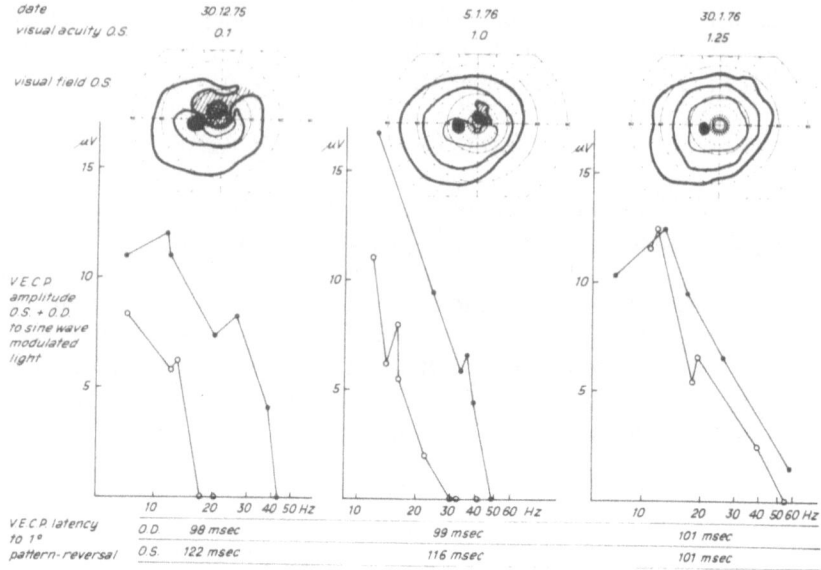

date 30.12.75   5.1.76   30.1.76

visual acuity O.S.   0.1   1.0   1.25

visual field O.S.

V.E.C.P. latency to 1° pattern-reversal

O.D. 98 msec   99 msec   101 msec
O.S. 122 msec   116 msec   101 msec

Fig. 4. Clinical and electrophysiological recovery in optic neuritis OS Simultaneous improvement of visual acuity, visual field, high frequency V.E.C.P. and latency to pattern reversal stimulus (1° Check size, 16° Field, 2/sec pattern reversal rate).

followed the improvement in de Lange curves and V.E.C.P. at two frequencies in a similar case. Instead of the psychophysical de Lange curve we plotted the electrophysiological one. Fig. 4 not only did the reduced high frequency responses improve during a complete clinical recovery including vision, visual field, color vision (Farnsworth 100 Hue) but also the latency of pattern evoked potentials (Courtesy Dr. Lehmann & Dr. Mir) improved to normal. This is somehow different from the results of Millner et al. Who never saw an abnormal delay at high frequencies and described a reduction of amplitude to luminance changes only in cases with grossly reduced vision. The recovery of high frequency responses is a gradual process and it is obvious that a single measurement in the frequency range below 20 Hz can be very misleading due to the high amplitude variability. The position of the curve along the frequency axis is however more or less constant for the right eye and gradually shifting to the right in the left eye. Pattern reversal responses are certainly more convenient and reliable for the diagnosis of RBN as only a few measurements can give a latency value with a high degree of confidence. In those patients, however, who due to the neuritis or to any other cause cannot see the pattern, the measurement of frequency dependent luminance responses is a tool sensible enough to follow the recovery of an acute RBN. At low frequency a response can be obtained when no pattern response is obtainable. Massive papillary stasis in subjects with cerebral tumor or occlusive hydrocephalus in three cases with normal central vision is in contrast to neuritis, compatible with the presence of high frequency responses.

74

AMBLYOPIA

The original aim of our study was to see if we could make the diagnosis of an amblyopia behind opacities of the ocular media. This however was not possible. From a group of 15 subjects with amblyopia, fig. 5 shows 3 patients with strong amblyopia in one eye due to very different causes (squint, congenital ptosis, macular aplasia). The vision in the amblyopic eyes is in the three cases reduced to finger counting the vision of the sound eye full. There are no massive differences between the amblyopic and the normal eye and the curves are similar to the luminance curves in amblyopes shown by van der Tweel (1974) and Abe, Kojima, Namba, Iwata (1974).

RETINITIS PIGMENTOSA

The diagnosis of retinitis pigmentosa can be made very early with the ERG. The later evolution of the disease however cannot be followed with the ERG as the retinal responses under ganz feld stimulation are absent. The V.E.C.P. can still be recorded in the period between ERG extinction and blindness. Fig. 6 shows a group of 6 patients with no more recordable ERG.

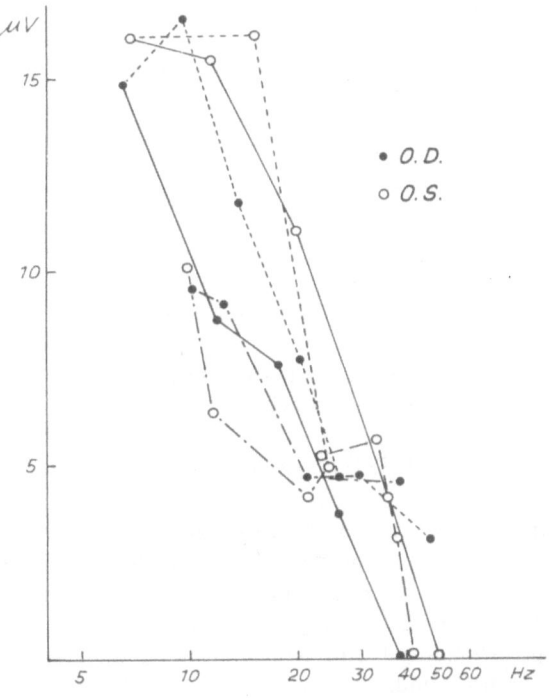

Fig. 5. Amblyopia V.E.C.P. to sine wave modulated light in one sided amblyopia of various origins. x- - -x squint amblyopia OS x ——— x Macular Aplasia OD x-.-.x Congenital ptosis (Occlusion Amblyopia) OS. No differences between sound an amblyopic eye.

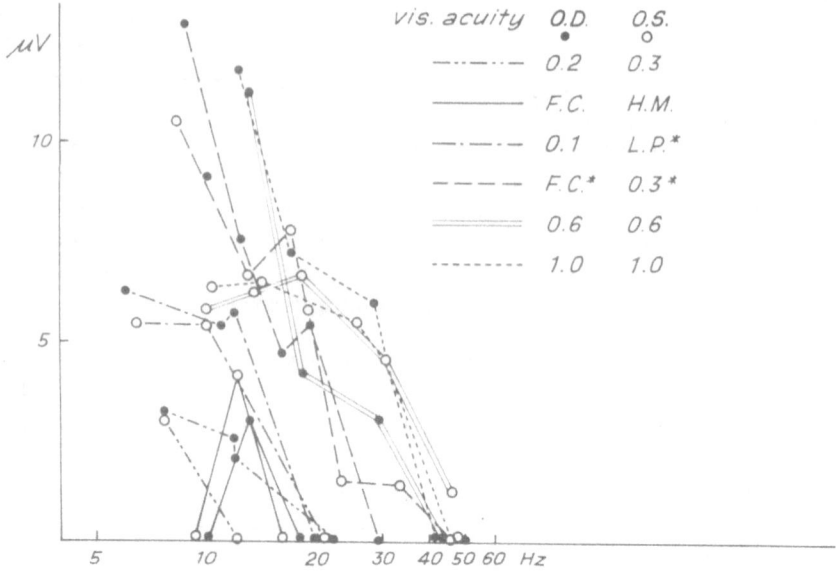

Fig. 6. Retinitis pigmentosa V.E.C.P. amplitudes in 6 patients with no measurable ganzfeld ERG F.C. = Finger counting, H.M. = Hand movement. L.P. = Light perception. *: Cataract The reduction of high frequency response is not correlated with the presence of a cataract.

The spread of the curves along the frequency axis reaches from normals to curves similar to those obtained in optic atrophy. The position of the curves are similar in both eyes and are not dependent on the presence of a cataract. A nearly normal curve can be obtained with very low vision in patients with cataract. There are however no cases with clear media, low vision and normal high frequency responses. An extremely reduced V.E.C.P. with no high frequency response may therefore contribute to a negative prognosis before the operation of a pigmentosa cataract.

PROGRESSIVE CONE DYSTROPHY

As a last example and as an alternative to psychophysical testing in children. Fig. 7 shows a 30 year old mother affected with a progressive cone dystrophy (Courtesy Dr. Wildberger) who was very anxious to know if her two year old daughter suffered already from the same disease. There was a suspicion of pepper and salt fundus alteration in the child but we did not want to make an ERG under general anesthesia as there were no therapeutic consequences. The V.E.C.P. of the mother and the child differ widely and the V.E.C.P. flicker fusion in the mother is reduced but not in the child. The examination is possible with the smallest infant whether cooperative or not. The high frequency deffect in the mother is similar to the de Lange curve alteration described by Breukink (1962) psychophysically.

DISCUSSION

Stimulus frequency as a variable parameter in V.E.C.P. measurements has the advantage of not being affected by refraction errors or opacities of the ocular media as are pattern movement or in a less amount modulation depth. The absolute amplitude of a V.E.C.P. to sine wave modulated light may vary widely individually or interindividually especially at low frequency, the position of the high frequency cut of is however reproducible and shows a smaller interindividual variability than do the amplitude values.

The disadvantage of measuring amplitude values instead of latencies is in our opinion compensated by the fact of being able to record V.E.C.P.'s at all in patients with very little vision.

We are now collecting material in patients with extreme opacities of the ocular media and uncertain retinal function who are planned for vitrectomy, keratoplasty or capsulectomy in the hope of getting a rough correlation between best attainable vision and the preoperative V.E.C.P. Although, we already know that we cannot detect amblyopia, or even macular oedema, which may be compatible with very low vision and a normal frequency range in the V.E.C.P.

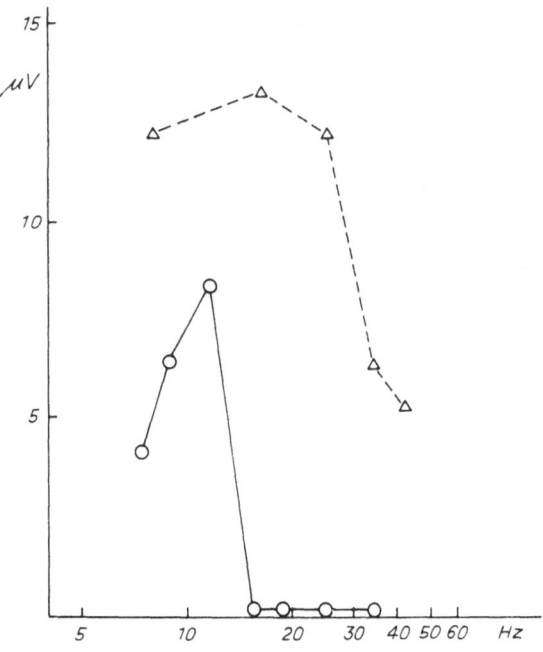

Fig. 7. V.E.C.P. amplitude in a 30 year old mother with a progressive cone dystrophy (0————0) and of her 2 year old daughter x-----x. No measurable high frequency response in the mother.

ACKNOWLEDGEMENTS

This work was subsidised by a material grant from the Schweizerischer Nationalfond zur Förderung der Wissenschaften (Nr. 3.020.73). I thank Dr. Lehmann and Dr. Mir for their help in the latency measurement to pattern reversal stimulation.

REFERENCES

Abe, H., Kojima, M. & Iwata, K., Flicker: VER studies on the flicker in normal subjects. *Acta soc. Ophthal. japonicae* 78, *4*, (1974).

Abe, H., Kojima, M. & Iwata, K., Flicker and VER studies on the flicker VER in patients with lesion of the visual pathways. *Acta ophtalmologicae japonicae* 78, *9* (1974).

Adachi-Usami, E., Kellerman, F. & Makabe, E.J.: VER threshold in different stages of optic neuritis. *Ophtalmic research* 4, *284-296* (1973).

Asselman, P., Chadwick, D.W. & Marsden, C.D.,: Visual evoked responses in the diagnosis and management of patients suspected of multiple scerosis. *Brain* 98, *261-282* (1975).

Breukink, E.W.: De frequentiekarakteristick van het menselijk oog onder normale en pathologische omstandigheden. Thesis. Drukkerij-Elinkwijk Utrecht (1962).

Halliday, A.M., McDonald, W.I. & Mushin Joan: Delayed visual evoked responses in optic neuritis. *Lancet* May 6, *982-985*, (1972).

Lehmann, D. & Mir, Z.: Zur Methodik und Auswertung visuell evozierter Potentiale bei Verdacht auf multiple Sklerose. *J. Neurol.*, in press (1976).

Milner Beryl, Regan, D. & Heron, J.R.: Differential diagnosis of multiple sclerosis by visual evoked potential recording. *Brain* 97, *755-772*, (1974).

Trimble, J. & Potts, A.: Ongoing occipital rythms and the VER. I Stimulation at peaks of the alpha rythm. *Invest. ophtal.* July (1975).

Regan, D.: A high frequency mechanism which underlies visual evoked potentials. *EEG et clin. neurophysiol.* 25, *231-237*, (1968).

Van Lith, G.H.M. & Mak, G.T.: A quantitative evaluation of the V.E.C.P. in optic neuritis.

Van der Tweel, L.H. & Verduijn Lunel: Human visual responses to sinusoidally modulated light. *Electroenceph. clin. neurophysiol.* 18, *587*, (1965).

Van der Tweel, L.H. & Estevez, O.: Subjective and objective evaluation of flicker. *Ophtalmologica* 169/1, *70-81*, (1974).

Author's address:
Universitäts-Augenklinik
Rämistrasse 100
8091 Zürich
Switzerland

THE VISUALLY EVOKED RESPONSE AND PSYCHOPHYSICAL TESTING IN OPTIC NEURITIS

C. BARBER & N.R. GALLOWAY

(Nottingham)

A delay in the latency of certain components of the Visually Evoked Response (V.E.R.) is now recognised as a feature of optic nerve damage. For this reason the use of the V.E.R. as a test for detecting a previous attack of optic neuritis is now being investigated in several clinics throughout the world. (Halliday A.M., McDonald W.I., Mushin J. 1975.). In this report we have compared the results of measuring latencies in the V.E.R. with the results of certain psychophysical tests in a series of twenty normal subjects and thirty patients with optic neuritis.

MATERIAL AND METHODS

Subjects

The twenty normal subjects had a mean age of 27.3 yr. with a range between 19 and 41 yr. The average age of the thirty patients was 31.7 yr. and their ages ranged between 19 and 64 yrs. The patients were referred for these special investigations after the diagnosis had been made in the Eye Clinic and confirmed by a neurologist. Although the V.E.R. was often measured in the acute phase, the results here were obtained after the eyes had recovered.

V.E.R.

An appearance-disappearance pattern was used with the grating size arranged to be smallest centrally increasing in size peripherally (Barber C. & Galloway N.R., 1974.). We have found this stimulus to give a larger and more clear cut response than an even sized chequerboard pattern. This pattern was back projected on to a screen situated one meter from the seated subject. It subtended an angle of 30° at the subjects eye. The stimulus cycle frequency was 1.06 Hz the pattern being illuminated for 100 ms. with a 10 ms. turn on time. Scalp electrodes of a conventional E.E.G. type were positioned at the vertex, 2.5 cm. above the inion and on the ear. After preliminary amplification the signals were averaged in a Data-Lab averager and continuously monitored on an oscilloscope. Final read out was recorded on an X—Y plotter.

Visual Fields. These were performed by a trained technician using the Goldmann perimeter.

Colour Vision. The Farnsworth 100 Hue test was used in the recommended manner. The coloured discs were illuminated by a Macbeth lamp. (For details see Farnsworth D. 1957.).

Other Investigations. All patients underwent routine ophthalmological and neurological examination and in particular the optic discs were examined after the instillation of mydriatic drops. Although many patients had fundus photography this was not found to be a reliable way of assessing optic atrophy and these results are not included here.

RESULTS

The V.E.R.

Normal Series. Fig. I. shows the distribution of the latency of the three major peaks in normal subjects. A typical normal response is shown in fig. 2 to demonstrate the different components that were measured. The first positive peak proved to be the most reliable one to measure and the scatter of values for its latency was smaller than for the other peaks and showed a clear Gaussian distribution. The mean value for the latency of P1 was 129.5 ms. for right eyes and 130.5 ms. for left eyes with a standard deviation of 12.1 and 11.8 respectively. The average age of our normal series was slightly less than the average age of the patients but it has been shown that a significant increase in latency is not usually seen until after the age of 60 yr. (Asselman P, Chadwick D.W. & Marsden C.D. 1975.). The amplitudes of the V.E.R. were very variable from person to person in normal subjects although a given subject's responses could be accurately reproduced at different times. In four of the normal subjects the V.E.R. was repeated three times over periods varying between one week and six months and the latency of P1 was shown to be very constant. In many cases it was identical from time to time and on no occasion was a difference of more than 5 ms. noted in any individual for this particular component.

Colour Vision. The colour scores as measured from the Farnsworth 100 Hue test showed a mean figure of 44.2 for right eyes and 35.5 for left eyes with a standard deviation of 28.3 and 21.5 respectively. In this test a higher score indicates poorer colour discrimination. The frequency distribution histogram shows a skew devation and a wide scatter of values which has also been demonstrated by other authors (see fig. 3.). (Kinnear P.R. 1970.). The subjective nature of colour vision testing made us suspect that an individuals score could be improved by practice and it is interesting to see that this appears to be borne out by repeated testing in one of our subjects but not in others. If the subjects vision was blurred by interposing fogging lenses then an increased colour score was obtained showing that the wearing of a correct spectacle prescription was just as important for this test as for the V.E.R. (see fig. 4). It also emphasizes the need for patients over the age of forty-five to wear their presbyopic correction when undertaking the Farnsworth 100 Hue test.

Abnormal Series Fig. 5 shows a comparison of the results obtained by measuring P1 latencies in eyes affected by retrobulbar neuritis and those obtained from the unaffected eyes of patients. The mean value of the latency for unaffected eyes was 119.1 ms. with a standard deviation of 15.3 (26 eyes) and the mean value for affected eyes was 147.0 ms. with a standard deviation of 32.9 (34 eyes). Although the mean of the unaffected group was comparable with the normal series figure, there was a wide scatter and it can be seen from figure 5 that there is considerable overlap between the two groups. If one examines the patients who showed clinically unilateral disease then more significant results are obtained by measuring the difference in P1 latency between the two eyes. Out of these fifteen patients

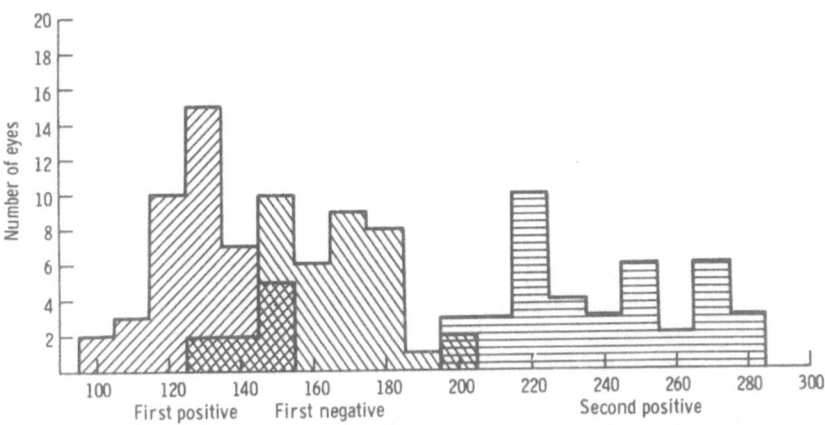

LATENCIES TO MAJOR COMPONENTS OF THE VER IN CONTROLS LATENCY (ms)

Fig 1.   Distribution of the latency of the three major peaks of the visually evoked response in normal subjects

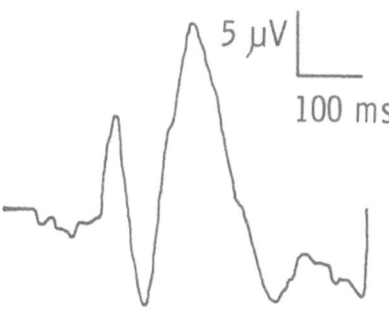

Fig 2.   A typical normal response.

DISTRIBUTION OF NORMAL COLOUR SCORES

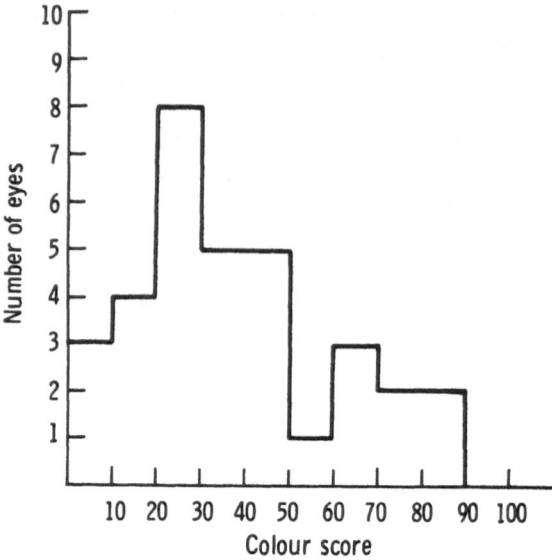

Fig 3. Frequency distribution of colour scores in normal subjects using the Farnsworth 100 Hue test.

only two showed no difference between the eyes and in these two cases a complete recovery had been made from their attack of optic neuritis. In all the other unilateral cases the affected eye showed a delayed response compared with the unaffected eye. The mean difference in latency was 26.8 ms. (S.D. 23 ms.).

Colour Vision. Although the mean value of the colour scores was considerably higher in the eyes affected by optic neuritis, 269 as opposed to 128 there was a wide scatter in both groups, with a standard deviation of 300 for the affected eyes and 67 for the unaffected eyes. It is interesting that the unaffected eyes had rather poor colour vision, but the subjective nature of the test makes this difficult to assess. It could be claimed that some of our normal subjects were more familiar with this type of test than the patients and hence gave better results than the supposedly normal eyes of the patients.

Visual Fields. Eleven of the 34 affected eyes showed defects in their visual fields and four of the fifteen unilateral cases showed field defects.

Pallor of the Disc. Sixteen of the 34 affected eyes showed definite pallor of the optic disc compared with the other eye. Of the unilateral cases, six out of the fifteen showed dic pallor.

Visual Acuity. The generally recognized good visual prognosis was borne out by the fact that only eight of the 34 eyes affected by optic neuritis had a visual acuity less than 6/6 and in general the poor visual outcome was limited to bilateral cases. This probably reflects the fact the bilateral cases tend to appear as more advanced cases of multiple sclerosis and many of them may have suffered several attacks of optic neuritis.

DISCUSSION

Comparison of abnormal V.E.R. with other signs of optic neuritis

If we take the fifteen unilateral cases and make a comparison of the results obtained from the affected eyes then Fig. 6 shows that the V.E.R. gives at least as many abnormal results as the other tests including the visual acuity and the visual fields. These last two tests were often normal in affected eyes. This of course depends on the criterion for abnormality of the V.E.R. which here was taken as a latency of more than 145 ms. This is only one standard deviation above the normal mean. If one compares the two eyes and adopts a difference of more than 15 ms. between them as being abnormal (normals— mean difference 4 ms. S.D. 3.5) then nine instead of six eyes are abnormal, making this particular test the most useful of all in detecting previous optic neuritis.

The V.E.R. has one outstanding advantage as a clinical test and that is its objectivity but its disadvantages, that of its cost and the time involved, must

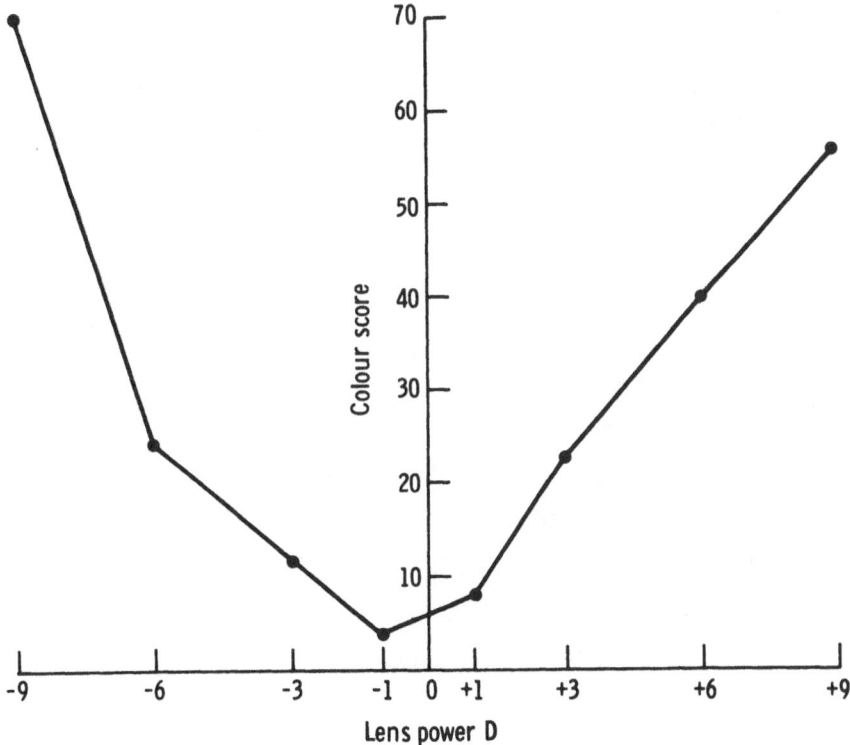

Fig 4. Graph to show the effect of interposing different strengths of fogging lens in the Farnsworth 100 Hue test.

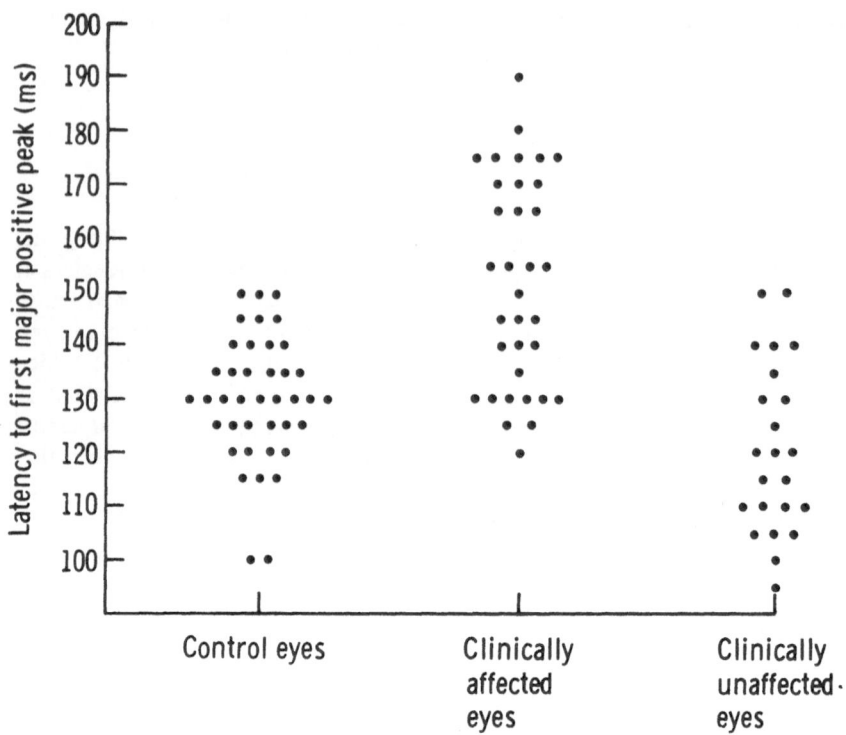

Fig 5. Comparison of the latencies of the first positive peak (P1) in normal subjects, and the affected and unaffected eyes of patients suffering from retrobulbar neuritis.

15 CASES OF UNILATERAL RETROBULBAR NEURITIS

V.E.R.	Latency > 145 ms		6
	Latency > 15 ms	between eyes	9
FIELD DEFECTS			4
COLOUR VISION SCORE > 40 between eyes (Farnsworth 100 Hue)			6
VISION < 6/6 in affected eye			3
DISC PALLOR			6

Fig 6. Table indicating the frequency of abnormal results for each individual method of examination. A difference in V.E.R. latency between the two eyes was the most useful index of a previous attack of retrobulbar neuritis.

be borne in mind. Another problem which applies to any electrodiagnostic technique is that of standardization. Because we do not yet know the best form of stimulus there is no standard one and results from different centres vary considerably. Asselman et al found a mean latency in the first positive peak of 90.5 ms., a much shorter latency than that found by Halliday et al. Both these groups of workers show shorter latencies than ours. These differences can probably be explained by differences in turn-on time and brightness of the stimulus. The technique used here differs from the above two in that 'on-off' rather than pattern reversal stimulation has been used, and it is possible that this also could affect the latency values.

Of the other investigations apart from the V.E.R. it is well recognized that the visual acuity may recover completely following an attack of optic neuritis and hence this alone is not a valid sign. The visual fields gave rather disappointing results in that in some cases when one would have expected to find a defect, none could be detected. However, coloured targets were not used and perhaps better results might have been obtained with more prolonged testing using small coloured targets. The colour of the optic discs is always difficult to assess and in particular must be looked at with caution when there is a difference in refractive error between the two eyes. Photography of the discs may be very misleading since the colour can be distorted by variations in film processing technique. The Farnsworth 100 Hue gave some interesting and useful results which seem to compare favourably with the V.E.R. as a means of detecting previous optic neuritis but the wide scatter of normal values was a disadvantage and perhaps an improvement in the scoring system could increase the validity of this test.

Although we have attempted to compare the value of these tests it is apparent that they all are needed to obtain the most accurate diagnosis. Indeed one might expect that the optic nerve could be damaged in different ways by optic neuritis so that colour vision for example or the V.E.R. might be altered to a different extent; this appeared to be the case in this series.

SUMMARY

A comparison has been made between the visually evoked response, the accurate assessment of colour vision and other more routine ophthalmological investigations in the detection of healed optic neuritis.

ACKNOWLEDGEMENTS

We wish to thank the Trent Regional Health Authority for their financial support in this work. We are especially grateful to Mrs. Christine Sills for her technical assistance.

REFERENCES

Asselman P., Chadwick D.W. & Marsden C.D. Visual Evoked Response in diagnosis and management of patients suspected of multiple sclerosis. *Brain* 98, *261-282*. (1975).
Barber C. & Galloway N.R. A pattern stimulus for optimal response from the retina.

Proc. XII ISCERG Symposium. Clemont Ferrand 1974, *Doc. Ophthal. Proc. Series* 10, *77-86* (1976).

Farnsworth D. (1957) The Farnsworth Munsell 100 Hue Test. Hunsell Colour Co. Inc. Baltimore. Maryland.

Halliday A.H., McDonald W.I. & Mushin J. Delayed Visual Evoked Response in Optic Neuritis. *Lancet* 1, *982*. (1972).

Kinnear P.R. Proposals for scoring and assessing the 100 Hue test. *Vision Research* 10, *423-433*. (1970).

Athor's address:
Middlebrook House
261 Alfreton Road
Underwood, Nottinghamshire NG 16 5GX
England

ON THE LACK OF CORRELATION BETWEEN
ERG AND EOG ALTERATIONS
IN MALIGNANT MELANOMA OF CHOROID*

F. PONTE & M. LAURICELLA

(Palermo)

Electrophysiological tests have not been considered of a relevant diagnostic value in malignant melanoma of choroid, because ERG and EOG alterations depend essentially on the retinal detachment caused often by the tumour.

Recently Bohár & Farkas (1973) reported their experience in 25 cases of intraocular tumour. They found that the tumour damages the electroretinogram and the electro-oculogram more than a recent retinal detachment of equal extent. If this is true, the electroretinogram and electro-oculogram could have a great diagnostic value in certain intricate diagnostic problems.

We had the opportunity to examine some patients affected by malignant melanoma of choroid and by metastatic tumour with or without retinal detachment and performed electrophysiological tests to verify the diagnostic value of ERG and EOG in tumour of choroid.

MATERIALS AND METHODS

A brief history of our 7 patients is reported in Tab. I. Four of them (cases 2, 3, 4 and 5) had a malignant melanoma of choroid histologically diagnosed, case 1 had a choroidal metastasis from a mammal cancer. Cases 1, 2 and 3 presented a tumour, without retinal detachment, limited to one quadrant of the fundus, while cases 4 and 5 had an extensive retinal detachment involving two more quadrants of the fundus surrounding the tumour. The last two cases (cases 6 and 7) were taken as controls: patient 6 was affected by a small peripapillar benign melanoma, while patient 7 was an high myope with chorioretinal distrophy and a large subretinal haemorrhage looking like a malignant melanoma of choroid.

In all patients we performed radio-phosphorus test, transillumination with optical fibers, ERG and EOG. The technique used for ERG and EOG registrations and normal data are described elsewhere (Wirth & Ponte, 1963; Ponte & Lauricella, 1975).

* This investigation was supported by Grant No. 72.00851.04 of the Consiglio Nazionale delle Ricerche.

87

Table 1. Clinical history of our 7 cases. Note that in fundus picture the dashed area indicates the tumour while the dotted area indicates the retinal detachment.

Fundus	Case No	Sex	Age	Diagnosis	Retinal detachment	Radio-phosphor test	Transillumination
	1	F	49	metastatic tumour	absent	positive	positive
	2	M	69	malignant melanoma of choroid	absent	positive	positive
	3	F	37	malignant melanoma of choroid	absent	positive	positive
	4	M	46	malignant melanoma of choroid	present	positive	positive
	5	M	54	malignant melanoma of choroid	present		positive
	6	M	47	peripapillar benign tumour	absent	negative	
	7	M	30	sub-retinal haemorrhage	absent	negative	negative

Fig. 1 shows ERG and EOG in cases 1, 2 and 3 in which the tumour of choroid was circumscribed to one quadrant of the fundus and no retinal detachment was observed. The photopic and scotopic ERG response was close to normal in cases 2 and 3 and subnormal in case 1 with a reduction of the photopic b-wave amplitude (dark adapted state). On the contrary the EOG was abnormal in all three patients: the electro-oculogram amplitude did not show any increase during light stimulation and consequently the ratio of maximum light-adapted to minimal dark-adapted response (LP/DT ratio) was 100 or less.

Patients 4 and 5 were affected by a tumour of choroid with a large retinal detachment involving two more quadrants of fundus. In these cases (Fig. 2) both ERG and EOG were pathological: the scotopic and the photopic response of electroretinogram was always extinguished and LP/DT ratio of EOG was 100 or less.

Cases 6 and 7, used as control, presented a fundus picture similar to the malignant melanoma of choroid although they were not affected by such disease. As the Fig. 3 shows, normal ERG and EOG records (LP/DT = 186) were obtained in case 6, who had only a small peripapillar benign tumour.

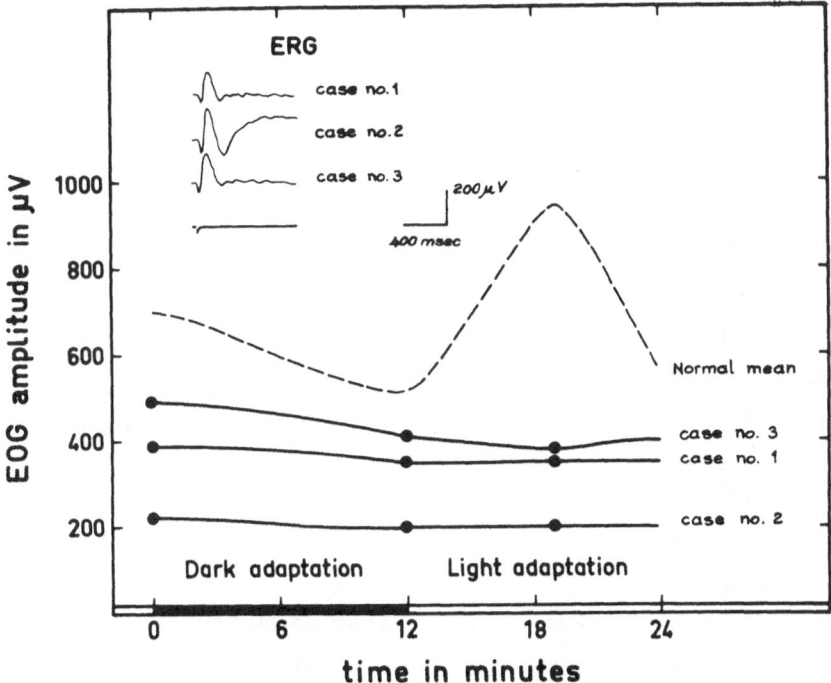

Fig. 1. A plot of the EOG amplitude of patients 1, 2 and 3 in comparison to the normal mean. Note that at the top of figure are reported the ERG recordings obtained in dark adapted state with stimulus of high intensity.

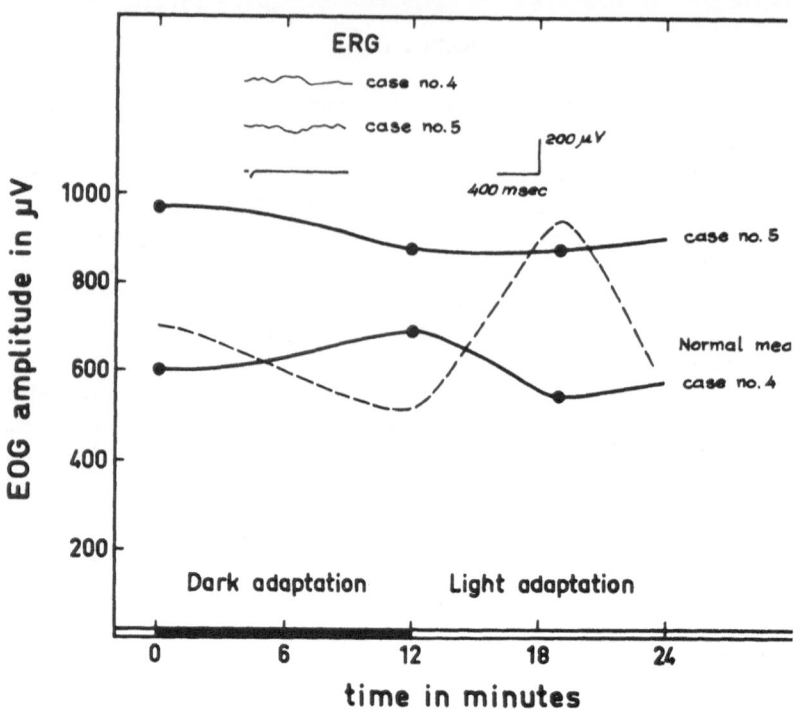

Fig. 2. A plot of the EOG amplitude in patients 4 and 5 in comparison with normal mean. Legends as in Fig. 1.

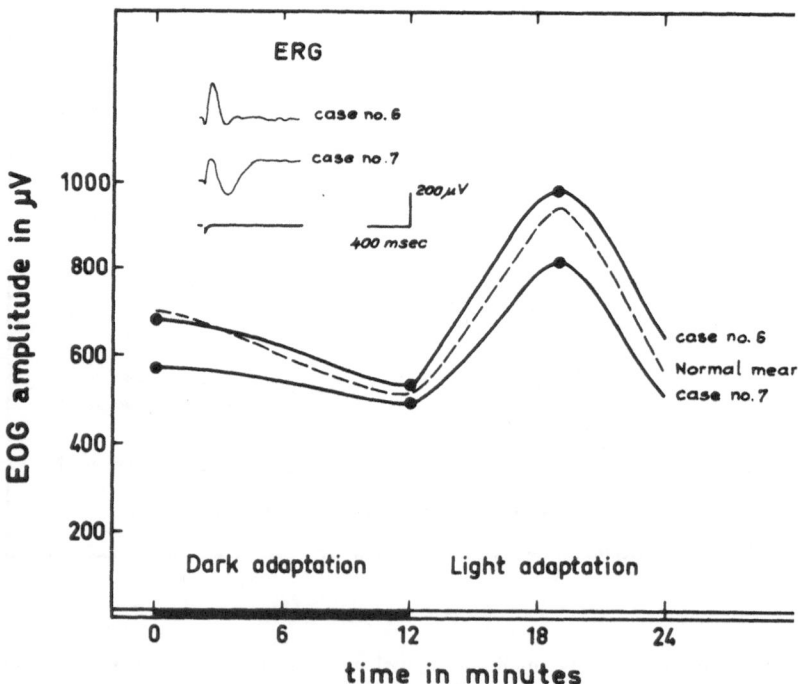

Fig. 3. A plot of the EOG amplitude in patients 6 and 7 in comparison with normal mean. Legends as in Fig. 1.

Patient 7 was affected by an high myopia with chorio-retinal dystrophy; a large dark mass extending along the infero-temporal quadrant of the fundus, looking like a malignant melanoma of choroid, was present. The radio-phosphor test and the transillumination were negative; the ERG response showed a slightly reduction of the scotopic b-wave; a normal LP/DT ratio of EOG (LP/DT = 162) was observed. Two months later the fundus picture and all the clinical observations did not show any change and the patient was discharged with a diagnosis of sub-retinal haemorrhage.

CONCLUSIONS

Our results confirm that in patients with malignant melanoma or metastatic tumour of the choroid with or without retinal detachment severe abnormalities of EOG are always present without any correlation with the extension of the tumour and the existence of retinal detachment.

In fact, all our patients showed a LP/DT ratio of EOG equal to 100 or less; while the EOG was normal in case 6, affected by a small benign melanoma of choroid, and obviously in case 7 which showed only the typical myopic ERG alterations. On the contrary, the ERG changes are strictly related to the extension of the retinal damage: it is almost normal when only one quadrant of the fundus is involved whereas it is subnormal or extinguished when the lesion involves a larger retinal area or when a retinal detachment is present.

This type of EOG changes is similar to that observed in macular vitelliform degeneration where the EOG modifications are the most important functional sign although the ophthalmoscopic lesion appears to be circumscribed to a small central area of the retina (François & De Rouck, 1967).
The following conclusions can be drawn:
— no correlation between ERG and EOG alterations is detected in malignant melanoma of choroid without retinal detachment. While the EOG is always flat, the ERG shows alterations strictly related to the extension of lesion;
— the existence of severe EOG abnormalities in association with minor ERG changes is in agreement with the choroidal origin of the tumour involving primarily the chorio-capillaris tissue, Bruch's membrane and pigment epithelium of the retina;
— the EOG alterations do not seem to be related with the ophthalmoscopic picture. This fact indicates that probably the lesion is not circumscribed to the area of the tumour but involves a larger retinal area as in macular vitelliform degeneration.

SUMMARY

Electrophysiological tests have been performed in patients affected by malignant melanoma or by metastatic tumour of choroid with or without retinal detachment in order to verify the diagnostic value of ERG and EOG in this affection of the eye.
The results are briefly summarized as follow:

— in patients without retinal detachment a normal or a slightly subnormal ERG amplitude was found; on the contrary, the EOG showed always a pathological light-peak/dark-through ratio (100 or less);

— in patients with an extensive retinal detachment both ERG and EOG were involved: the ERG was absent and the EOG showed a pathological LP/DT ratio (100 or less).

The lack of correlation between ERG and EOG findings in patients without retinal detachment is discussed.

REFERENCES

Bohár, A. & Farkas, A. Comparative electrophysiological observations of intraocular tumour and retinal detachment. 12th ISCERG Symposium, Clermont Ferrand, 1974. *Doc. Ophthal. Proc. Series* 10, *399-404* (1976).

François, J. & De Rouck, A. Compared EOG and ERG in some retinal diseases affecting the posterior pole. 6th Symposium ISCERG, Erfurt, Germany (1967).

Ponte, F. & Lauricella, M. Limiti tra normalità ed anormalità in elettro-oculografia clinica. *Ann. Ottal. e Clin. Ocul.*, 101, *413-424* (1975).

Wirth, A. & Ponte, F. Fisiopatologia e clinica dell'elettroretinogramma. In. Gra. Na., Palermo, Italy (1964).

Author's address:
Clinica Oculistica Università
Policlinico
Via L. Giuffre 13
Palermo
Italy

NORMAL EOG VALUES OF YOUNG SUBJECTS

ROBERT MICHAEL JONES, THOMAS S. STEVENS & SHIRLEY GOULD

(Madison)

ABSTRACT

Electro-oculograms were recorded from fifty normal subjects between fifteen and thirty years of age, 25 males and 25 females. Refractive error distributions were the same in both sex groups. Average EOG ratio for the male subjects was 2.28, for the females 2.49; this difference was statistically significant. Twenty subjects were retested on another day to establish limits on the intersession variability of the tests. 95% of the eyes retested were found to have an intersession variability of less than 0.6.

INTRODUCTION

Since the Electro-oculogram was first introduced in its clinical form (Arden *et. al.* 1962) several studies have been published on the normal range of test results and factors influencing that range. Only one, (Adams, 1973) found a statistically significant difference in normal limits between males and females. Other studies either found no difference (Reeser *et. al.* 1970) or did not explore for a possible difference. In order to resolve the question of whether males and females have a difference in normal values, we tested a carefully matched group of 25 males and 25 females between the ages of 15 and 30.

METHOD

After the subject's pupils were dilated, the subject was seated in front of a square x-ray viewing box. The box was 1 meter from the subject and subtended an angle of 22 degrees. When the fluorescent tubes inside the viewing box were turned on, the retinal illumination was approximately 7,000 trolands. Attached to the box were two small red fixation lights, each 30 degrees from the center of the viewing box. Ag-AgCl subminiature skin electrodes were placed on the inner and outer canthi of each eye. A silver disc ear clip electrode was used as a ground electrode. After the electrodes had been atached, the room lights were turned off, and the fluorescent viewing box lights were turned on for 5 minutes of 'preadaptation'. Next, the viewing box lights were turned off, and the subject was dark adapted for 20 minutes. Finally, the viewing box was relit, and the subject was light adapted for 15 minutes.

During each minute of dark and light adaptation, the subject was asked

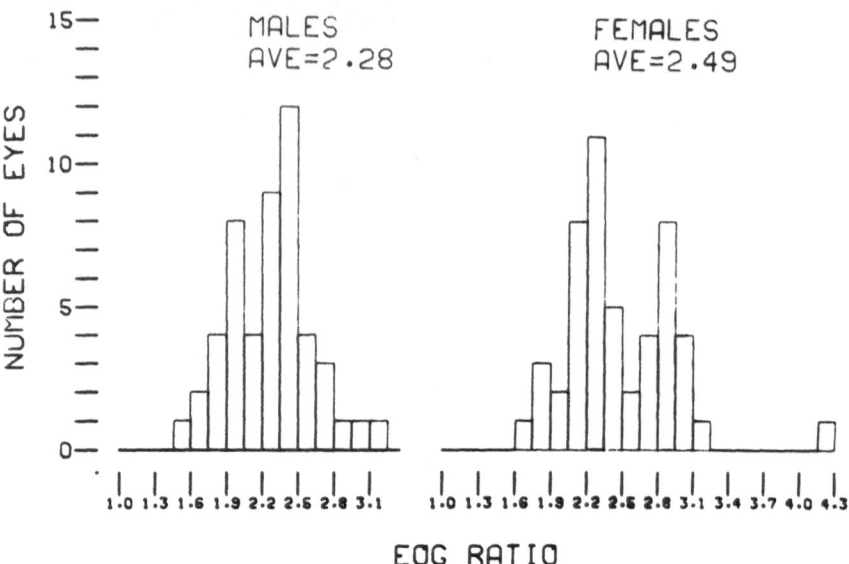

Fig. 1. The frequency distribution histograms of the EOG ratio for the 25 males and 25 female subjects. The difference in averages for the two groups was found to be statistically significant.

to alternately fixate the two red lights several times. The electrical signal was amplified and recorded on a Beckman strip chart recorder. The amplifiers were D.C. coupled with a frequency response up to 15 Hz. The deflections for each minute were measured, and the ratio of the peak value in the light to the trough in the dark was calculated.

MATERIAL

Fifty normal volunteers between the ages of 15 and 30 were tested, 25 males and 25 females. The distribution of refractive error was matched between the male and female groups by selecting 13 for each group with refractive errors between +2 and −2 diopters (spherical equivalent), 7 with a refractive error between −2 and −6 diopters, and 5 with a refractive error greater than −6 diopters.

The volunteers were given an eye examination, including ophthalmoscopy. All volunteers could be corrected to 20/20 at distance and J1 at near. Subjects were questioned regarding family history of retinal disease, personal history of eye disease, and personal history of systemic disorders, especially diabetes or hypertension. All volunteers with a positive history were excluded from the study.

Twenty of the fifty volunteers were asked to return on a seperate day to be retested. Attempts were made to retest these subjects at the same time of the day as on their initial visit.

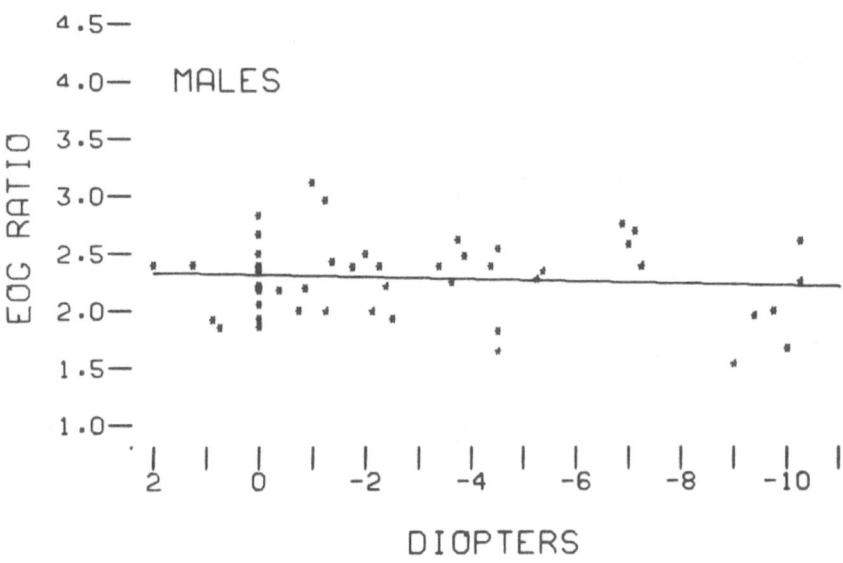

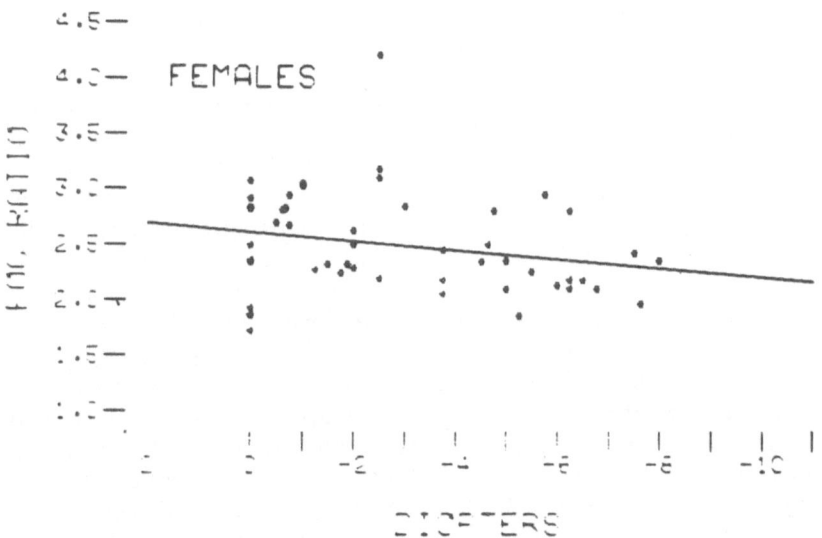

Fig. 2. The EOG ratio is plotted against the refractive error (spherical equivalent). A. Males. B. Females. The straight line is the best linear fit to the data. The small negative slope is not statistically significant in either graph.

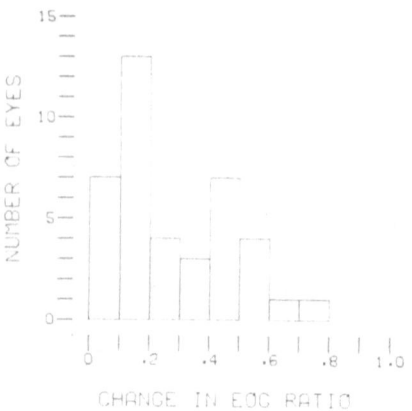

Fig. 3. The frequency distribution histogram of the change in EOG ratio when 20 subjects were retested on another day.

RESULTS AND DISCUSSION

The frequency distribution histogram of the EOG ratios for the male and female subjects are shown in Fig. 1. For the male subjects the ratios ranged from 1.54 to 3.12 with an average of 2.28. For the female subjects the ratios ranged from 1.72 to 4.21 with an average of 2.49. Using a Wilcoxon rank sum test, the difference between groups was statistically significant at the 5% level. This is in agreement with the results reported by Adams, but disagrees with the results reported by Reeser *et al.*

A myopic refractive error, especially when accompanied by chorioretinal degeneration, has been shown to have a lowered EOG ratio (Blach *et al.* 1966). To study the effect of myopia on the EOG ratio and to determine whether the male-female difference in the EOG might be due to the influence of myopia, the EOG ratio was plotted against refractive error for the male and female groups. These data are shown in Fig. 2A and 2B with the best straight line fit to the data. The linear fit has a small negative slope for both groups. In neither group is the negative slope statistically significant.

The intersession variability of the EOG ratio is an important consideration when patients are being followed to determine a change in retinal status, such as in cases of retinotoxic drugs or intraocular foreign bodies. Twenty subjects were retested on a different day to provide data on the intersession variability. The frequency distribution histogram of the change in their EOG values is shown in Figure 3. While variations as high as 0.75 were found in one eye, 95% of the eyes tested had intersession variation of less than 0.6. In only 1 of the 40 eyes retested did the ratio change from normal to abnormal. This value of intersession variability and the fact that the variations are within normal limits is in good agreement with that reported previously by Kelsey 1967 and Van Lith & Balik 1970.

96

CONCLUSION

1) Males have a statistically significant lower EOG light peak dark trough ratio than females.

2) Myopia without apparent chorioretinal degeneration does not influence the EOG.

3) 95% of subjects retested on different days have a no greater than 0.6 ratio difference, and in only 1 of the 40 eyes retested did the ratio change from normal to abnormal.

ACKNOWLEDGEMENTS

The authors would like to acknowledge the assistance of Karen Brown in locating normal volunteers.

This study was supported in part by a gift from Research to Prevent Blindness, Inc.

REFERENCES

Adams, A. The normal electro-oculogram (EOG) *Acta Ophthal.* 51: *551-561* (1973).

Arden, G.B. & Barrada, A. & Kelsey, J.H. New clinical test of retinal function based upon the standing potential of the eye. *Brit. J. Ophthal.* 46, *449-467* (1962).

Blach, R.K., Barrie, J. & Kolb, H. Electrical activity of the eye in high myopia. *Brit. J. Ophthal.* 50, *629-641* (1966)

Kelsey, J.H. Variations in the normal Electro-oculogram. *Brit. J. Ophthal.* 51, *44-49* (1967)

Reeser, F., Weinstein, G.W., Felock, K.B. & Oser, R.S. Electro-oculography as a test of retinal function. *Am. J. Ophthal.* 70, *505-514* (1970).

Van Lith, G.H.M. & Balik, J. Variability of the electro-oculogram (EOG). *Acta. Ophthal.* 48, *1091-1096* (1970).

Author's address:
Dept of Ophthalmology
University of Wisconsin
Madison, Wis. 53706
USA

VARIATIONS OF THE DIRECTLY RECORDED STANDING POTENTIAL OF THE HUMAN EYE IN RESPONSE TO CHANGES IN ILLUMINATION AND TO ETHANOL[1]

SVEN ERIK G. NILSSON & KLAS-OLAV SKOOG

(Linköping)

SUMMARY

The standing potential (SP) of the human eye was studied by means of a newly developed method including a suction contact lens, calomel electrodes and d.c. amplification. In this way stable and reproducible long-term direct registrations of the SP could be obtained without the use of general anaesthesia. An abrupt alteration of the illumination gave rise to characteristic cyclic variations of the SP.

A sudden change in illumination from darkness to 16 Lux almost immediately provoked a comparatively fast, transient negative change of the SP, reaching its maximum after 0.5-1 min. Thereafter, starting in a positive direction, a much slower variation of the SP in the form of damped oscillations with a frequency of about 2/hour appeared. The maximum amplitude of the first slow oscillation was of the order of 5 mV. When the illumination was changed in the opposite direction, the oscillations were reversed as to polarity and they were smaller in amplitude. With respect to phases and frequencies the results correspond well to findings in EOG measurements.

In response to a small dose of ethanol, given orally, the SP showed variations similar to those after a change in illumination from darkness to light.

INTRODUCTION

Because of its vital importance to the visual process the pigment epithelium is now being subjected to an increasing scientific interest. The SP (Noell 1954, Heck & Papst 1957 and Gouras 1969) as well as the *c*-wave of the ERG (Noell 1954, Brown & Wiesel 1961, Steinberg, Schmidt, & Brown 1970, Schmidt & Steinberg 1971, Miller & Steinberg 1975, Oakley & Green 1975) are known to be generated mainly in the pigment epithelium (or in the pigment epithelium — receptor complex). A method for d.c. registration of the human *c*-wave has been developed (Knave, Nilsson & Lunt 1973, Nilsson & Knave 1974, Skoog & Nilsson 1974 a, b, Skoog 1974). In animal experiments stable SP recordings were performed by Kika-

[1] This investigation was supported by grants from the Swedish Medical Research Council (Project No 12X-734), Ollie and Elof Ericsson's Research Foundation and the Research Committee of the Östergötlands läns landsting.

99

wada (1968) (a variety of animals) and by Knave, Persson & Nilsson (1974 a, b) (sheep). So far the standing potential (SP) of the human eye has been measured only indirectly, with the electrooculogram (EOG) technique. For several reasons it would be of interest to study the human SP also in direct registrations, which would enable simultaneous recordings of the SP and the *c*-wave of the ERG. However, electrode problems, eye movements etc. have so far made it very difficult to obtain stable direct recordings (Dewar & McKendrick 1876, Solé, Alfieri & Dumas-Perrier 1971).

The present paper describes a new method for direct recordings of the human SP under stable conditions and in long-term experiments, without the use of general anaesthesia, and the variations of this potential in response to changes in illumination. See also Skoog (1975). As an example of drug effects on the human SP the influence of ethanol has been investigated. See also Skoog, Textorius & Nilsson (1975). The effects of ethanol on the human *c*-wave have been demonstrated by Skoog (1974).

MATERIAL AND METHODS

1. Experiments concerning the effect of changes in illumination

The method used (Skoog 1975) represents a further modification of the method developed for d.c. registration of the human *c*-wave (Knave, Nilsson & Lunt 1973, Skoog & Nilsson 1974 a,b).

Five healthy volunteers, females aged 22 to 28 years, were chosen. After dilatation of both pupils and topical anaesthesia a scleral contact lens, connected to the recording electrode by means of a saline bridge in an agar-filled polyethylene tube, was applied to one of the eyes (Fig. 1) and kept still in relation to the eye by means of gentle suction. (A saline-filled polyethylene tube connected the lens to a beaker with saline, the surface of which was placed 20 cm below the level of the eye.) Applanation tonometry before application and immediately after removal of the lens did not reveal significant changes in intraocular pressure. Pretests also showed that this gentle suction did not affect the *a*- and *b*-waves of the d.c. recorded ERG. Two plastic chambers were placed on the forehead using pieces of ring-shaped, two-sided adhesive tape as shown in Fig. 1. The chamber above the investigated eye was connected to the reference electrode by means of a saline-agar bridge. In the same way the other chamber was connected to the ground electrode. The contact lens as well as the chambers were filled with Methocel®. Temperature stabilized (± 0.1° C, by means of circulating water) and matched calomel half-cells were used as recording and reference electrodes, and the ground connection was equipped with a calomel electrode as well (Fig. 2). A wire-net cage shielded the volunteer and the electrode system from alternating current etc. The potentials from the electrodes were fed into the differential inputs of a low-drift d.c. amplifier, lowpass-filtered (220 Hz cut-off, 18 dB/octave) and forwarded to a Tandberg analogue tape recorder and a Hewlett-Packard 5480 S signal analyzer, where the measurements were displayed. The d.c. drift of the electrode system was less than 15 μV, and the stability of the total system was continuously checked on a separate oscilloscope.

The eyes of the volunteer were exposed either to darkness or a constant illumination for 80 min. During the first 20 min of this period the contact lens etc. was applied. (In case of dark adaptation the later procedure was carried out in an illumination of the eyes not exceeding 1 Lux.) After the adaptation the base-line was checked for stability during 10 min, and the average potential level during this period is referred to as zero potential. Then the illumination was suddenly changed, either from darkness to 16 Lux, or from 16 or 1100 Lux to darkness.

The SP was recorded for five seconds every minute except for the first 5 min after the change in illumination, when 30 sec intervals were used. During recordings the volunteer was made to fix with her free eye upon a very weak deep red light in the ceiling. Fifteen experiments were carried out, each registration lasting 50-60 min. In a few experiments particularly designed to describe the initial fast change, continuous recordings were made during 15 min. This procedure, in which the free eye was closed, required a great deal of co-operation from the volunteer.

2. Experiments concerning the effect of ethanol

(Only discrepancies from the above described technique are mentioned.) Five healthy volunteers, aged 22-31 years, weighing 56-70 kg, and not under

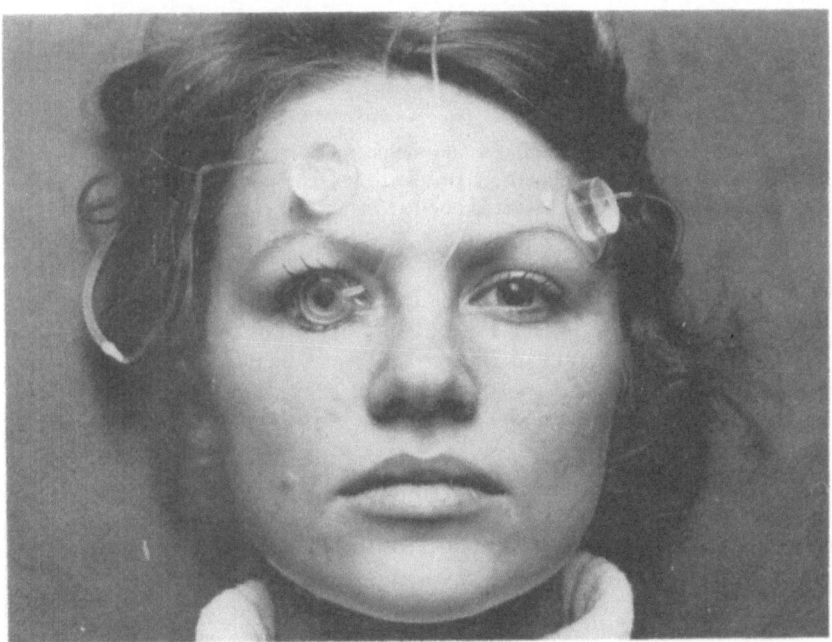

Fig. 1. The contact lens (for the tip of the recording electrode) and the two plastic chambers (for the tips of the reference and ground electrodes respectively) attached to a volunteer. Saline bridges in agar-filled polyethylene tubes lead to the electrodes. The contact lens is equipped with a second tube through which suction was applied. (From Skoog 1975.)

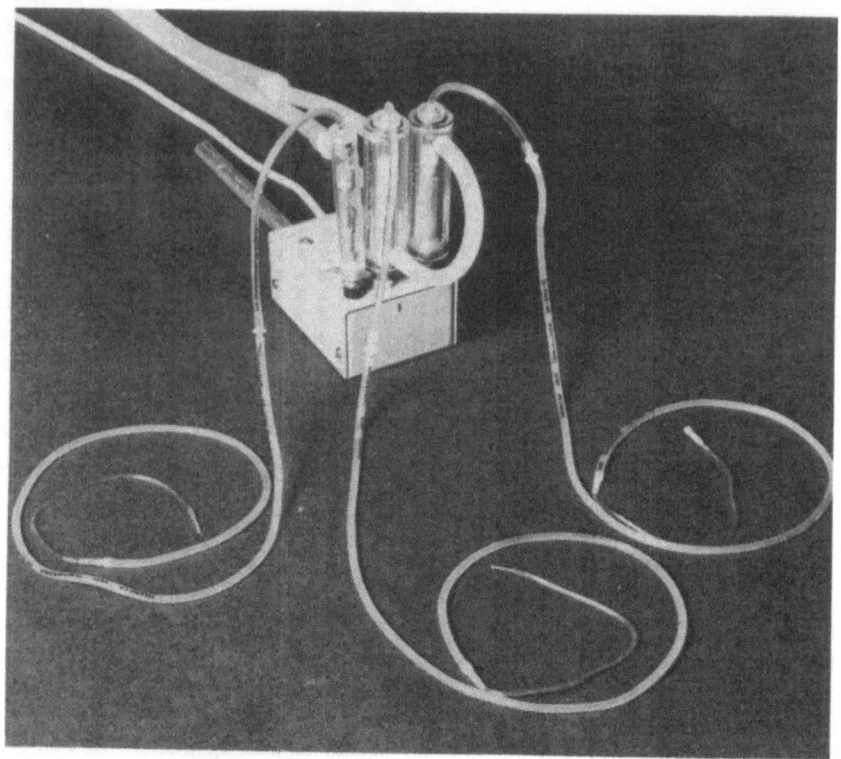

Fig. 2. Two temperature stabilized and matched calomel half-cells used as recording and reference electrodes respectively (to the right). The third calomel electrode mediates the ground connection. (From Skoog 1975.)

the influence of any previous intake of alcoholic beverages, participated in this study. They were fasting for 4 hours prior to the intake of alcohol, and before the fasting they had had only a very light meal. The eyes were adapted to darkness or to 1100 Lux. Recordings were carried out twice a minute. The SP variations were traced on a Hewlett-Packard 7402 A ink writing recorder.

0.4 g ethanol/kg body weight was given orally in the form of brandy with an addition of 95 vol% ethanol to make 50 vol%. The dose was taken in less than one min, during which the electrodes were kept in place. Blood alcohol analyses were carried out by means of gas chromatography.

RESULTS

1. Experiments concerning the effect of changes in illumination

The effect on the SP of a sudden change in illumination from darkness to 16 Lux is shown in Fig. 3. A comparatively fast, transient negative change was followed by a much slower variation of the SP in the form of damped oscillations, which were very small after 1 hour and should be negligable after 80 min. The maximum amplitude of the initial transient was about 2 mV and occurred 0.5-1 min after the change in illumination. The frequency of the slower oscillation was about 2/hour and the full amplitude of the first oscillation, which started in a positive direction, was of the order of 5 mV. In some experiments the oscillations seemed to be superimposed upon a small and much slower change.

Fig. 4 shows on an expanded time scale a continuous recording of the first part of the SP variations after a change from darkness to 16 Lux from a a volunteer, who managed to keep her eyes still without fixation. The initial, negative transient is easily seen, as well as an indication of a small plateau where the slow oscillation has started but still seems to be influenced by the first, fast component. Thus also the fast component appears to by cyclic in nature.

In Fig. 5 the effect of a sudden change from 1100 Lux to darkness is illustrated. The initial transient is here positive and the slower oscillation begins in a negative direction. Thus, as to polarities the curve is more or less

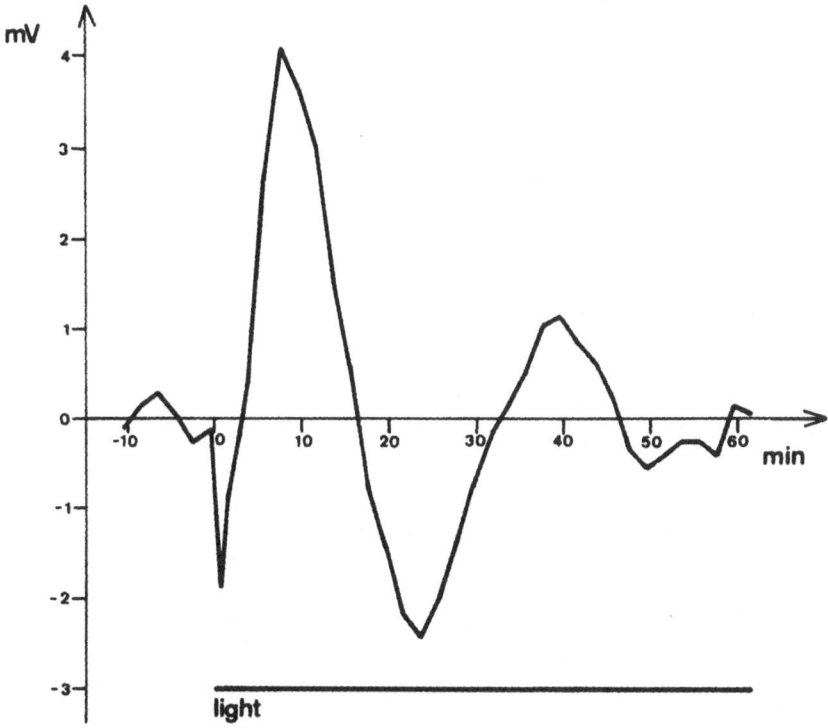

Fig. 3. The result of a typical experiment showing SP oscillations in response to a change in illumination from darkness to 16 Lux. SP recorded every min, except from 0 to 5 min, when 30 sec intervals were used. Each point of the curve represents the average of two consecutive measurements. (From Skoog 1975).

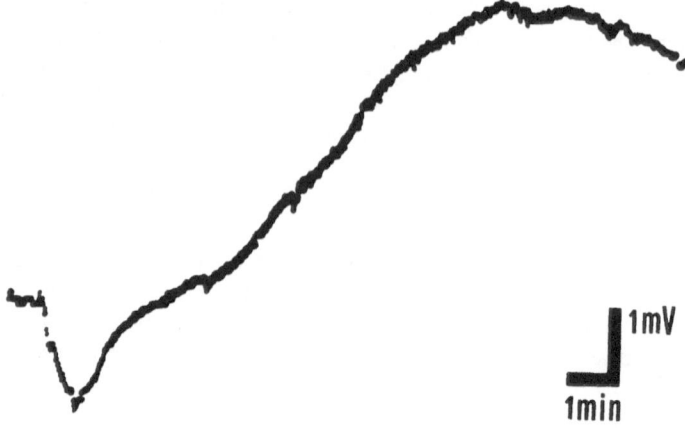

Fig. 4. Continuous registration of SP changes following a change in illumination from darkness to 16 Lux. (From Skoog 1975.)

a mirror image of that in Fig. 3. The amplitudes of these variations were slightly less than half of those when the illumination was changed from darkness to 16 Lux. (When the illumination was altered from 16 Lux to darkness the amplitudes were even smaller.) The other experiments fully confirmed the above findings.

2. Experiments concerning the effect of ethanol

Oral administration of ethanol provoked cyclic variations of the SP in the dark adapted eye in the form of damped oscillations with a frequency of about 2/hour (Fig. 6) and, with respect to amplitudes and polarities, very much resembling the above described oscillations seen after a change in illumination from darkness to light. The average latency of the first positive peak was about 10 min, and the full amplitude of the first oscillation was 4-5 mV on an average. When the ethanol experiment was carried out in an illumination of the eyes of 1100 Lux, the polarity of the oscillations were the same as when performed in darkness, although the amplitudes were slightly smaller.

The blood alcohol concentration was rapidly increasing during the first 25 min, after which the curve began to level off. At 10 min the concentration was about 0.1 g/litre and at 25 min it was about 0.15 g/litre.

DISCUSSION

1. Experiments concerning the effect of changes in illumination

Eye movements, sliding contact lenses, variations in polarizing currents of ordinary ERG electrodes and thus considerable d.c. drift disturbed earlier attempts to follow directly the human SP. In the present investigation these disadvantages were avoided to a very great extent by the use of fixation light, suction contact lens, matched and temperature stabilized calomel electrodes and d.c. amplification.

Because the effects of electrical shunting in the body tissues, a somewhat variable positioning of the reference electrode, and perhaps also changes at the electrode − body junctions have so far not been evaluated, the SP is not given in absolute but in relative values. Also in EOG technique a relative value, the light peak/dark trough ratio, is generally used (Arden & Kelsey 1962).

Gouras & Carr (1964), using 4/sec flicker stimuli, were able to follow the SP in the monkey for about 1 hour and demonstrated 2/hour oscillations.

The timing and the general shape of the directly measured SP oscillations of the present investigation, the initial faster as well as the slower damped oscillation with a frequency of about 2/hour, are in close agreement with the indirectly studied SP changes (EOG variations) after sudden light and dark steps (Kris 1958, Kolder 1959, Täumer, Hennig & Pernice 1974 and others).

Also the amplitude of the c-wave of the ERG shows damped oscillations with a frequency of about 2/hour (Calissendorff, Knave & Persson 1974 (sheep), Skoog & Nilsson 1974 b and Nilsson & Skoog 1976 (man)). This

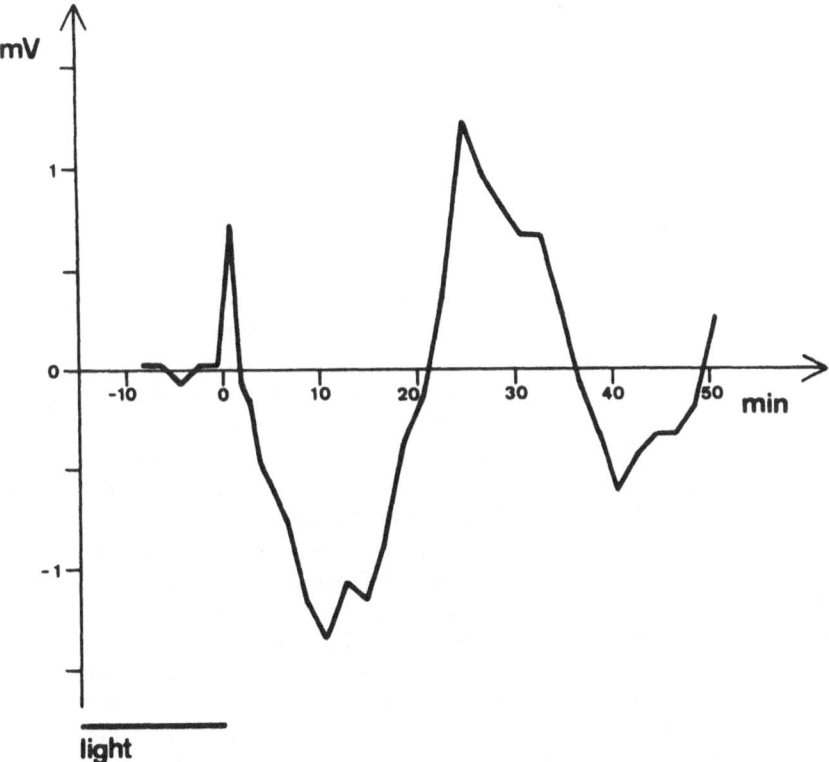

Fig. 5. SP oscillations in response to a change in illumination from 1100 Lux to darkness. Recording procedure and plotting as for Fig. 3. (From Skoog 1975.)

105

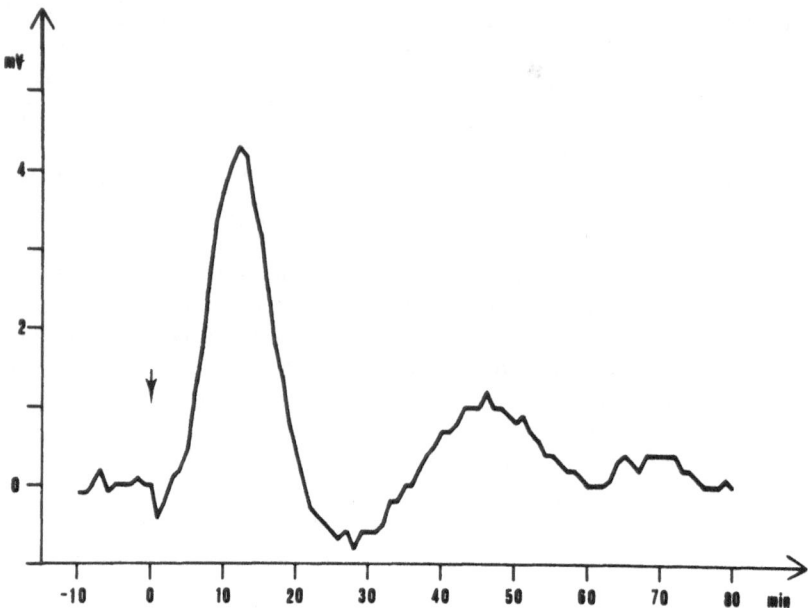

Fig. 6. The result of a typical experiment performed in darkness, showing SP oscillations provoked by the oral administration (arrow) of 0.4 g ethanol/kg body weight. SP recorded twice a minute. Each point on the curve represents the average of two consecutive measurements. (From Skoog, Textorius & Nilsson 1975).

similar behaviour of the *c*-wave and the SP is not surprising, since the pigment epithelium (or the pigment epithelium — receptor complex) is a major source of both potentials. It also ought to be of importance to report that simultaneous recordings of the SP and the *c*-wave recently were performed in our laboratory. These experiments demonstrated that the oscillations of the SP and the *c*-wave were parallel in time (Nilsson & Skoog 1975). The findings are an additional strong support of the conception that the SP and the *c*-wave are closely related. In some of the experiments it seemed that the 2/hour SP oscillations were superimposed upon a small and much slower variation, the exact nature of which could not be determined. In this connection it is interesting to note, that Calissendorff, Knave & Persson (1974) (sheep) convincingly showed that the 2/hour oscillations of the *c*-wave amplitude were superimposed upon slower, 0.5/hour oscillations. Very slow EOG variations were reported by Davis & Shackel (1960) and by Jacobs, Feldman, Rabinowitz & Bender (1973). In all electrophysiology concerning the SP and the *c*-wave (and perhaps the pigment epithelium in general) it is of importance to take the oscillations with time into close consideration. It should be remembered that every change in illumination of the eye provokes such oscillations. For this reason the illumination of the eyes of the volunteer in the present study, also in the ethanol experiments, was kept constant for 60-80 min.

Stepanik (1958) demonstrated an alteration in SP in response to a rise in intraocular pressure (IOP), provoked by the use of a special suction contact lens with strong negative pressures (40-300 mm Hg below atmospheric pressure). Also the *b*-wave of the ERG is known to be sensitive to an increase in IOP (Wulfing 1963, Henkes, Usami & van Lith 1968). In the present study only a very moderate negative pressure of about 15 mm Hg below atmospheric pressure was applied, and this suction did not significantly affect either the IOP, as controlled with applanation tonometry before and after the experiments, or the *b*-wave of the ERG.

2. Experiments concerning the effect of ethanol

It is somewhat surprising that even a small, single oral dose of ethanol provokes dramatic and long-term effects on the SP in the form of damped 2/hour oscillations. Repeated venous blood samples revealed that the maximum SP amplitude occurred while blood alcohol concentrations were still increasing. The same was true for the *c*-wave maximum (Skoog 1974). Psychophysical experiments have demonstrated that a certain blood alcohol level exerts a greater influence on test parameters during the rising than during the falling phase (Goldberg 1943 and others).

Ethanol effects on the *a*- and *b*-waves of the human ERG were extensively studied by Straub (1957), Ikeda (1963) and Jacobson, Hirose & Stokes (1969). A large increase in *c*-wave amplitude after *i.v.* injection of ethanol was found in animal experiments (sheep) by Knave, Persson & Nilsson (1974 a). Skoog (1974) demonstrated that a small oral dose of ethanol provoked 2/hour oscillations of the amplitude of the human *c*-wave, and that the amplitude of these oscillations was larger than that of oscillations provoked by stimulus light flashes. The *c*-wave is sensitive also to other substances, which has been demonstrated in animal experiments: epinephrine (Therman 1938), sodium azide and sodium iodate (Noell 1954), rifampicin (Knave, Persson, Calissendorff & Nilsson 1973), quinine and chloroquine (Calissendorff 1976 a) and phenothiazines (Calissendorff 1976 b).

In animal experiments the SP has been shown to be affected by several drugs. It was dramatically decreased by sodium iodate, while sodium azide caused an increase (Noell 1954 and Heck & Papst 1957). Small doses of barbiturates caused a negative shift in the SP, while larger doses provoked a negative-positive, damped cyclic variation of the SP (Knave, Persson & Nilsson 1974 a, b).

For the sheep it was demonstrated by Knave, Persson & Nilsson (1974 a) that *i.v.* injected ethanol gave rise to SP changes in the form of an initial negative transient followed by a large positive change. The transient was not so clearly seen in our experiments, probably because of the slower, oral route of administration of ethanol. The positive change resembled the first part of the oscillations of the present study.

The SP variations in response to ethanol observed in the present study correlate well with the oscillations of the *c*-wave amplitude after corresponding doses of ethanol shown by Skoog (1974). The frequency of the oscillations as well as the latency of the first maximum were of the same magnitude in both types of experiments. The results strongly favour the idea that the SP and the c-wave are derived, at least partly, from the same structures and/or physiological processes. The SP response to ethanol was the same under scotopic as well as under photopic conditions. Thus these SP oscillations do not seem to be dependent on the level of rod sensitivity to light. The c-wave is considered to be rod-dependent (Steinberg, Schmidt & Brown 1970 and others). In experiments now in progress in our laboratory no c-waves could be obtained at a photopic level of adaptation, at which ethanol-induced SP oscillations were easily elicited.

In response to a variety of stimuli (changes in illumination, ethanol, drugs) the SP as well as the c-wave of the ERG react in a stereotype way with damped cyclic variations. It thus seems, that all these stimuli affect a certain mechanism, which is closely related to the generation of the SP as well as the c-wave. This mechanism is most likely located in the pigment epithelium. Further studies of this problem are necessary in order to help clarify the exact origin of the oscillations and the mechanisms for toxic effects on the pigment epithelium.

REFERENCES

Arden, G.B. & Kelsey, J.H. Changes produced by light in the standing potential of the human eye. *J. Physiol. (Lond.)* 161, *189-204* (1962).

Brown, K.T. & Wiesel, T.N. Localization of origins of electroretinogram components by intraretinal recording in the intact cat eye. *J. Physiol. (Lond.)* 158, *257-280* (1961).

Calissendorff, B. Melanotropic drugs and retinal functions. I. Effects of quinine and chloroquine on the sheep ERG. *Acta Ophthal. (Kbh.)* 54, *109-117* (1976 a).

Calissendorff, B. Melanotropic drugs and retinal functions. II. Effects of phenothiazine and rifampicin on the sheep ERG. *Acta Ophthal. (Kbh.)* 54, *118-128* (1976 b).

Calissendorff, B., Knave, B. & Persson, H.E. (1974) Cyclic variations in the c-wave amplitude of the sheep ERG. *Vision Res.*, In press.

Davis, J.R. & Shackel, B. Changes in the electro-oculogram potential level. *Brit. J. Ophthal.* 44, *606-618* (1960).

Dewar, J. & McKendrick, T.G. The physiological action of light. *Royal Inst. of Great Britain Proc.* 8, *137-149* (1876).

Goldberg, L. Quantitative studies on alcohol tolerance in man. *Acta physiol. scand.* 5, *Suppl. 16* (1943).

Gouras, P. Clinical electro-oculography. In: Straatsma, B.R., ed. *The Retina*, pp.565-581. University of California Press, Berkeley & Los Angeles (1943).

Gouras, P. & Carr, R.E. Primate retinal responses: slow changes during repetitive stimulation with light. *Science* 145, *413-414* (1969).

Heck, J. & Papst, W. Über den Ursprung des corneo-retinalen Ruhepotentials. *Bibl. ophthal. (Basel)* 48, *96-107* (1957).

Henkes, H.E., Usami, E. & van Lith, G.H.M. Flicker-electro-dynamography. In: Schmöger, E., ed. *Proc. VIth ISCERG Symposium*, pp. 391-401. Georg Thieme, Leipzig (1968).

Ikeda, H. Effects of ethyl alcohol on the evoked potential of the human eye. *Vision Res.* 3, *155-169* (1963).

Jacobs, L., Feldman, M., Rabinowitz, M. & Bender, M.B. Alterations of the corneofundal potential of the eye during sleep. *Electroenceph. clin. Neurophysiol.* 34, *576-586* (1973).

Jacobson, J.H., Hirose, T. & Stokes. P.E. *Ophthalmologica (Basel)* 158, *Suppl.*, pp. 669-677 (1969).

Kikawada, N. Variations in the corneo-retinal standing potential of the vertebrate eye during light and dark adaptations. *Jap. J. Physiol.* 18, *687-702* (1968).

Knave, B., Nilsson, S.E.G. & Lunt, T. The human electroretinogram: d.c. recordings at low and conventional stimulus intensities. Description of a new method for clinical use. *Acta ophthal. (Kbh.)* 51, *716-726* (1973).

Knave, B., Persson, H.E., Calissendorff, B. & Nilsson, S.E.G. Selective effect of a new antituberculous drug, rifampicin, on the c-wave of the sheep electroretinogram. *Acta ophthal (Kbh.)* 51, *371-374* (1973).

Knave, B., Persson, H.E. & Nilsson, S.E.G. A comparative study on the effects of barbiturate and ethyl alcohol on retinal functions with special reference to the c-wave of the electroretinogram and the standing potential of the sheep eye. *Acta ophthal. (Kbh.)* 52, *254-259* (1974 a).

Knave, B., Persson, H.E. & Nilsson, S.E.G. The effect of barbiturate on retinal functions. II. Effects on the c-wave of the electroretinogram and the standing potential of the sheep eye. *Acta physiol. scand.* 91, *180-186* (1974 b).

Kolder, H. Spontane und experimentelle Änderungen des Bestandpotentials des menschlichen Auges. *Pflügers Arch. ges. Physiol.* 268, *258-272* (1959).

Kris, C. Corneo-fundal potential variations during light and dark adaptation *Nature (Lond)* 182, *1027-1028* (1958).

Miller, S.S. & Steinberg, R.M. An electrophysiological analysis of the frog retinal pigment epithelium. *Invest. Ophthal.* In press (1975).

Nilsson, S.E.G. & Knave, B. A new method for d.c. registration of the human ERG at low and conventional stimulus intensities. *In* Dodt, E. and Pearlman, J.T. (Eds.): XIth ISCERG sympos. Bad Nauheim 1973. *Documenta Ophthal. Proc. Ser.* 4, *229-235* (1974).

Nilsson, S.E.G. & Skoog, K.-O. Covariation of the simultaneously recorded c-wave and the standing potential of the human eye. *Acta Ophthal. (Kbh.)* 53, *721-730* (1975).

Nilsson, S.E.G. & Skoog, K.-O. Intensity-amplitude relationships and cyclic variations of the c-wave of the human d.c. registered ERG. *Documenta Ophthal. Proc. Ser.* 10, *255-265* (1976).

Noell, W.K. The origin of the electroretinogram. *Amer. J. Ophthal.* 38, *78-90* (1954).

Oakley, B. & Green, D.G. The ionic basis of the c-wave of the electroretinogram. *Invest. Ophthal.* In press (1975).

Schmidt, R. & Steinberg, R.H. Rod-dependent intracellular responses to light recorded from the pigment epithelium of the cat retina. *J. Physiol. (Lond.)* 217, *71-91* (1971).

Skoog, K.-O. The c-wave of the human d.c. registered ERG. III. Effects of ethyl alcohol on the c-wave. *Acta ophthal. (Kbh.)* 52, *913-923* (1974).

Skoog, K.-O. The directly recorded standing potential of the human eye. *Acta ophthal. (Kbh.)* 53, *120-132* (1975).

Skoog, K.-O. & Nilsson, S.E.G. The c-wave of the human d.c. registered ERG. I. A quantitative study of the relationship between c-wave amplitude and stimulus intensity. *Acta ophthal. (Kbh.)* 52, *759-773* (1974 a).

Skoog, K.-O. & Nilsson, S.E.G. The c-wave of the human d.c. registered ERG. II. Cyclic variations of the c-wave amplitude. *Acta ophthal. (Kbh.)* 52, *904-912* (1974 b).

Skoog, K.-O., Textorius, O. & Nilsson, S.E.G. Effects of ethyl alcohol on the directly recorded standing potential of the human eye. *Acta Ophthal. (Kbh.)* 53, *710-720* (1975).

Sole, P., Alfieri, R. & Dumas-Perrier, N. An original technique of retinal electrodiagnosis in the child: coupled electro-oculogram and electroretinogram. In: Basar, D. &

109

Bengusi, *U.*, eds. *Proc. VIIth ISCERG Symposium*, pp. 143-146. Faculty of Medicine, University of Istanbul, Istanbul (1971).

Steinberg, R.H., Schmidt, R. & Brown, K.T. Intracellular responses to light from cat pigment epithelium: origin of the electroretinogram *c*-wave. *Nature (Lond.)* 227, *728-730* (1970).

Stepanik, J. Das Bestandpotential des Auges und die experimentelle Steigerung des intraocularen Druckes beim Menschen. *Albrecht v. Graefes Arch. Ophthal.* 160, *226-235* (1958).

Straub, W. Untersuchungen über die Beeinflussung des Elektroretinogramms beim Menschen durch Athylalkohol. *Albrecht v. Graefes Arch. Ophthal.* 159, *353-358* (1957).

Therman, P.O. The neurophysiology of the retina. *Acta Soc. Sci. Fenn. Nova Series B. II.* 1, *1-74* (1938).

Täumer, R., Hennig, J. & Pernice, D. The ocular dipole – a damped oscillator stimulated by the speed of change in illumination. *Vision Res.* 14, *637-645* (1974).

Wulfing, B. Clinical evaluation of electroretino-dynamography. *Acta ophthal. (Kbh.) Suppl. 73* (1963).

Author's address:
Department of Ophthalmology
University Hospital
S – 58185 Linköping
Sweden

THE ERG AND EOG DURING THE COURSE
OF SYMPATHETIC OPHTHALMIA

WILLIAM R. BIERSDORF

(Columbus, Ohio)

INTRODUCTION

Not much literature exists on the electroretinogram in sympathetic ophthalmia (Georgiades, *et al.*, 1967; Bogoslovsky, *et al.*, 1973). ERG amplitudes have been reported abnormally reduced in the sympathising eye beginning early in the course of the disease. The peak latency of the scotopic b-wave was also reported delayed (Georgiades, *et al.*, 1967). Generally in uveitis the ERG is normal. although it can be subnormal or even extinguished (Francois, 1953) In one report on chronic uveitis, the scotopic b-wave was found subnormal in 8 of 29 cases (Algvere, 1967). Animal studies on experimental uveitis have also shown ERG's ranging from normal to extinguished (Lawwill, *et al.*, 1972; Algvere *et al.*, 1968).

In the present case of sympathetic ophthalmia, photopic and scotopic ERG's and the electro-oculogram (EOG) have been recorded from the outset on seven different occasions over a period of twenty-six months.

METHOD

Recording of the ERG utilized a xenon flash tube (Grass) illuminating the inside of a 18in. diameter ganzfeld to obtain uniform full field stimulation (Berson, *et al.,* 1968). The patient was seated at the ganzfeld in a shielded room with his head in position on a chin rest. ERG's were recorded with a Riggs contact lens with a chlorided silver electrode. The other active electrode was attached to the skin overlying the zygoma and a ground electrode was attached to the mastoid. Amplification was provided by Tektronix 122 amplifiers with band pass of 0.2 to 250 Hz. To reduce interference from blinking and eye movements, the responses were averaged by a Hewlett-Packard 5480 signal analyzer, and displayed on an x-y recorder. Photopic ERG's were recorded with flicker stimulation at 9 Hz, and scotopic ERG's at 1.1 Hz.

The photopic ERG was recorded first at an adaptation level of 8ft-L in the ganzfeld with three intensities of test flash. Fig. 1 illustrates a normal photopic electroretinogram under our recording conditions at an intensity of I 16. For I 16, a normal photopic b-wave was $\geq 80~\mu v$ as measured from the a-wave trough, with a peak latency of 30 msec or less. A photopic b-wave of less than 10 μv, or having a peak latency of more than 40 msec was classified as severely abnormal.

111

PHOTOPIC   SCOTOPIC

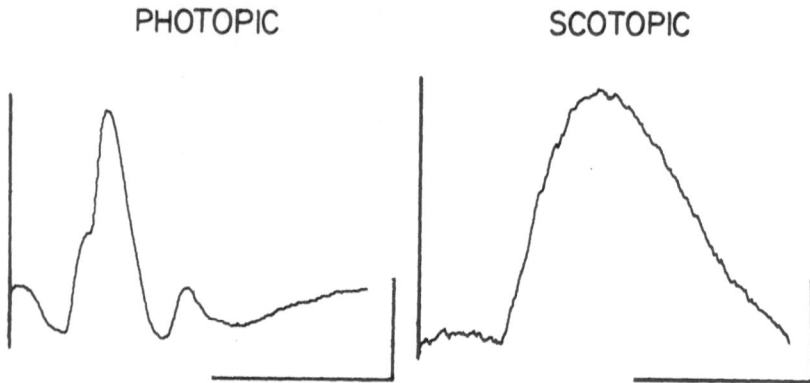

Fig. 1 Normal ERG's (undilated pupils). Photopic I 16 (Grass) in ganzfeld. Galib. 20 μv, 50 ms. Scotopic I 1 at 5 min. darkness. Galib. 20 μv, 100 ms.

After photopic testing, the adaptation light was turned off and the temporal course of dark adaptation was followed with white test flashes in the ganzfeld. Testing was done once a minute with different test intensities, varied with photic stimulator settings and neutral density filters. Dark adaptation was usually complete within 10 minutes following this minimal pre-exposure. The scotopic ERGs illustrated were obtained at intensity I 1 with no neutral filters at 5 minutes of dark adaptation. A normal scotopic b-wave was $\geq$ 100 μv under these conditions. A b-wave of less than 15 μv, or a negative waveform, was classified as severely abnormal.

The macular ERG was recorded with a 4° diameter red test patch against a rod-saturating luminance of blue adaptation following previous procedures (Biersdorf & Diller, 1969). The EOG was recorded with Arden's method. Borderline light rise values were from 165-185 with normal above and abnormal below this range.

CASE REPORT

On 12-21-73 the patient, a 19 year old male, was involved in an automobile accident and suffered laceration of the right eye, involving sclera, cornea and iris. Surgical repair was performed the same day with excision of the incarcerated iris. Following surgery, visual acuity was 20/70 in the injured eye. Six weeks later the patient began experiencing headaches and blurred vision. He was placed on systemic steroids and given an injection of retrobulbar steroids.

He was first seen at Ohio State University on 2-11-74. Visual acuity was hand movement O.D. and 20/400 O.S. Examination of the injured O.D. showed a healed corneo-scleral scar with adherent iris. The fundus was not seen O.D. because of a cataract but ultrasonography showed a subtotal retinal detachment. Ophthalmoscopic examination of the sympathising O.S. showed a grayish retina, choroidal thickening and a shifting posterior pole detachment. Anterior uveitis was also present. Intensive treatment was given including prednisone and Imuran.

Electrical testing was begun the following day. The results of the sequential testing are shown in Table I, including photopic and scotopic ERG's, the electro-oculogram and visual acuities in the sympathising eye. Representative scotopic ERG's are illustrated in Fig. 2. On initial examination Feb. 12, the scotopic ERG was very abnormal in the injured O.D., of entirely negative waveform (showing no b-wave) for moderate intensity stimulation. For brighter test flashes, a short latency positive wave was present. The scotopic ERG for the sympathising eye was also very abnormal with only a short latency positive wave present. For brighter test flashes, a small a-wave also appeared. The electro-oculogram light rise was abnormal O.U. (O.D.-110%, O.S.-133%), and the absolute level of the resting potential was abnormally low O.U.

On the second ERG exam 3-7-74, the scotopic ERG in the injured eye had improved to a very low positive amplitude with abnormally long latency. In O.S., the scotopic ERG had improved to showing an abnormal split b-wave with both early and late peaks. For brighter test flashes, an a-wave was also present for both eyes. The EOG light-rise was still abnormal O.D. (116%) with abnormally low resting potential. In O.S., the resting potential had improved to within normal limits, and the light-rise had improved to borderline (165%). At this time visual acuity was 20/200 O.S. Ophthalmoscopic examination showed a reduced, but still present retinal detachment O.S., and a fine peppered pigmentation in the macular and perimacular area.

On the third exam 3-21-74, not much change was seen in the scotopic ERG's. The EOG light-rise had increased to normal O.D. (192%), although the resting potential was still abnormally low. At this time, the patient's color vision was tested and found to be protanomalous by the D. & H. Color Rule (Biersdorf). The patient got 12 of 14 correct on the A.O. H-R-R plates, but could not read the demonstration plates. Examination, including ultrasonography O.D., showed that the retinal detachments O.U. had resolved.

Table I.

	Injured O.D.			Sympathising O.S.			
	Phot. ERG	Scot. ERG	EOG	Phot. ERG	Scot. ERG	EOG	v.a.
2-12-74	Abn. ***	Abn. ***	(119)	Abn. *	Abn. **	(133)	20/400
3- 7-74	Abn. **	Abn. **	(116)	Nl/abn.	Abn. *	165	20/200
3-21-74	Abn. *	Abn. **	(192)	Abn. *	Abn. *	150	20/100
4- 4-74	Abn/nl.	Abn. *	(208)	Abn. *	Abn. **	159	20/ 30
6-24-74	Abn. *	Norm.	(168)	Abn. *	Norm.	210	20/ 25
12-23-74	Abn. *	Norm.	(165)	Abn. *	Abn. *	205	
2-25-76	Abn. *	Abn. *	(265)	Abn. *	Nl/abn	257	20/ 25

Abn. ***   severely abnormal (amplitude and/or latency)
Abn. **   moderately ,,
Abn. *   mildly   ,,
(---)   Abnormally low resting potential

Not much change on the average was seen on the ERG exam of April 4 although acuity O.S. had improved to 20/30. On June 24, the scotopic ERG's in both eyes had improved to the normal range. The EOG light-rise O.S. improved to normal (210%), but O.D. regressed to borderline (168%). At this time, color vision had improved to normal on the D. & H. Color Rule.

Six months later (12-23-74), findings were similar. Scotopic ERG's were normal O.U. (Fig. 2). The two eyes differed on the EOG, results being normal O.S. (205%), and borderline normal O.D. (165%). The absolute level of the resting potential O.D. remained abnormally low.

A period of 14 months elapsed before the ERG's were tested again. On 2-25-76, the scotopic ERG's regressed in amplitude to mildly abnormal O.D. and borderline O.S. EOG light-rises in both eyes had improved (normal

SCOTOPIC ERG

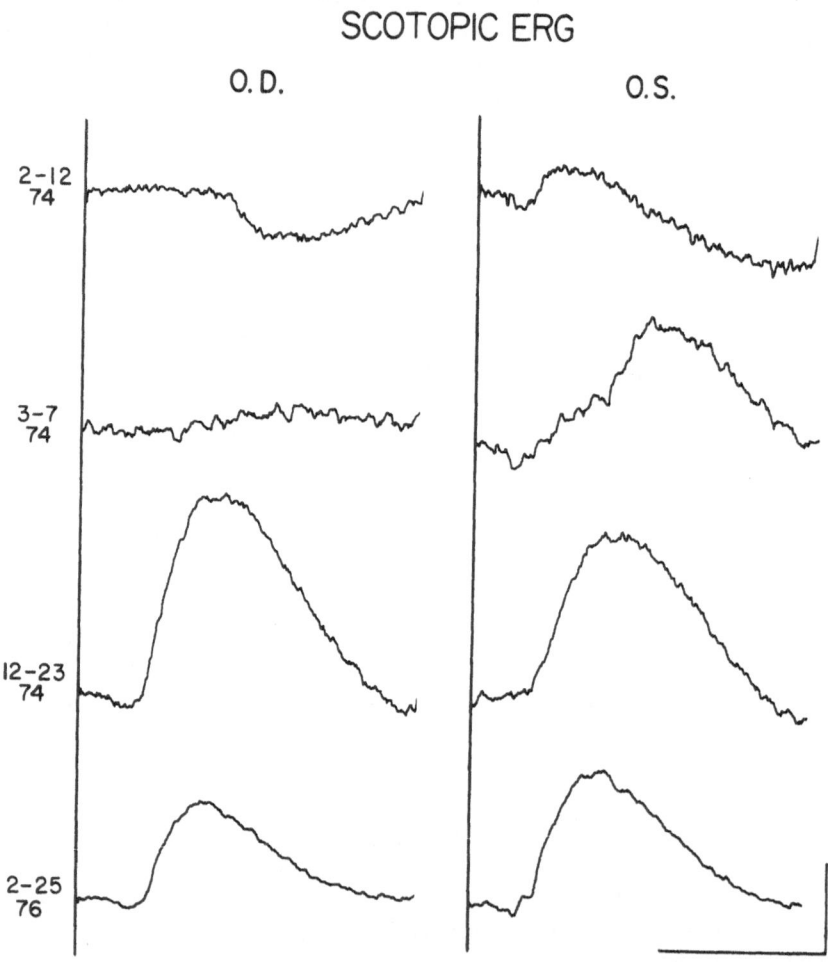

Fig. 2 Scotopic ERG's in case of sympathetic ophthalmia. Conditions as in Fig. 1. Galib. 20 μv, 100 ms.

range) while the absolute resting potential remained abnormally low O.D. Ophthalmoscopic exam O.S. showed diffuse mottling of the posterior pole and peripapillary atrophy of the choroid and pigment epithelium. The patient's medications had previously been reduced to topical steroids. Treatment was continuing.

Photopic ERG's of the patient showed a somewhat different course (Fig. 3). On initial exam 2-12-74, the photopic ERG was very abnormal in the injured O.D., similar to the scotopic. In the sympathising eye, however, the photopic ERG was only mildly abnormal (reduced amplitudes, slightly prolonged peak latencies of 31 msec). On subsequent exams, the photopic ERG O.D. improved (Table 1) to the third exam 3-21-74 when it was also mildly abnormal (reduced amplitudes, slightly prolonged latencies of 33 msec). On all subsequent exams, photopic ERG peak latencies O.U. re-

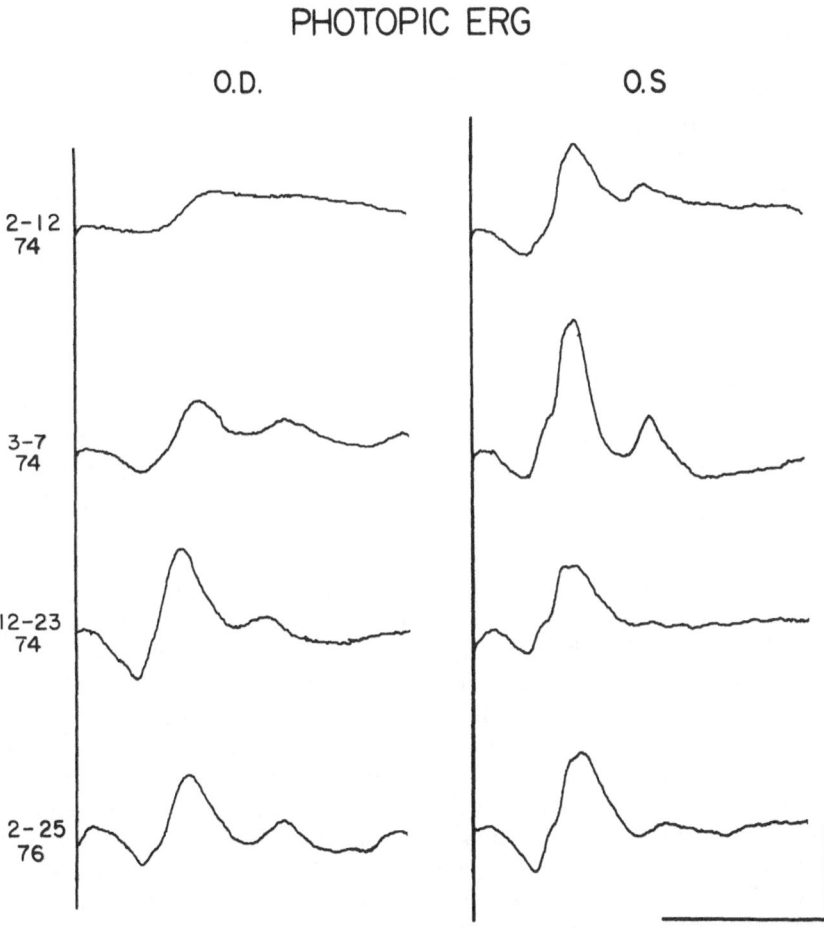

Fig. 3 Photopic ERG's in case of sympathetic ophthalmia. Conditions as in Fig. 1. Galib. 20 μv, 50 ms.

115

mained in the mildly abnormal range of 31-34 msec with reduced amplitudes. A macular ERG on the sympathising O.S., June 24 proved within normal limits (Biersdorf & Diller, 1969). At this time, visual acuity was 20/25.

In addition to the patient's electrical responses showing improvements and decrements during this time, the clinical course also showed periodic regressions when steroids had to be increased in spite of the general trend of improvement.

COMMENT

At the height of the disease when first tested, the scotopic ERG's were severely abnormal with only a long latency negative response or a short latency positive response. This latter is probably actually a photopic b-wave, as indicated by the b-waves present in photopic conditions. These results are consistent with previous reports of early ERG abnormality in sympathetic ophthalmia (Georgiades, et al., 1967; Bogoslovsky, et al., 1973). The initial EOG's also were abnormal O.U. (both absolute level and lightrise values).

There is a significant difference, however, in the photopic and scotopic b-waves in the sympathising eye at the outset. While the scotopic ERG was severely abnormal, the photopic b-wave was only mildly abnormal with slightly reduced amplitudes and slightly delayed latencies. We can reasonably conclude that the scotopic b-wave was affected first and most severely in comparison to the photopic b-wave by the inflammatory process. Presumably the disease was arrested by medical treatment before the photopic b-wave in the sympathising eye could be severely affected. This points up the low correlation between the photopic b-wave and the visual acuity which was 20/400 at the outset in the sympathising eye. Of course the visual acuity is not dependent on the approximately 97% of the retinal cones outside the fovea which are tested by the photopic ERG. Actually, there was a better correlation between the scotopic ERG (very abnormal) and the clinical state (including visual acuity) in the sympathising eye. A good correlation between the scotopic ERG and post-operative visual acuity has also been reported in retinal detachment (Jacobson, et al., 1958; Rendahl, 1961). This must be a correlation mediated by some metabolic factor in the eye, as of course there is no direct relation between rods and foveal visual acuity. Although there was a poor correlation between photopic b-wave and clinical state at the outset, photopic b-waves on the final exam were mildly abnormal consistent with incomplete clinical recovery.

There was a improvement in the scotopic ERG's and EOG's with treatment, as the clinical state of the eyes improved. This was not a continuous improvement, but a course showing periodic regressions both in the clinical state and in the electrical findings. On some occasions, the ERG improved somewhat while the EOG regressed somewhat, and vica versa. About 6 weeks after the start of treatment, the retinal detachments had resolved O.U. The gradual improvement in ERG and EOG following reattachment is consistent with the literature (Blach & Behrman, 1967).

Other tests also showed improvement in function. The macular ERG was

116

normal on 6-24-74, but as the sensitivity of this test is limited to about 20/60 (9), is doesn't tell us whether there was complete recovery. Color vision testing (D. & H. Color Rule) indicated recovery to within normal limits between 3-21 to 6-24-74.

No consistent difference between the EOG light-rise and the scotopic ERG was found, as is consistent with previous work showing that the light-rise involves the retina as well as the pigment epithelium (Gouras, 1969). The absolute level of the resting potential in the injured O.D. remained abnormally low, however, while the scotopic ERG returned to normal for some period of time. The absolute level has been shown to be abnormally low in circulatory occlusions in the eye as well as in retinal detachment.

On the final exam, both photopic and scotopic ERG's were mildly abnormal, indicating incomplete recovery of function. While the EOG light rise was normal in both eyes, the absolute level was abnormally low in the injured eye. Ophthalmoscopic examination of O.S. also indicated abnormal retina and choroid.

The results in this case indicate that scotopic ERG's and EOG's are very abnormal early in the course of sympathetic opthalmia and support Georgiades suggestion that ERG or EOG testing might be a good way of following trauma cases for early detection of sympathetic ophthalmia. The ERG also appears useful in following the treatment of sympathetic ophthalmia to assist in the evaluation of recovery.

ACKNOWLEDGEMENT

The author wishes to express his appreciation to Frederick H. Davidorf, M.D. for making available the clinical records and his patient for electrophysiological testing.

NOTE FROM DISCUSSION

It has been reported that oral steroids increase ERG amplitudes (Zimmerman, T.J. et al. Ann. Ophthal. 5, 757, 1973). Thus the decline in this patient's ERG between the last two exams could have resulted from his intervening removal from systemic prednisone threapy.

REFERENCES

Algvere, P. Electroretinographic studies on posterior uveitis. Acta Ophthal. 45, 299 (1967).

Algvere, P. et al. The electroretinogram and histopathology in experimental uveitis of the pigeon. Acta Ophthal. 46, 920 (1968).

Berson, E.L., et al. Rod responses in retinitis pigmentosa, dominantly inherited. Arch. Ophth. 80, 58 (1968).

Biersdorf, W.R. & Diller, D.A. Local electroretinogram in macular degeneration. Amer. J. Ophthal. 68, 296 (1969).

Biersdorf, W.R. The D. & H. Color Rule as a color vision screening test (inpreparation).

Blach, R.K. & Behrman, J. The electrical activity of the eye in retinal detachment. Trans. Ophthal. Soc. U.K.. 87, 263 (1967).

Bogoslovsky, A.I. *et al.* (Electrophysiological investigations in sympathetic ophthalmia) *Vestn. Oftalmol.* 1, *33* (1973). (Russian).

François, J. L'electroretinographie dans les uveites. *Ophthalmologica* 125, *137* (1953).

Georgiades, G., *et al.* E.R.G. au cours d'un cas d'ophtalmie sympathique a localisation posterieure. *Ann. d'Ocul.* 200, *817* (1967).

Georgiades, G., *et al.* Etude des signes electro-retinographiques dano quatre cas d'ophtalmie sympatheque. *Ann.d'Ocul.* 200, *917* (1967).

Gouras, P. Clinical electro-oculography. In B.R. Straatsma, *et al.*, eds., The Retina. Morphology, Function and Clinical Characteristics. Berkeley: Univ. of Calif. 1969.

Jacobson, J.H., *et al.* The electroretinogram as a prognostic aid in retinal detachment. *Arch. Ophth.* 59, *515* (1958).

Lawwill, T., *et al.* The role of electroretinography in evaluating posterior uveitis. *Amer. J. Ophthal.* 74, *1086* (1972).

Rendahl, I. The clinical electroretinogram in detachment of the retina Acta Ophth. Suppl. 64 (1961).

Author's address:
Institute for Research in Vision
1314 Kinnear Road
Columbus, Ohio 43212
USA

ISCHEMIC RETINOPATHY: REDUCED LIGHT PEAK- AND DARK TROUGH AMPLITUDES IN ELECTROOCULOGRAPHY*

A. THALER, P. HEILIG & M.R. LESSEL

(Vienna)

ABSTRACT

In 10 adult subjects with occlusion of the central retinal artery and in 2 children with surgically transsected retinal artery, the standing potential as well as the light peak and dark through were found to be reduced.

In ischemic retinopathy the pathological changes are confined to the inner retinal layers. Pigment epithelium and receptors remain unaffected (Popp, 1875). This well defined retinal lesion leads to disturbances of bioelectric activity. Hence the location of the generators of ERG- and EOG-potentials can be determined inferentially. In 1964 Nagaya reported a normal dark trough amplitude in a clinical electrooculographic recording in a case of long standing ischemic retinopathy. No light induced increase of the standing potential was recorded. Based on these observations it was assumed that the EOG dark trough is generated in the retinal pigment epithelium/receptor layer whereas the light induced potential is controlled by more proximal retinal structures. It is the purpose of this study to prove whether a component analysis of EOG oscillations can be applied for the localization of retinal defects.

METHODS

In 10 adult subjects with ischemic retinopathy the EOG was recorded under steady state conditions (Thaler & coworkers, 1974). The dark trough was preceded by a steady state in 20 asb; the light peak was initiated following a steady state in darkness (time of adaptation 35 min.). In 2 children with surgically transsected central retinal artery electrooculographic examination was performed following the same protocol. Gliomas of the optic nerve had been excised 8 and 10 months prior to the EOG-examination. Normal choroidal circulation in the operated eyes of the children warranted normal electrophysiological function of the pigment epithelium/receptor layer.

RESULTS

In all affected eyes dark trough- and light peak- as well as standing potential-

* Supported by 'Fonds zur Förderung der Wissenschaftlichen Forschung' Grant Nr.: 2455.

Table I. Single values, mean values(m) and standard deviation(s) of dark trough(DT)- and light peak amplitudes(LP) in normal eyes(N) and in eyes with central retinal artery occlusion(P).

AGE/SEX	DT		LP	
	N	P	N	P
46/M	67	99	238	138
54/F	72	96	202	130
62/M	71	94	174	106
65/F	89	98	231	168
67/M	76	99	202	140
68/F	82	97	170	105
71/F	82	97	174	114
75/F	73	87	218	135
75/M	82	97	204	138
75/F	88	94	180	99
M	78	96	199	127
S	7,5	3,6	24,5	21,2
05/F	85	98	182	151
08/F	86	98	186	162

Table II. Mean values(m) and standard deviation(s) of standing potential(st.pot.) in 20 asb and in darkness in normal eyes(N) and in eyes with central retinal artery occlusion(P).

	20 asb st.pot.		dark st.pot.	
	N	P	N	P
m	432	226	441	232
s	143.8	75.7	154.4	83.3

10 subjects

amplitudes were reduced. The EOG amplitudes of the unaffected fellow eyes were within normal limits (Tab. 1 and Tab. 2).

DISCUSSION

Disintegration of inner retinal layers due to ischemia causes reduced amplitudes of standing potential, dark trough and light peak. Consequently standing potential as well as dark trough and light peak are not controlled by the pigment epithelium/receptor layer exclusively. Intact inner retinal layers are also requisite for normal EOG oscillations.

Because of these facts it has to be concluded that a localization of the level of retinal defects cannot be based on a component analysis of clinical electrooculography solely.

REFERENCES

Nagaya, T. The standing potential of the eye in vascular and degenerative disease of the retina. *Bull. Yamaguchi Med. Sch.* 11, *187-201* (1964).

Popp, F. Über Embolie der Arteria centralis retinae. Inaugural-Dissertation Regensburg 1875. Ref. in: Elschnig. A. Über die Embolie der Arteria centralis retinae. *Knapp-Schweigger's Arch. L. Augenheilk.* 24, *1-82* (1891).

Thaler, A., Heilig, P. & Gordesch, J. Clinical electrooculography: interference of the dark oscillation with the light-induced potential. *Bibl. Ophthal.* 85, *110-114* (1976).

Authors' address:
2nd Eye Department
School of Medicine
University of Vienna
Alserstr. 4
A-1090 Vienna, Austria

THE CORRELATION OF ELECTROPHYSIOLOGICAL AND PSYCHOPHYSICAL MEASURES: THE ELECTRORETINOGRAM*

JOHN C. ARMINGTON

(Boston, Mass.)

INTRODUCTION

In broad historical context psychophysics is a branch of psychology that studies the effect of physical processes upon mental processes of an organism. Its early goal was to develop a scientific means of investigating relations between the mind and the body or, in other words, between the psychical and physical realms. But this is not the concern today. Now, psychophysics refers to a set of behavioral methods for investigating sensory function and to the data that are produced. Furthermore, the results are interpreted in physiological, not mentalistic, terms.

Psychophysics has been concerned with methodology from the outset. Its techniques, always sophisticated, have reached a high level of development in the century that has elapsed since Fechner's initial work (Fechner, 1966). A broad spectrum of psychophysical methods, all of which provide exact data regarding visual function, now exists, but the present report will be concerned with those aspects of psychophysics which seem to have the widest application to electroretinography: specifically, the relations between electroretinographic and psychophysical measures of visual function.

Although not a new field, psychophysics remains an active branch of science, with much current interest in scaling (Marks, 1974), signal detection theory (Green & Swets, 1966), etc., but the more traditional and classical methodologies are the ones that have found the most application to electroretinography. There are good reasons for this. Classical methods reduce the experimental situation to one of utmost simplicity both with respect to the stimulus presented to the subject and the response judgment required from him. Examples of classical psychophysical experiments are those in which the subject adjusts one patch of light so that it is indistinguishable from a standard patch of light with respect to luminance, color, or some other stimulus parameter, or experiments in which the subject reports when he can just detect a patch of light that is set at predetermined values by the experimenter, or experiments in which the stimulus is raised and lowered above and below the region where it can just be seen. The procedures for collecting and analyzing the data obtained with these methods are so well established that they have been given names such as the method of adjustment, the method of constant stimuli, the method of

* Supported by PHS Grant EY00589

limits, and others. Significantly, the concept of a visual threshold is an important feature of all of them. The stimulus is manipulated so that it lies at the subject's 'threshold' or else a 'threshold' match is made between stimuli.

In addition to their operational simplicity and their reliance on the threshold concept, classical psychophysical experiments have several other features that are worthy of note. One is that the data are expressed in terms of stimulus settings, so that the results may be graphed with physical units on both axes. As Boring has emphasized (Boring, 1963), there is a distinct advantage in expressing data on physical scales even when the data are primarily of psychological interest. In the present case, it is not just a matter of objectivity, however; it is also a matter of expressing the data in a form that permits comparison with the results of electrophysiological and photochemical investigations.

Yet another important characteristic of classical psychophysics, and one that is often overlooked, is the nature of the subject's observation. He responds to some aspect of the stimulus that is abstracted from the whole. For example, threshold stimuli of different wavelengths may differ in color, but in making his response, the subject only responds to their luminance; or as another example, two patches of light which appear to be equally bright may differ in their size, their shape, and their retinal location. The fact that threshold stimuli do not always look alike is one that belies psychophysics' apparent simplicity. A similar complication is inherent in work with the electroretinogram. When comparing it with psychophysical data, it is also necessary to abstract some feature of the response waveform such as amplitude, latency, or implicit time for measurement. Responses that have the same amplitude may not be alike in overall waveform.

In its quest for accurate measurement, psychophysics usually makes use of rather elaborate testing devices. Stimulus apparatus of equal quality should be used when recording the electroretinogram. Some studies use a stimulator so designed that it may be used for psychophysical as well as for electrical recording purposes.

The following is the gist of the points already made. An improved understanding of visual function may be obtained by comparing electroretinographic and psychophysical data obtained under comparable conditions, and this is facilitated when the data from both forms of investigation are expressed on similar scales and when the experimental situation is reduced to one of simplicity. Comparison is effected by expressing relations among stimulus parameters that produce constant effects on both response measures. Furthermore, careful measurement is the cardinal characteristic of good psychophysics. Thus, when many refer to psychophysics and the electroretinogram, they are not referring to actual comparisons of data but merely to the desirability of recording under carefully controlled stimulus conditions and of obtaining precise response measurements. The discussion that follows will first consider specific examples of electroretinographic-psychophysical comparison. Then some new electroretinal data that may have an effect on psychophysics will be reviewed.

Comparing Electrophysiological and Psychophysical Data: Many

124

stimulus dimensions may be taken into account when comparing electro-retinal and psychophysical data, but not all of these need be considered when reviewing the steps taken in making comparisons. The current discussion will be limited to spectral sensitivity. The pioneering spectral investigations with the human eye were conducted by Riggs, Berry & Wayner (1949), and several important studies with minor modifications of procedure have been conducted subsequently by others (Armington, 1974). Some of the steps taken to determine spectral sensitivity in these early studies are outlined (using hypothetical data) in Figure 1. First, an apparatus is assembled for presenting the eye with stimulus flashes of selected wavelengths and luminances, other conditions being held constant. A recording system that has adequate response characteristics and that ensures the safety of the subject is used. During the experiment responses are recorded to stimuli that span a range of luminances and that are distributed throughout the visual spectrum. The amplitudes of the responses (or some other feature of their waveform such as their latency or implicit time) is measured, and then (Section 2), a family of curves is plotted which relates the measures to the stimulus intensities that produced them at each test wavelength. A logarithmic intensity scale is generally used. From these curves, it is possible to determine those combinations of stimulus intensity and wavelength which produce criterional responses, ie., responses that have the same amplitude. The broken horizontal line indicates criterion in the present case. The verticals dropped from the intersection of this line with the curves for each test wavelength provide intensity values that, when corrected with stimulator calibrations, show the amount of light required to produce a fixed amplitude at each wavelength. Finally, the reciprocals of the corrected values, plotted against stimulus wavelength, describe spectral sensitivity as shown by the straight lines that connect the points in Section 3.

values, plotted against stimulus wavelength, describe spectral sensitivity as shown by the straight lines that connect the points in Section 3.

Both axes on the sensitivity plot are marked off in physical units. Thus, the result is in a form where it can be directly compared with psychophysical measures. The CIE photopic luminosity curve, actually a standardized psychophysical relation, is drawn through the points as a smooth line for this purpose. When making comparisons, however, it is desirable to go even further and to obtain additional psychophysical data with the same stimulus equipment used for the electroretinogram. Data from other laboratories, even though standardized, may have been obtained under conditions that differed in some important way from those of the ERG study.

Sensitivity as plotted here is based on an energy scale, the same sort of a scale that has been used for many psychophysical investigations. Strictly speaking, however, spectral sensitivity refers to a quantum intensity scale. It is particularly important to take this into account when relating the electroretinogram to photochemical data (Dartnall & Goodeve, 1937). In all events, caution must be taken to be certain that sensitivity is defined on similar scales when comparing different sets of data.

Although the methodology just described is quite sophisticated and has been useful in investigating theoretical problems as well as practical prob-

125

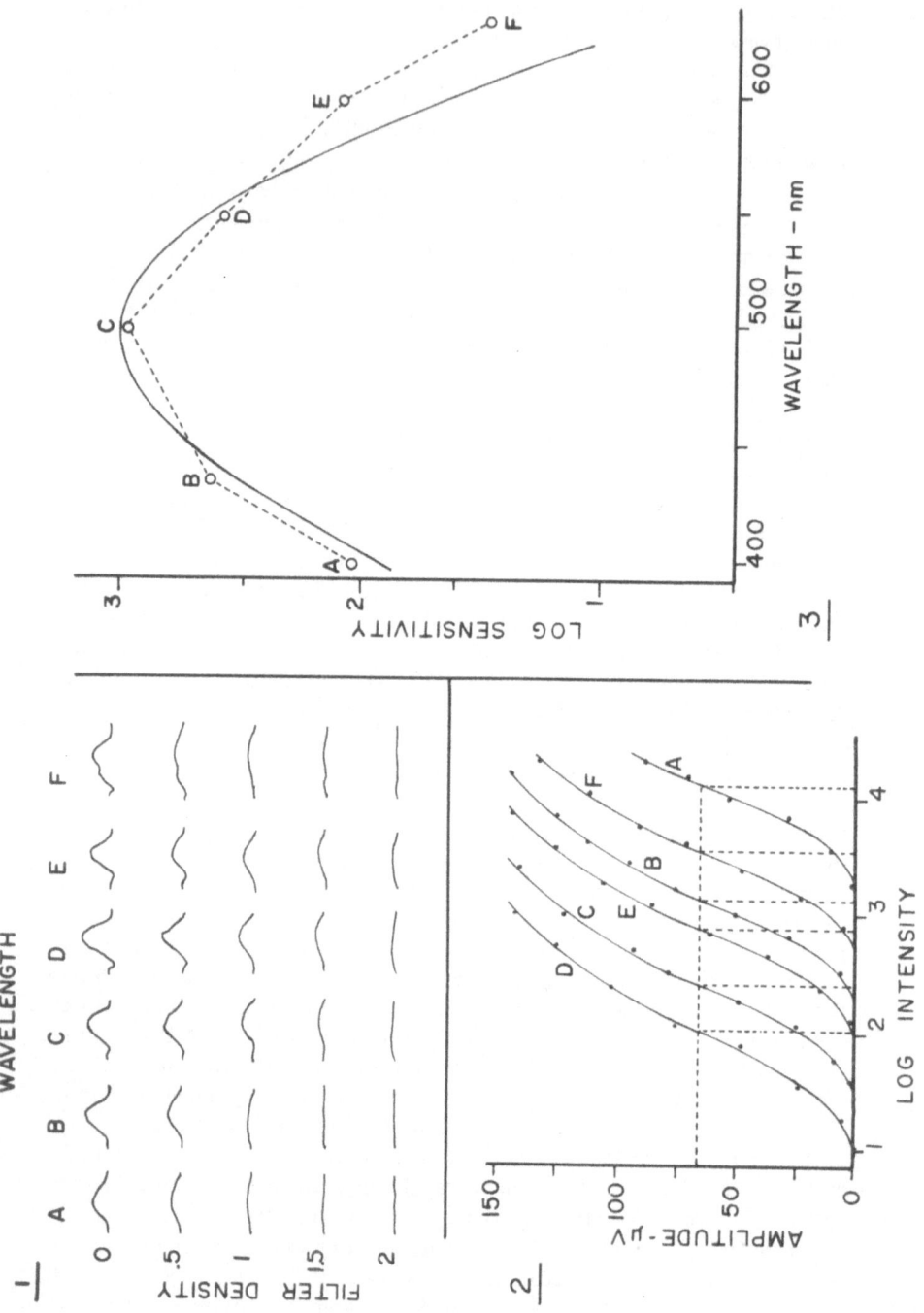

Fig. 1.   Steps taken to determine spectral sensitivity.

lems of color blindness (Armington, 1952), night blindness (Armington & Schwab, 1954), and others (Boynton & Riggs, 1951), it presents problems in its application. These are illustrated by the lack of exact correspondence between the psychophysical and electroretinal spectral data shown in Section 3 of Figure 1. One reason for a lack of agreement is that photopic and scotopic activities are confounded in the electroretinal measures. Further difficulty results from the fact that more intense stimuli are needed to elicit the electroretinogram than to obtain psychophysical responses when simple stimulus flashes are used. Thus, there is the problem of comparing sets of data that were obtained at differing levels of retinal illumination. Associated with all this is the problem of stray light. When a stimulus flash is imaged on a circumscribed area much of its energy is distributed to other parts of the retina by reflection and scatter. This stray light is the primary stimulus for the electroretinogram (Fry & Bartley, 1935), but not for the psychophysical response. The experimenter is presented with the difficulty of comparing the sensitivities of retinal areas with unequal properties. The problem becomes even more complicated because the distribution of stray light seems to depend on stimulus wavelength (Boynton, 1953; Dodt, Copenhaver & Gunkel, 1959). Hence, the lack of agreement between the two kinds of data in Section 3 of Figure 1 is not surprising.

Stray light remained as a major problem for electroretinography until recently. Nevertheless, some progress was made with the simple techniques just described, and in addition, they drew attention to the potential seriousness of stray light for visual experimentation in general.

Stimulation Alternation: With the inception of average response computers, a bit over a decade ago, it became possible to avoid the stray light problem. There are two reasons for this. With averaging, the luminance of the test stimuli and adaptation stimuli could be reduced to levels that approached those of psychophysics (Armington, Tepas, Kropfl & Hengst, 1961). More important, averaging revealed the responses produced by alternating stimuli (Johnson, Riggs & Schick, 1966; Spekreijse, 1966). These are stimuli in which the subject is presented with a repetitive interlaced pattern such as one of stripes or a checkerboard. Responses are produced by periodically interchanging the elements of the pattern.

Brief consideration will clarify the way in which alternating stimuli control stray light. Picture a pattern of alternate bright and dark stripes of equal area whose luminances are reversed periodically. A response is produced within the retinal image area because some receptors receive an increment and others a decrement in illumination with each alternation, but no response is produced by the stray light extending beyond the image area because it does not change. The total flux entering the eye is constant. Thus, the response is localized. Averaging is required when stray light is under control because the response from a limited stimulus area is small. But, although alternation requires rather complicated recording techniques, it provides effective control of stray light.

Not all problems are solved, however. Alternating stimuli differ in an essential way from the flashes, matching stimuli or increments that are used for most of psychophysics. The alternating stimulus that elicits the electro-

127

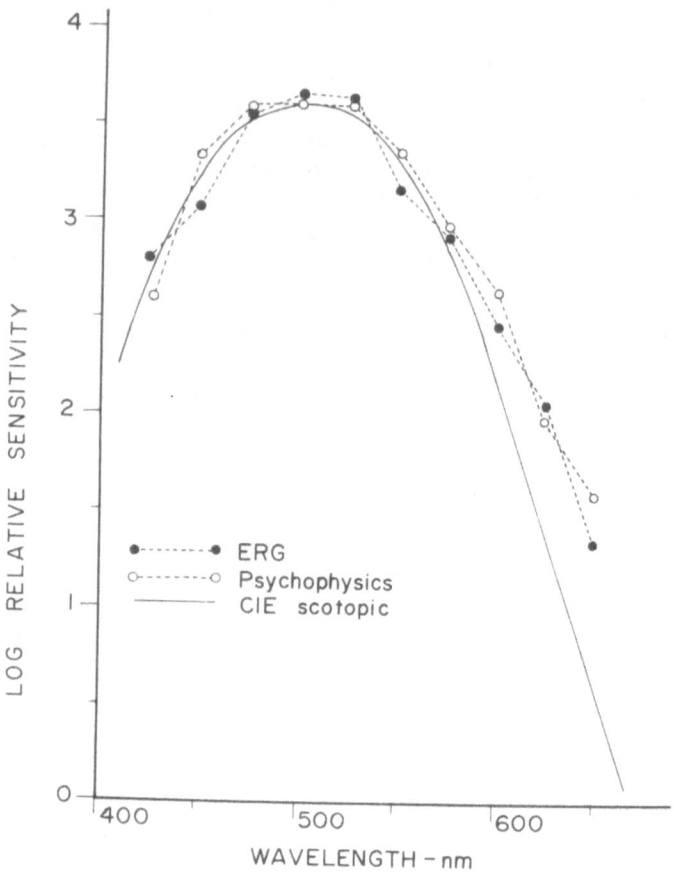

Fig. 2. A comparison of psychophysical and electroretinal spectral sensitivity.

retinogram also determines the state of the eye's adaptation. Thus, in investigations of spectral sensitivity, the eye necessarily is adapted successively to the several wavelengths of the spectrum at which determinations are being made. In introducing the method of alternation to the study of spectral sensitivity, Johnson, Riggs & Schick (1966) set up a special procedure to obtain psychophysical data suitable for comparison with that of the electroretinogram. Good agreement was found.

Most work with alternating stimuli has been conducted under photopic conditions, but it is possible to work at low levels. A study comparing electroretinal and psychophysical spectral sensitivity has been completed by the present author using alternating stimuli and scotopic levels (Armington, 1976). The results, summarized in Figure 2, show a close agreement between the two forms of measurement. Experimental points, the average of two subjects, are connected by straight lines in this figure. The smooth curve is the scotopic CIE function. Note that the CIE curve falls below both the psychophysical and the electroretinal data in the long wavelength part of the spectrum. The light adaptation produced by the alternating stimulus was sufficient to prevent pure scotopic function in that part of the spectrum. The figure thus exemplifies the desirability of obtaining psychophysical data and electroretinal data in the same setting.

Stimulus alternation methodology, although relatively new, clearly holds much promise for future research, and has already been applied in studies of stimulus fields (Armington, 1976), the Stiles-Crawford effect (Armington, 1967), retinal focus and acuity (Millodot & Riggs, 1970), pattern effects (Armington, Corwin & Marsetta, 1971), and other phenomena.

Responses Accompanying Eye Movement: A new recording technique that has grown out of stimulus alternation takes advantage of the natural displacements of the retinal image that accompany micro-saccadic eye movements (Armington & Bloom, 1974). Whenever a saccade occurs, the retinal image is abruptly displaced. If the subject is viewing a striped or checked pattern, stimulation takes place in much the same way as it does with alternation, and hence, an electroretinogram is produced. It may be observed by recording eye movements and potentials across the eye simultaneously. The sharp rise of the saccade triggers the computer that is used to average the electroretinogram. Examples of the electroretinograms obtained this way are shown in Figure 3. The waveform is essentially the same as found with other recording methods, and as the figure shows, is independent of the direction of eye movement. In fact, analysis shows that these responses behave the same way with respect to several common stimulus variables as do responses to stimulus alternation (Armington, 1976). A conclusion drawn from this work is that the peak amplitude of the photopic electroretinogram when recorded with the eye movement method is approximately proportional to the number of cone receptors that are stimulated — a phenomenon also true of electroretinograms obtained with alternation (Armington, 1968). Thus under certain conditions, at least, the electroretinogram can be interpreted in terms of a simple additive model.

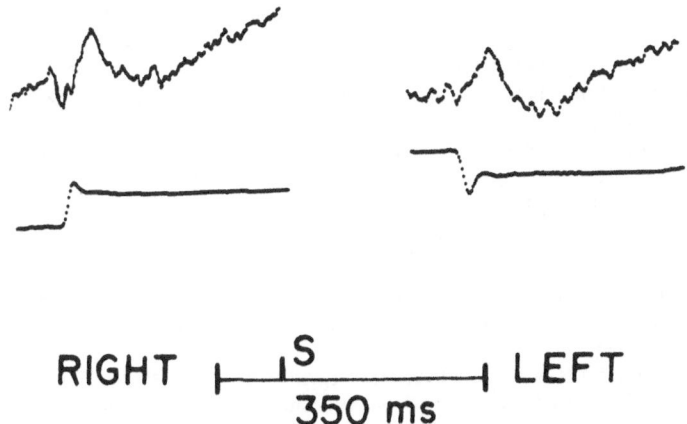

Fig. 3. Electroretinograms accompanying left and right microsaccadic eye movements.

Summary and Review: A series of experiments concerned with psychophysical problems has been briefly surveyed. Early experiments concerned with the comparison of electroretinographic and psychophysical measures met with limited success because high test luminances were needed and because stray light exerted a strong influence on the results, but the advent of computers has made it possible to circumvent these difficulties with two new stimulus methods, the method of stimulus alternation and the eye movement method. These methods ultimately may lead to new applications to psychophysics as well as in electroretinography. Electroretinography and psychophysics already are powerful compliments for investigating visual function. There is every sign they will be more so in the future.

REFERENCES

Armington, J.C. A component of the human electroretinogram associated with red color vision. *J. opt. Soc. Am.* 42, *393-401* (1952).

Armington, J.C. & Schwab, G.J. Electroretinogram in nyctalopia. *A.M.A. Arch. Ophthal.* 52, *725-733* (1954).

Armington, J.C., Tepas, D.I., Kropfl, W.J., & Hengst, W.H. Summation of retinal potentials. *J. opt. Soc. Am.* 51, *877-886* (1961).

Armington, J.C. Pupil entry and the human electroretinogram. *J. opt. Soc. Am.* 57, *838-839* (1967).

Armington, J.C. The electroretinogram, the visual evoked potential and the area-luminance relation. *Vision Res.* 8, *263-276* (1968).

Armington, J.C., Corwin, T.R. & Marsetta, R. Simultaneously recorded retinal and cortical responses to patterned stimuli. *J, opt. Soc. Am.* 61, *1514-1521* (1971).

Armington, J.C. The Electroretinogram, Chap. 8, New York: Academic, 1974.

Armington, J.C. & Bloom, M.B. Relations between the amplitudes of spontaneous saccades and visual responses. *J. opt. Soc. Am.* 64, *1263-1271* (1974).

Armington, J.C. Spectral sensitivity of low level electroretinograms. *Vision Res.* 16, *31-35* (1976).

Armington, J.C. Visual cortical potentials and electroretinograms triggered by saccadic eye movements. in The Visual Evoked Potential, Cerebral Evoked Potentials, J.E. Desmedt, editor. London, Oxford University Press, scheduled to appear 1976.

Boring, E.G. The Physical Dimensions of Consciousness. New York: Dover, 1963.

Boynton, R.M. & Riggs, L.A. The effect of stimulus area and intensity upon the human retinal response. *J. exper. Psychol.* 42, *217-226* (1951).

Boynton, R.M. Stray light and the human electroretinogram. *J. opt. Soc. Am.* 43, *442-449* (1953).

Dartnall, H.J.A. & Goodeve, C.F. Scotopic luminosity curve and the absorption spectrum of visual purple. *Nature, Lond.* 139, *409-411* (1937).

Dodt, E., Copenhaver, R.M. & Gunkel, R.D. Electroretinographic measurement of spectral sensitivity in albinos, Caucasians, and Negroes. *AMA Arch. Ophthal.* 62, *795-803* (1959).

Engen, T. Psychophysics: 1. Discrimination and detection, Chapter 2 in Kling, J.W. and Riggs, L.A. Experimental Psychology, 3rd ed. New York: Holt, Rinehart, and Winston, 1971.

Fechner, G. Elements of Psychophysics, vol 1, Adler, H.E., translator, Howes, D.H. and Boring, E.G., editors. New York: Holt, Rinehart and Winston, 1966.

Fry, G.A. & Bartley, S.H. The relation of stray light in the eye to the retinal action potential. *Am. J. Physiol.* 111, *335-340* (1935).

Green, D.M. & Swets, J.A. Signal Detection Theory and Psychophysics. New York: Wiley, 1966.

Johnson, E.P., Riggs, L.A. & Schick, A.M.L. Photopic retinal potentials evoked by phase alternation of a barred pattern. in Clinical Electroretinography. H.M. Burian and J.H. Jacobson (EDS.) Oxford, Perganon, 1966, 75-91

Marks, L.E. Sensory Processes: The New Psychophysics. New York: Academic, 1974.

Millodot, M. & Riggs, L.A. Refraction determined electrophysiologically. *A.M.A. Arch. Ophthal.* 84, *227-228* (1970).

Riggs, L.A., Berry, R.N. & Wayner, M. A comparison of electrical and psychophysical determinations of the spectral sensitivity of the human eye. *J. opt. Soc. Am.* 39, *427-436* (1949).

Spekreijse, H. Analysis of EEG Responses In Man, Evoked By Sine Wave Modulated Light. Academisch Proefschrift, Universiteit van Amsterdam, 1966.

Author's address:
Dept of Psychology
Northeastern University
360 Huntington Avenue
Boston, Mass. 02115
USA

DYNAMIC ELECTRORETINOGRAPHY AND ABSOLUTE PHOTOPTOMETRY IN SHORT WAVE-LENGTH ULTRAVIOLET LIGHT AFTER ORAL ADMINISTRATION OF SODIUM FLUORESCEINATE IN MAN

RINALDO ALFIERI, BERNADETTE NORMAND AND PIERRE SOLE

(Clermont-Ferrand)

ABSTRACT

The ingestion of sodium fluoresceinate increases the luminous efficacy of near ultra-violet light: the ultraviolet photons, which are almost without visual effect, are in fact converted by means of fluorescence into visible photons of a longer wave-length. This effect is proven by two methods; one objective method: fluorescence electroretino-graphy which shows the appearance of an electrical response after administration of sodium fluoresceinate; one subjective method: absolute photoptometry in ultraviolet light shows that the absolute threshold of luminance is lowered after ingestion of a fluorescent product which acts as a 'photonic adapter'.

INTRODUCTION

The transmittance of ultraviolet photons in the wave-length range of 320 nm to 400 nm by the ocular media is low but does exist: these 'near' ultraviolet photons may therefore reach the retina but they elicit very little sensorial excitement. Thus, for a photostimulation at 365 nm, one can say that the objective result is electrical tracings which are practically flat and the subjective result is a scotopic spectral luminous efficiency of around 10^{-4}. The purpose of our study was to increase the luminous efficacy of near ultraviolet light by bringing the ocular tissues into contact with a fluorescent substance: the ultraviolet rays are thus converted by means of electronic stimulation into rays of longer wave-length and consequently greater efficiency. We used two techniques to evaluate the action of the fluorescent substance: dynamic electroretinography and absolute photoptometry.

I – DYNAMIC ELECTRORETINOGRAPHY

A. Procedure

We used the technique of fluorescence electroretinography (Alfieri & Solé, 1971): this is dynamic electroretinography in ultraviolet photostimulation. *1° – Equipment.* Two systems of measurement were used: one based on a transient averager the ART 1000 (Société des Applications Industrielles de la Physique); the other is a homogeneous and polyvalent electroretinograph, the PANTOPS 200 (Société FERLUX). The photostimulation is effected by means of a xenon discharge tube and an ultraviolet interferential filter

(Schott): the maximum transmission is 40% at 365 nm with a band pass of 10 nm; the stimulation frequency is 4 Hz. The dazzling is obtained either by setting the photostimulator at 1500 Hz for the first system, or by means of a semi-cylindrical cupola lit by four incandescent bulbs for the Pantops 200; the light-level, maintained for 3 mn is of 3000 lux. The electrodes are of Ag-AgCl; the active electrode is held on the cornea by means of a contact lens (Keracolor) whereas the indifferent electrode is a small disc fixed on the temple with conduction paste. Total amplification can vary between 2000 and 40 000, the band pass between 0.8 and 160 Hz and the time constant is 0.2 s. Normally 100 measurements are necessary for summation; the analysis time is 250 ms with the ART 1000 and 200 ms with the Pantops 200. The averaged electrical tracing appears on a cathode ray oscilloscope screen and is photographed by means of a camera which develops the picture immediately (Polaroid).

$2°$ – *Method*. For each subject, two comparative measurements were made. The first measurement was made before administration of the fluorescent substance; the cornea was anaesthetised and the pupil dilated (mydriaticum); the subject is dazzled for 3 mn, then dark-adapted for 16 mn with electroretinographic recordings every 2 mn (monochromatic stimulation at 365 nm). We then administered 1 gram of sodium fluoresceinate; this total amount was divided into 4 doses of 250 mg taken at times t_o, $t_o + 15$ mn, $t_o + 30$ mn and $t_o + 45$ mn; the second electroretinographic measurement was taken at time $t_o + 2h30$ mn; this specific time was chosen following the results of test carried out on samples of human blood taken at varying times after ingestion of sodium fluoresceinate (Normand, 1975). We obviously used the same system of measurement for each comparative test.

B. Results

Figure 1 represents the results obtained for Dominique M...; the recordings made just after the subject was dazzled being practically indistinguishable from the isoelectric line, we are only showing those obtained after the 16th minute of dark-adaptation. For tracing (1) recorded before ingestion of sodium fluoresceinate we did not obtain a response; for tracing (2), recorded after ingestion of sodium fluoresceinate, a scotopic b_2 wave appears distinctly.

C. Discussion

We have proved here by an objective method that ultraviolet photons are converted into blue-green photons; these latter provoke a scotopic electric response by means of their wave-length and the resulting weak retinal light flux. This confirms the electrophysiological results we reported previously with fluorescein administered intraveinously (Alfieri & Solé, 1969). But does a subjective improvement of scotopic vision correspond to this objective electrical response? In order to answer this question we also measured absolute visual thresholds in ultraviolet light.

II – ABSOLUTE PHOTOPTOMETRY

A. Procedure

We used the technique of constant stimuli: this consists of submitting the subject to varying light-levels and taking as the absolute visual threshold the one which, on average, can be perceived every other time.

$1°$ – *Equipment.* We used the absolute photoptometer of Baumgardt (Ferlampin, 1968) which we adapted for measurement in ultraviolet light. The instrument (Fig. 2) is constituted as follows:

a) an optical part made up of the alignment of a xenon arc source (S), 3 achromatic lenses (L_1, L_2, L_3) giving an image (S') of the light source in the pupillary plane of the subject (condition of maxwellian vision), a diaphragm (D) which fixes the apparent diameter of the light-spot presented at $9°$ (geometric condition of GAUSSIAN approximation and sensorial condition of lack of spatial summation), a set of neutral density filters (FL_1, FL_2) allowing the adaptation of the energy flux for each subject (about one nanowatt, measured by a thermopile), an anticalorific filter (FL_3), a neutral wedge (C) allowing the patient to be presented automatically with 5 different light-levels, 2 interferential filters (FL_4, FL_5) giving a monochromatic ray of 365 nm (with a resulting band pass of 4 nm); lastly, a device (PF) gives a fixation beam with a red colouring so as not to disadapt the retinal rods.

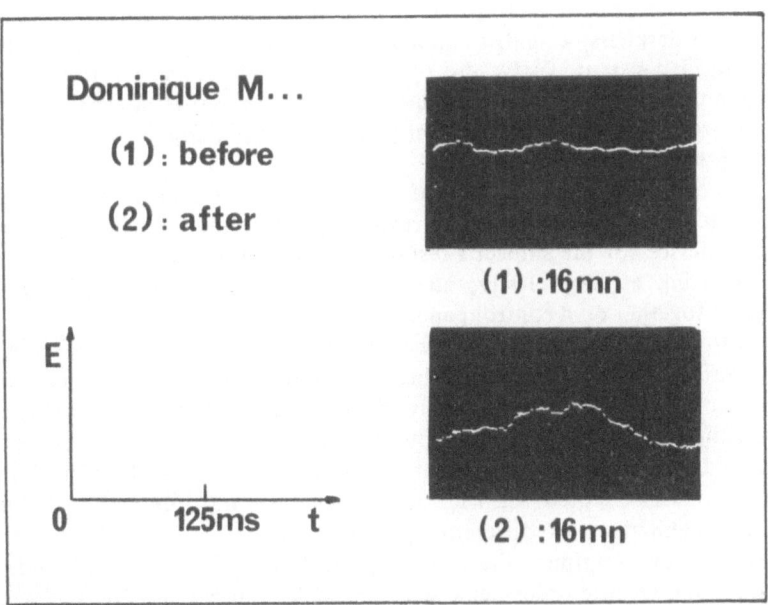

Fig. 1. Fluorescence electroretinography before (1) and after (2) oral administration of sodium fluoresceinate.
E: potential; t: time.

135

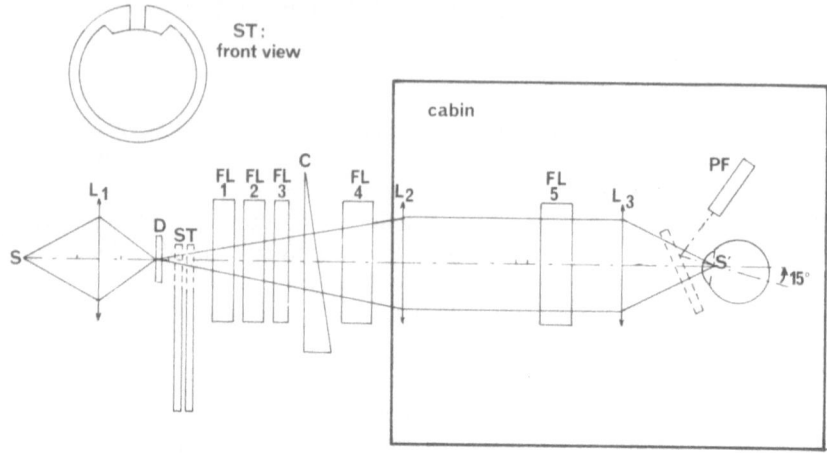

Fig. 2. Absolute photoptometer of BAUMGARDT: schematic representation of the optic path.

b) a mechanical part made up of an optical bench, two revolving sectors (ST) which fix the stimulation time at 104 ms (sensorial condition where temporal summation still exists), a metallic shutter placed between (L_1) and (D) which allows the operator to present the light-spots at a chosen time (one can also present a 'trap' i.e. a zero light-level), a cabin to keep the subject in darkness, a dentist's mould which keeps the position of the subject's head constant; lastly, the optical system producing the fixation ray being on a metallic plate, the operator can move from foveal vision to extra-foveal vision with an exentricity of 15° on the temporal side (maximal rod density on the retina).

c) an electrical part composed of stabilising power supply for the xenon arc lamp, electrical motors for the revolving sectors and the neutral wedge, a display device for the subject's responses ('seen' or 'not seen') with a device for resetting at zero; lastly, all the controls and checking systems are grouped together on a control panel.

2° – Method. Our experiment was carried out on 4 subjects: a series of 5 measurements for 2 of these subjects were recorded firstly after ingestion of sodium fluoresceinate and followed up 15 days later by another series of 5 measurements without sodium fluoresceinate; for the other 2 subjects the order was reversed. In order to determine the absolute visual threshold, the subject is dark-adapted for 1 hour; he then bites into the dentist's mould and is presented with 6 different light-levels (one being zero and therefore a trap), each one 40 times: these 240 presentations which take about an hour are randomised, the order being determined by a program (TAGUE's algorithm) written in PAL assembly language on a PDP-8E computer; for each position of the neutral wedge on the X-axis, the percentage of 'seen' responses is marked on the Y-axis: the sigmoid curve of frequency-of-seeing is then traced using the interpolation method of Lagrange-Sylvester (program written in BASIC higher-level language); by definition, the absolute visual threshold corresponds to 50% of the 'seen' responses: a radiometric calibration gives the results in joules per steradian (J/sr). As for the electroretinographic measurements, the total dose of 1 g of sodium fluoresceinate was spread over 4 doses of 250 mg taken at times t_o, $t_o + 15$ mn, $t_o + 30$ mn and $t_o + 45$ mn; the beginning of dark-adaptation took place at time $t_o + 1h15$ mn and the beginning of light-spot presentation at $t_0 + 2h15$ mn.

B. Results

Figure 3 shows the curves obtained for Dominique M...; the absolute thresholds obtained before ingestion of sodium fluoresceinate are between 0.81×10^{-10} and 1.44×10^{-10} J/sr; after ingestion of sodium fluoresceinate, the thresholds fall to between 0.66×10^{-10} and 0.81×10^{-10} J/sr. The average subjects was from 1.30×10^{-10} J/sr before fluoresceinate to 0.96×10^{-10} J/sr after ingestion of the fluorescent product.

C. Discussion

The variance analysis of this three-factor experiment (order, subject and treatment) shows that only the treatment factor is significant at the one per cent level: the value of the absolute threshold is lowered and is indeed due

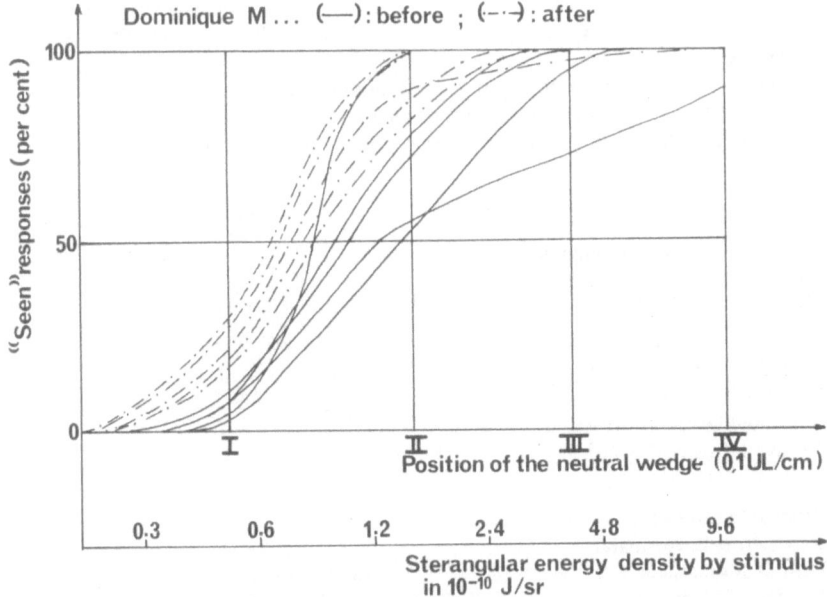

Fig. 3. Frequency — of — seeing curves before (——) and after (.–.–) oral administration of sodium fluoresceinate.

to the ingestion of sodium fluoresceinate. Thus this objective method fully confirms the electroretinographic results.

CONCLUSION

We gave the name 'photonic adapters' to those substances capable of increasing luminous efficacy by a fluorescence phenomenon (Alfieri & Solé, 1971). Here we have shown the reality of this effect both from an electrophysiological point of view (objective proof) by obtaining an electroretinogram in ultraviolet stimulation after ingestion of sodium fluoresceinate, and from a psychophysical point of view (subjective proof) by showing that the absolute threshold of luminance is lowered after ingestion of a fluorescent substance.

ACKNOWLEDGMENTS

We would like to express our thanks to Mrs Hill and Messrs Bonnemoy, Chiron, Danne, Flamant, Giraud, Heydel, Jouan, Rouaisnel for their suggestions and technical assistance.

REFERENCES

Alfieri, R. & Solé, P.: On very short wave-length electroretinography: an original technique of diagnosis in infraclinical synthetic antimalarial retinopathies. In: Occupational and medicative hazards in ophthalmology; Proc. 3rd Congress Europ. Soc. Ophthal., Amsterdam 1968. *Ophthalmologica additamentum ad vol.* 158: *661-668* (1969).

Alfieri, R. & Solé, P.: Electroretinographie de fluorescence. Principe et applications. In: C.R. symp. int. Angiographie fluorescéinique, Albi 1969. Karger, Basel: 670-674 (1971).

Ferlampin, F.: Etude d'un dispositif permettant des recherches psychophysiques sur la vision. Diplôme d'études supérieures de sciences, Paris (1968).

Normand, B.: Vision de fluorescence. Thèse de sciences, Clermont-Ferrand: 168-173 (1975).

Keywords:
Electroretinography (Dynamic ...)
Fluoresceinate (of sodium)
Fluorescence
Luminous efficacy
Photoptometry (Absolute ...)
Scotopic b_2 wave
Threshold (Absolute visual ...)
Ultraviolet (wave-length)

Authors' addresses:
R. Alfieri & B. Normand
Dept of Biomathematics
Faculty of Medicine
138 P.O. Box 38
63001 Clermont-Ferrand Cedex
France

P. Solé
Dept of Ophthalmology
Faculty of Medicine
P.O. Box 38
63001 Clermont-Ferrand Cedex
France

THE EFFECTS OF PHOTOCOAGULATION ON THE ELECTRORETINOGRAM AND DARK ADAPTATION IN DIABETIC RETINOPATHY

BARRY WEPMAN, S. SOKOL & J. PRICE

(Boston)

INTRODUCTION

The use of laser photocoagulation as a treatment for diabetic retinopathy provides the opportunity to examine changes in the human electroretinogram (ERG) and dark adaptation after a specified area of the retina has been destroyed. The purpose of our investigation was to measure the ERG following fixed increments of laser treatment in patients with diabetic retinopathy. In one group of patients the ERG was measured after 15-18% of the retina had been treated and in a second group the ERG was measured periodically as the photocoagulated area was increased from 3% to 18%. In addition, dark adaptation thresholds were measured before and after treatment.

METHODS

The patient population consisted of 25 patients with retinopathy staged between B to $N_1 F_0 H_0$ of the Airlie House classification. All patients classified under B (background retinopathy) had at least grade 1 classification of soft exudates, grade 1 retinal edema, grade 1 intra retinal microvascular abnormalities, and grade 2 hemorrhages and/or microaneurysms. All of these patients had approximately symmetrical retinopathy. Those with vitreous hemorrhages were excluded from the study. There were 21 males and 4 females. All were white, and with the exception of 3 patients in their early 20's, their ages ranged from 45 to 60 years.

An argon laser photocoagulator was used for treatment, which was accomplished in the standard fashion through a coated contact lens. The conditions of exposure were a shutter set at 0.1 and 0.2 seconds, a retinal beam diameter of 500 μ, and variable corneal power measurements to produce a uniform burn under observation. A counter was incorporated in the delivery system so that each exposure was registered.

All burns were placed in a grid pattern extending from the maculopapillary bundle to just beyond the equator (Aiello, Beetham, Balodimos, et al. 1969). One eye of 25 patients was treated and the untreated eye served as a control. The ERG's of 10 patients were recorded within one month before the initiation and after the completion of laser therapy. In this group the total number of laser burns varied between 500 and 1000. Baseline ERGs were determined for a second group of 15 patients and then ERGs were recorded one week following each of 4 weekly laser treatments consisting of 250 burns each (1000 total). Final ERG recordings were made 2-4 weeks after laser treatments were completed. This allowed the recording of the ERG at 4 levels of retinal destruction. Estimates of the area of retina destroyed at these levels were calculated based on the average retinal image diameter of the laser and the number of burns placed. The estimated percentage of retina treated was then calculated taking the average adult retinal area to be 1100 mm^2 (Taylor & Jennings, 1971).

The ERG was recorded from each eye with a Burian-Allen contact lens electrode. Stimuli were presented using a ganzfeld stimulator measuring 90 cm in diameter. The phototube of a photostimulator was mounted on top of the ganzfeld and filters were inserted to control the intensity and wavelength of the stimulation. Signals were processed through polygraph preamplifiers, driver amplifiers, and displayed on an oscilloscope. Low and high frequency cutoffs were 1 and 500 HZ respectively.

Pupils were dilated (average size 8 mm) with 1% tropicamide and 10% phenylephrine hydrochloride and corneas were anesthetized with 0.5% proparacaine hydrochloride. ERG's were recorded with a maximal intensity single flash white (W16 on photostimulator), first without, and then with a background of 8 foot-Lamberts. Following 2 minutes of light adaptation subjects were dark adapted for 10 minutes, and the ERG to dim blue (Wratten 47a) was recorded at 2 minute intervals. The ERG amplitudes for the W16 flash and the photopic condition were measured from the trough of the A-wave to the peak of the b-wave. The scotopic ERG (dim blue condition) was measured from the baseline to the peak of the b-wave. A-wave amplitude (W16 flash) was measured from the baseline to the trough of the a-wave. In addition, the implicit time (time from stimulus onset to peak amplitude of the b-wave) was measured for the W16 flash without background illumination.

A Goldmann-Weekers adaptometer was used to determine the dark adaptation curves. Thresholds were measured within one month before treatment and 2-4 weeks following treatment. The front opening of the adaptometer at the level of the chin rest was modified by fitting an opaque screen with 2 openings for the eyes. An occluder on a pivot could be swung back and forth so that complete dark adaptation curves could be simultaneously obtained from both eyes.

Two stimulus presentation conditions were utilized to measure dark adaptation thresholds. In one condition, 12 patients were tested with an 11° test spot viewed by the subject 15° from the fovea. In the second condition (the ganzfeld condition) 13 patients were tested with an opaque white placard placed in front of the 11° test spot. This provided even illumination of the entire hemisphere, simulating the ganzfeld used in recording the ERG. All subjects were preadapted for 5 minutes (2.25 log foot Lamberts) and thresholds were then measured at 1-minute intervals for 30 minutes. Fifteen subjects with no observed ocular abnormalities and who matched the experimental group with respect to age and sex were tested under identical stimulus conditions.

RESULTS

Dark Adaptation

Figures 1 and 2 show the mean dark adaptation curves for the normal controls and the diabetics under both testing conditions. Throughout dark adaptation, thresholds were elevated for the diabetics at the 1% level of significance (Mann-Whitney U test). Results with the 11° test spot (Figure 1) showed that the rod-cone break occurred at 5 minutes for the controls and at 10 minutes for the diabetics. With the ganzfeld condition (Figure 2), the diabetic group showed a well defined rod-cone break, while no break was observed for normals. This was not an artifact of averaging since individual curves from the control subjects also show the absence of a rod-cone break.

Following the completion of treatment, no changes in the mean dark adaptation curves for either stimulus condition were observed in the treated or untreated eyes. Individual curves from 4 patients showed small changes (½ log unit in either direction) following laser treatment but these changes were found in the untreated, control eye as well.

Electroretinogram

A reduction in the ERG a and b-wave amplitude was observed in all treated eyes following completion of laser treatments. Table 1 shows the mean percentage decrease in amplitude for the ERG following destruction of 15-18% of the retina (750-1000 burns). As the a-wave changes paralleled those of the b-wave, though smaller in magnitude, only the b-wave changes are presented. These data represent the change in ERG amplitude for both groups of patients regardless of the degree of retinopathy. The most pronounced change occured in the scotopic b-wave with a mean decrease of 61% while that of the photopic b-wave and maximal intensity white flash (W16) was 35 and 39% respectively. No changes in the general waveform or implicit times were found following treatment. ERGs from untreated eyes showed no significant change in amplitude.

Figure 3 shows the change in amplitude of the ERG for the bright flash (W16) condition as the total area of retinal destruction is increased. We have arbitrarily equated patients who received increasing areas of photocoagulation by deviding them into 3 groups according to their pre-treatment ERG amplitudes: (1) less than 200 μv (2) 200 to 300 μv; and, (3) greater than 300 μv. The resulting 3 curves show that eyes with large initial signals (greater than 300 μv) exhibit the greatest decrease in ERG amplitude as the amount of retinal destruction increases while those eyes with small pre-treatment amplitudes (less than 200 μv) show the least change in amplitude. In addition, eyes with initial signals greater than 200 μv, showed no difference between the treated and untreated eyes until at least 7-10% of the retina had been destroyed. Eyes with small initial signals (less than 200 μv) did not show an amplitude drop until 11-14% of the retina had been destroyed.

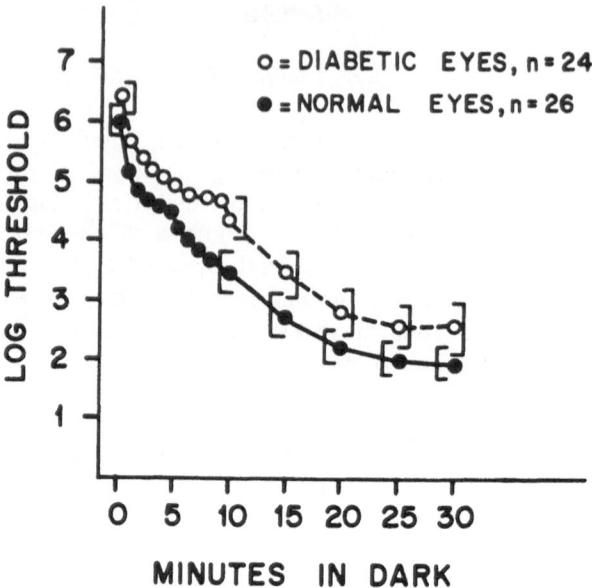

Fig. 1. Mean dark adaptation curves for diabetic and non-diabetic subjects determined with the 11° test spot viewed 15° from the fovea. Vertical bars represent ± one standard deviation. Thresholds were measured after 5 minutes light adaptation (2.25 log ft. Lamberts).

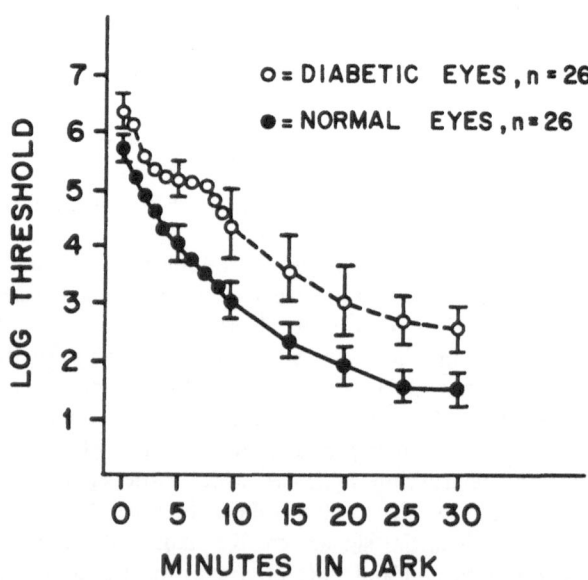

Fig. 2. Mean dark adaptation curves for diabetic and non-diabetic subjects determined with ganzfeld presentation. Vertical bars represent ± one standard deviation. Thresholds were measured after 5 minutes light adaptation (2.25 log ft. Lamberts).

DISCUSSION

Dark Adaptation

Our finding that diabetics have elevated dark adaptation thresholds with the 11% test field is in agreement with reports of other investigators (Chkoniya, 1965; Zetterstrom & Gjotterberg, 1973). In one study (Chkoniya, 1965), this impairment of dark adaptation was correlated with the severity of the retinopathy, duration of diabetes and quality of diabetic control. Although the cause of abnormal dark adaptation in diabetics is not fully understood, there is evidence of abnormal vitamin A metabolism in diabetes mellitus (Brazer & Curtis, 1939). The exact mechanisms involved remain to be elucidated.

Dark adaptation testing with the ganzfeld has not, to our knowledge been reported in patients with diabetic retinopathy. In addition to finding elevated thresholds in our diabetics tested with the ganzfeld, we found that the curves from the normal subjects do not show a rod-cone break while the curves from the diabetics do. Data from the 11° test field condition show that both normals and diabetics exhibit a rod-cone break, but the break is delayed by 5 minutes for the diabetics. The absence of a rod-cone break in normal subjects with the ganzfeld condition may be due to inadequate pre-adaptation luminance to completely desensitize all the rods (Hecht, Haig & Chase, 1937). A possible explanation for the presence of a rod-cone break in the diabetic curves using the ganzfeld may be that during the additional 5 minutes needed by the diabetic for rod adaptation the cone threshold is lower. As a result, the initial 5 minutes of dark adaptation may reflect a greater sensitivity of the cones. Results with the ganzfeld condition thus provide additional evidence of abnormal dark adaptation in patients with diabetic retinopathy.

No changes in dark adaptation were found following laser treatment and the same finding has been reported in another recent study (Zetterstrom & Gjotterberg, 1973). This is not surprising since the 11° test spot condition does not necessarily evaluate the region of retinal destruction and thresholds determined by ganzfeld stimulation are probably a reflection of the most sensitive areas of the retina (Alpern, 1972). Specific testing of those areas that have been lasered might be expected to show threshold changes.

Electroretinogram

Recently, Lawwill & O'Connor (1973), Frank (1975), Ogden, et al., (1976), and Carr (Pers. communication) have all reported ERG attenuation following xenon arc and argon laser panretinal photocoagulation (PRP) for diabetic retinopathy. We too find reductions in the ERG amplitude following treatment but differences between our results and those of other investigators deserve further comment.

Among diabetics, Ogden, et al.(1976), and Frank (1975) noted wide variability in the percentage reduction of the ERG following photocoagulation. Ogden found that no reliable correlation between the area of retina

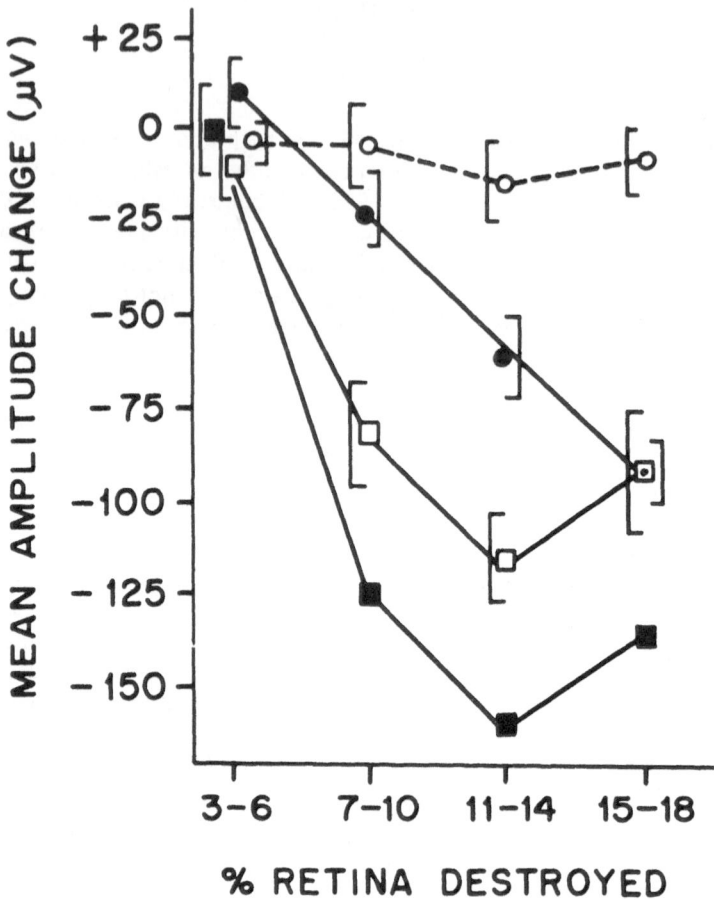

Fig. 3. Mean b-wave changes after photocoagulation using the W16 stimulus condition. Open circles-untreated eyes (N = 25), closed circles-pretreatment b-wave amplitude less than 200 μv (N = 9), open squares-pretreatment b-wave amplitude between 200 and 300 μv (N = 11), closed squares-pretreatment b-wave amplitude greater than 300 μv (N = 5). Vertical bars represent ± one standard error of the mean.

treated and ERG reduction could be demonstrated. As this variable effect was not found in a similar study on normal monkey eyes (Ogden, Riekhof & Benkwith, 1976), it was suggested that individual differences in retinopathy among diabetics might account for the variation. In the present study we find that the attenuation of the b-wave amplitude correlates with the area of retina destroyed. This relationship is only evident however after the size of the ERG prior to treatment is taken into account. Patients with large pre-treatment amplitudes show a greater amplitude reduction than patients with small pre-treatment signals even though they may have had equivalent amounts of retina destroyed. This may indicate that those patients with the smaller amplitude signals have pre-existing retinal damage secondary to microangiopathy. Laser treatment to functionally inactive retina would not

144

materially affect the ERG, resulting in a smaller net change in the ERG following treatment. Thus, it is not the total area treated that determines the degree of attenuation of the ERG, but the size of the ERG prior to treatment. This factor may account for the apparent wide variability in the ERG response to equal treatment reported by other investigators, and should be considered when standardizing treatment among patients.

The scotopic b-wave showed greater change than the photopic b-wave. This might be expected if one considers the retinal location of the treatment. Lesions were placed in the mid-periphery, where the rod density is much greater than the cone density. Ogden, et al. (1976), report similar findings with both monkeys and humans.

We find that the W16 b-wave is reduced an average of 39% when an estimated 15-18% of the retina has been treated. Ogden, et al. (1976), and Frank (1975) also note a disproportionately large percentage reduction in the ERG. This suggests a greater area of retinal damage than that predicted by calculation. Lawwill & O'Connor (1973), on the other hand, find only a 10% reduction in the ERG following treatment of about 20% of the retina. The explanation for this dicrepancy between these studies is presently unclear.

Histologic studies are necessary to eliminate the possibility that the unexpected large reductions in the ERG are the result of a larger area of retinal destruction than that estimated during treatment. Histologic examination by Ogden, et al. (1976) of normal rhesus monkey eyes following PRP, demonstrated that in fact less retina was destroyed than had been predicted on the basis of the amount of treatment administered. Ogden had suggested that intraretinal shunting of the ERG current may explain the disproportionately large reduction in ERG amplitude compared to the area of retina treated. The possibility of impaired function of histologically normal

Table I.

CHANGES IN ERG AMPLITUDE

FOLLOWING PHOTOCOAGULATION

B-WAVE	MEAN PERCENTAGE CHANGE	
	TREATED EYES	UNTREATED EYES
SCOTOPIC B-WAVE	−61%	−5%[+]
PHOTOPIC B-WAVE	−35%	−2%
BRIGHT FLASH ERG (W16)	−39%	·2%

* P<.01 Compared with change in photopic B-wave.
+ no significant differences between untreated eyes.

145

tissue surrounding a lesion might also explain this finding.

In summary, the attenuation of the ERG following laser treatment is correlated with the total area of retina destroyed, providing at least 7-10% of the retina has been treated. If the ERG is to be used as a clinical tool in the standardization and evaluation of the functional effects of argon laser photocoagulation, the pre-treatment ERG should be used to equate patients with diabetic retinopathy.

ACKNOWLEDGEMENTS

This research was supported in part by National Institutes of Health Career Development Award EY70275, National Eye Institute Research Grant EY00926 (Dr. Sokol), and NIH Training Grant EY0054 (Dr. Wepman), and Veteran's Administration Basic Institutional Support (Dr. Price).

REFERENCES

Aiello, L.M., Beetham, W.P. & Balodimos, M.C., *et al.*: Ruby laser photocoagulation in treatment of diabetic proliferating retinopathy: Preliminary report in Goldberg, M.F., Fine, S.L. (eds): Symposium on the Treatment of Diabetic Retinopathy, Bulletin 1890, Public Health Service, pp. *437-463* (1969)

Alpern, M.: Rod Vision, in Potts, A.M. (Ed) Assessment of visual function, CV Mosby, St.Louis, 1972, pp. 59-82.

Brazer, J.G. & Curtis, A.C.: Vitamin A deficiency in diabetes mellitus, a photometric study. *J. Clin. Invest.* 18, *495-496* (1939).

Carr, R., Personal Communication.

Chkoniya, E.A.: To the question of dark adaptation in diabetes mellitus. *Oftalm. Zhurnal* 20, *96-99* (1965).

Davis, M.D., Norton, E.W.D. & Myers, F.L.: The Airlie classification of diabetic retinopathy, in Goldberg, M.F., Fine, S.L. (eds)): Symposium on the Treatment of Diabetic Retinopathy, Bulletin 1890, Public Health Service (1969).

Frank, R.N.: Visual Fields and Electroretinography Following Extensive Photocoagulation. *Arch. Ophthalmol.* 93, *591-598* (1975).

Hecht, S., Haig, C. & Chase, A.M.: The influence of Light Adaptation on Subsequent Dark Adaptation of the Eye. *J. Gen. Physiology* 20, *831-850* (1937).

Lawwill, T. & O'Connor, P.R.: ERG and EOG in Diabetics Pre and Post Photocoagulation, in Pearlman, J. (Ed): X ISCERG Symposium, Vol. II, Junk, The Hague, 1973, pp. 17-23.

Ogden, T.E., Callahan, F. & Riekhof, F.T.: The Electroretinogram after Peripheral Retinal Ablation in Diabetic Retinopathy. *Am. J. Ophthalmol.* 81, *397-402* (1976).

Ogden, T.E., Riekhof, P.T. & Benkwith, S.M.: Correlation of Histologic and Electroretinographic Changes in Peripheral Retinal Ablation in the Rhesus Monkey. *Am. J. Ophthalmol.* 81, *272-279* (1976).

Taylor, E. & Jennings, A.: Calculation of the total retinal area. *Br. J. Ophthalmol.* 55, *262-265* (1971).

Zetterstrom, B. & Gjotterberg, M.: Photocoagulation in diabetic retinopathy with special reference to its effect on dark adaptation. *Acta Ophthalmol.* 51, *512-519* (1973).

Authors' addresses:
B. Wepman & S. Sokol
Dept of Ophthalmology
Tufts – New England Medical Center
Boston, Mass. 02111
USA

J. Price
Texas Tech University
School of Medicine
Dept. of Ophthalmology
Lubbock, Texas
USA

Requests for reprints to S. Sokol

HEREDITARY RETINAL DISEASES: CLASSIFICATION WITH THE FULL-FIELD ELECTRORETINOGRAM*

ELIOT L. BERSON

(Boston)

Hereditary retinal diseases can be separated with the electroretinogram (ERG) into those that involve the cone system, the rod system, or both. Representative responses will be presented to show that ERGs can be used as an aid not only in establishing diagnoses but also in determining long-term visual prognoses of affected patients.

Electroretinographic testing is performed with a full-field or Ganzfeld system (Gouras, 1970; Rabin & Berson, 1974; Gunkel, Bergsma & Gouras, 1976) (Fig. 1). The patient is stimulated with a relatively homogeneous full-field flash of light under stabilized conditions of dark adaptation or in the presence of a steady full-field background light. With this system, the problem of stray light falling on the retina is minimized, and ERG waveforms become remarkably reproducible, even in young children with variable fixation. With attention to stimulus wavelength, stimulus intensity, frequency of stimulus presentation, and the state of retinal adaptation, cone and rod contributions to the ERG can be monitored. (Gouras, 1970; Rabin & Berson, 1974; Berson, 1975). The interval between stimulus onset and the peak of the major cornea-positive component of the cone or rod ERG response has been considered exclusively for the measurement of implicit time in these studies.

I. HEREDITARY RETINAL DISEASES THAT INVOLVE EITHER CONE OR ROD FUNCTION ACROSS ALL OR NEARLY ALL THE RETINA

Examples of hereditary retinal diseases that affect either cone or rod function across the retina are dominant stationary night blindness and congenital rod monochromacy. The dominant stationary night blind patient (Nougaret type) (François, Verriest, De Rouck & Dejean, 1956) has normal cone function and no detectable rod function, and the congenital rod monochromat has normal rod function and no detectable cone function. Scotopically

* This work was supported by Research Grant EY00169 and Research Career Development Award EY70800 from the National Eye Institute and by grants from the National Retinitis Pigmentosa Foundation, Baltimore, Maryland, and the George Gund Foundation, Cleveland, Ohio.

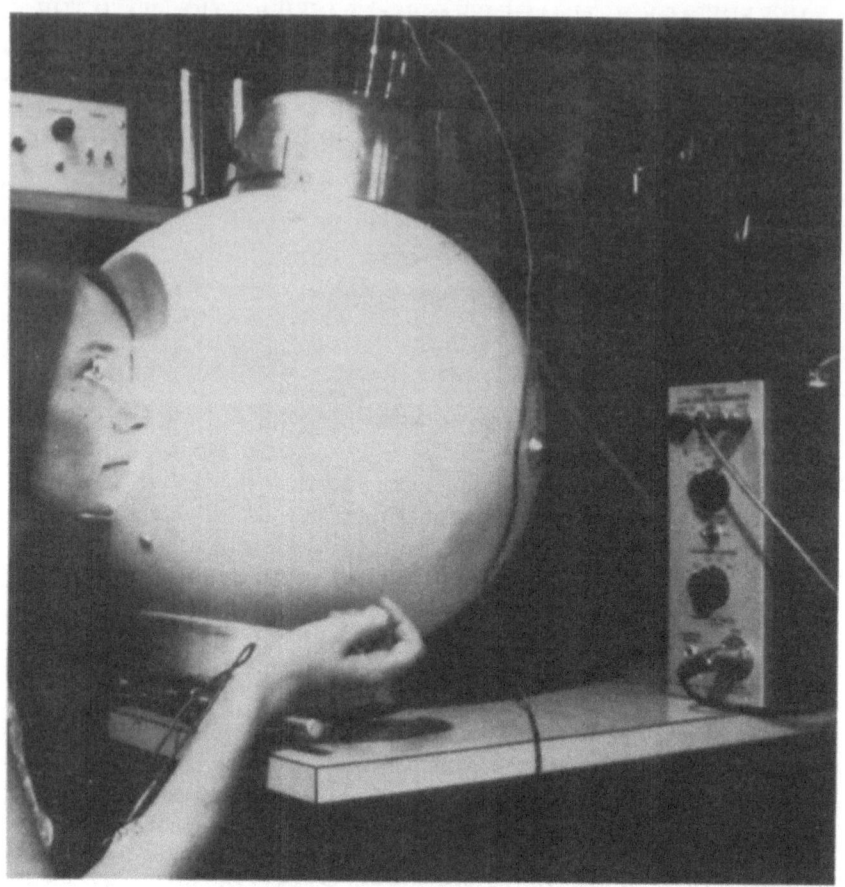

Fig. 1. Ganzfeld system. Stroboscope light (Grass PS 2) enclosed in case and attached to top of diffusing sphere illuminates inner white surface of this dome (40 cm in diameter) providing a full-field stimulus. Stimulus flash duration is about 10 μsec. Lights are recessed in top of dome so that patient can be tested in presence of steady full-field white background light. Wavelength of test flash can be modified by filters interposed between light source and dome. Responses are amplified (x 1000) by AC coupled (0.8 to 250 Hz bandpass) battery-powered amplifier (right in photograph) and displayed on oscilloscope. Under usual recording conditions ERGs as low as 10 μV in amplitude (peak to peak) can be resolved from background noise. For analysis of responses less than 10 μV in amplitude, a computer of average transients is required. (From Rabin, A.R. & Berson, E.L.: Arch. Ophthalmol. 92 : 59, 1974.)

balanced light stimuli (i.e., long wavelength and short wavelength lights matched in brightness under conditions of complete dark adaptation to elicit equal amplitude rod ERG b-waves near threshold from normal subjects), when presented well above threshold, elicit (Fig. 2) equal amplitude ERG responses from the rod monochromat (bottom, columns 1 and 2) but elicit unequal responses from the patient with dominant stationary night blindness (top, columns 1 and 2) and the normal subject with cone and rod function (middle, columns 1 and 2) (Berson, Gouras & Hoff, 1969). Figure 2 (right column) illustrates that the rod monochromat (bottom) has no detectable cone responses to white light stimuli presented at 30 cycles per second (cps) in contrast to the responses of the normal subject (middle) and the patient with dominant stationary night blindness (top). Long wavelength and short wavelength light stimuli can also be photopically balanced (i.e., matched in brightness to elicit equal amplitude 30 cps responses from a normal subject near threshold). Single flashes of these photopically balanced lights, presented in the presence of a full-field white background light sufficient to eliminate the rod contribution to the ERG (Fig. 2, columns 3 and 4, bottom row), elicit matched responses from the normal subject (middle row) and the patient with dominant stationary night blindness (top row). Cone and rod b-wave implicit times are normal respectively for the patient with dominant stationary night blindness and the rod monochromat.

Other examples of hereditary retinal diseases that affect the cone or rod system include recessive nyctalopia without myopia, sex-linked blue cone (π_1) monochromacy, and dominantly inherited progressive cone degeneration. Patients with recessive nyctalopia without myopia retain only a cone ERG with normal implicit time. Patients with advanced dominantly inherited progressive cone degeneration (Berson, Gouras & Gunkel, 1968) show ERG responses similar to those of the autosomal recessive congenital rod monochromat; their rod b-wave implicit times are normal. Since the blue cone system contributes normally only a few microvolts to the normal dark-adapted rod ERG of 300 μV, (Norren & Padmos, 1973; Mehaffey &

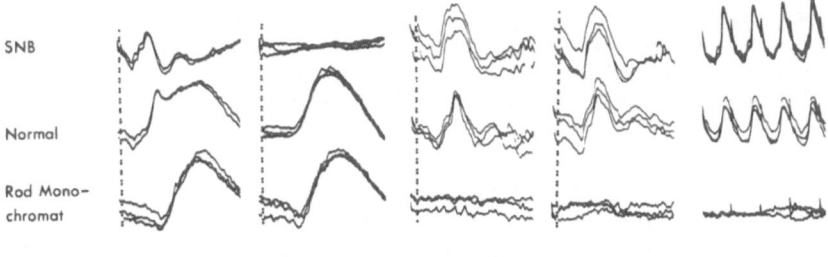

Fig. 2. ERGs to scotopically balanced red ($\lambda > 600$ nm, column 1) and blue ($\lambda < 470$ nm, column 2) light stimuli, to photopically balanced orange ($\lambda > 550$ nm, column 3) and blue-green ($\lambda < 550$ nm, column 4) stimuli in presence of 10 ft-L white background light, and to flickering (30 cps) white (8 ft-L) stimuli without a background (column 5) are shown successively from top to bottom for patient with stationary night blindness (Nougaret type), normal subject, and congenital rod monochromat. Two or three responses to same stimulus are superimposed; calibration symbol (lower right) signifies 60 msec horizontally and 50 μV vertically for columns 1 and 2, 30 msec horizontally and 50 μV vertically for columns 3 and 4, and 60 msec horizontally and 100 μV vertically for column 5; corneal positivity is an upward deflection; stimulus onset, vertical hatched line for columns 1 to 4, and shock artifacts for column 5. (From Berson, E.L., Gouras, P. & Hoff, M.: Arch. Ophthalmol. 81: 207, 1969.)

151

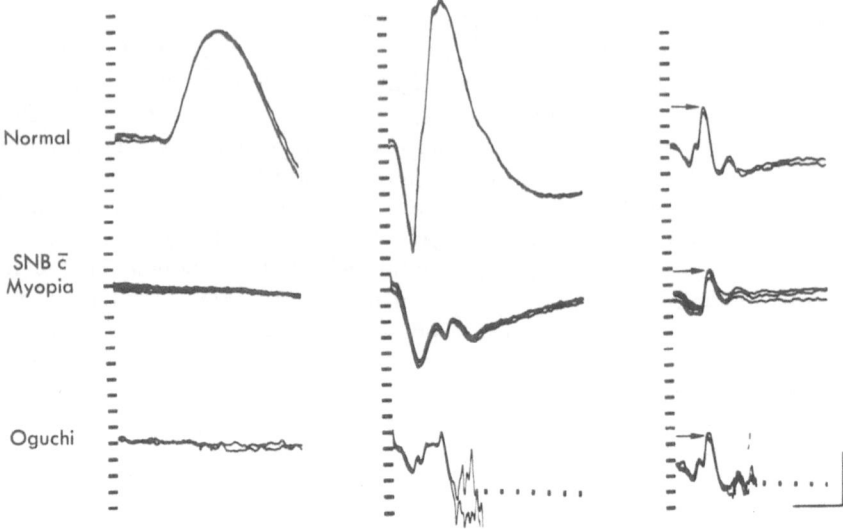

Fig. 3. ERGs from normal emmetropic subject (top row), patient with congenital stationary night blindness (SNB) with moderate myopia (middle row), and emmetropic patient with Oguchi's disease (bottom row). Responses were obtained to dim blue ($\lambda <$ 470 nm) light (left) and white (8 ft-L) flashes (middle) after 1 hour of dark adaptation. Responses to white (8 ft-L) flashes in presence of steady 10 ft-L white background sufficient to eliminate rod contribution are illustrated in right column. Horizontal arrows (right column) designate cone b-wave implicit times. Responses from the patient with Oguchi's disease are often interrupted by reflex blinking, so latter part of some responses cannot be illustrated. Calibration symbol (lower right corner) designates 50 msec horizontally and 100 μV vertically for all tracings. (From Berson, E.L.: Electrical phenomena in the retina. Adler's Physiology of the Eye, 6th edition. ed. R.A. Moses, C.V. Mosby, St. Louis, 1975, pp. 453-499).

Berson, 1974) dark-adapted recordings of the sex-linked blue cone (π_1) monochromat (Alpern, Lee & Spivey, 1965) are also virtually identical to those of the congenital rod monochromat shown in Figure 2.

Patients with congenital nyctalopia with myopia (Schubert & Bornschein, 1952; Auerbach, Godel & Rowe, 1969; Völker-Dieben, Van Lith, West & De Vries-De Mol, 1973; Hill, Arbel & Berson, 1974) (autosomal recessive or sex-linked) and autosomal recessive Oguchi's disease (Gouras, 1970; Berson, 1975; Carr & Gouras, 1965) have abnormalities within the rod system and are included in this first group. Patients with congenital nyctalopia with myopia show no rod ERG b-wave in response to dim blue light stimuli and have a characteristic deep cornea-negative a-wave to white light in the dark-adapted state and a small cornea-negative a-wave and a cornea-positive b-wave in the light adapted state (Fig. 3). The waveforms of congenital nyctalopia with myopia can be explained by preservation of the a-wave and b-wave from the cone system and the a-wave from the rod system with an absence of the b-wave from the rod-system; the ERG is a

152

summation of all three components in the dark-adapted state and only the cone a- and b-wave in the light adapted state. (Carr & Siegel, 1964), Rhodopsin kinetics measured by retinal densitometry are normal (Carr, Ripps, Siegel & Weale, 1966). The defect appears to involve intraretinal transmission of the response from the rod photoreceptors through more proximal retinal cells. These patients cannot attain normal rod thresholds even after prolonged dark adaptation. ERG amplitudes are reduced in recessive nyctalopia with myopia compared with those from normal emmetropes. These decreases in amplitudes may be associated with the known reduction of ERG amplitudes seen in patients with moderate axial myopia as the only finding. (Dhanda, 1966; Krill, 1972) Nevertheless, their cone ERG b-wave implicit times are within the normal range (Hill, Arbel & Berson, 1974) (Fig. 4).

Patients with Oguchi's disease require 2 to 12 hours to attain normal dark-adapted rod thresholds and show a characteristic change from a golden brown fundus in the light adapted state to a normal color fundus in the dark adapted state (Mizuo phenomenon). Following one hour of dark adaptation (Fig. 3), patients with Oguchi's disease have no rod b-wave in response to dim blue light and a cornea negative response to white light. They show a normal cone response to white light in the presence of a background light.

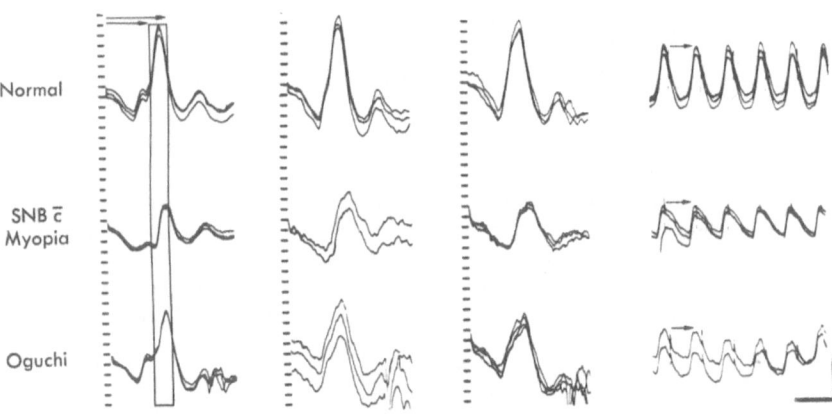

Fig. 4. Cone ERGs from normal, stationary night blindness (SNB) with myopia, and Oguchi's disease. Responses were obtained in the presence of 10 ft-L white background to single flashes of white light (first column) and long wavelength ($\lambda > 550$ nm, second column) and short wavelength ($\lambda < 550$ nm, third column) light stimuli. Responses (right column) were obtained to 30 cps flickering white light stimuli without background light. Vertical bar defining range of b-wave implicit times (mean ± 2 S.D.) in normal response to white light (left column) has been extended through tracings of patients with SNB with myopia and Oguchi's disease. Cone implicit times in column 4 are designated by arrows. Calibration symbol (lower right corner) signifies 25 msec horizontally for columns 1 to 3 and 50 msec for column 4, and 75 μV vertically for columns 1 and 4 and 30 μV vertically for columns 2 and 3. (From Berson, E.L.: Electrical phenomena in the retina. Adler's Physiology of the Eye, 6th edition, ed. R.A. Moses, C.V. Mosby, St. Louis, 1975, pp. 453-499.)

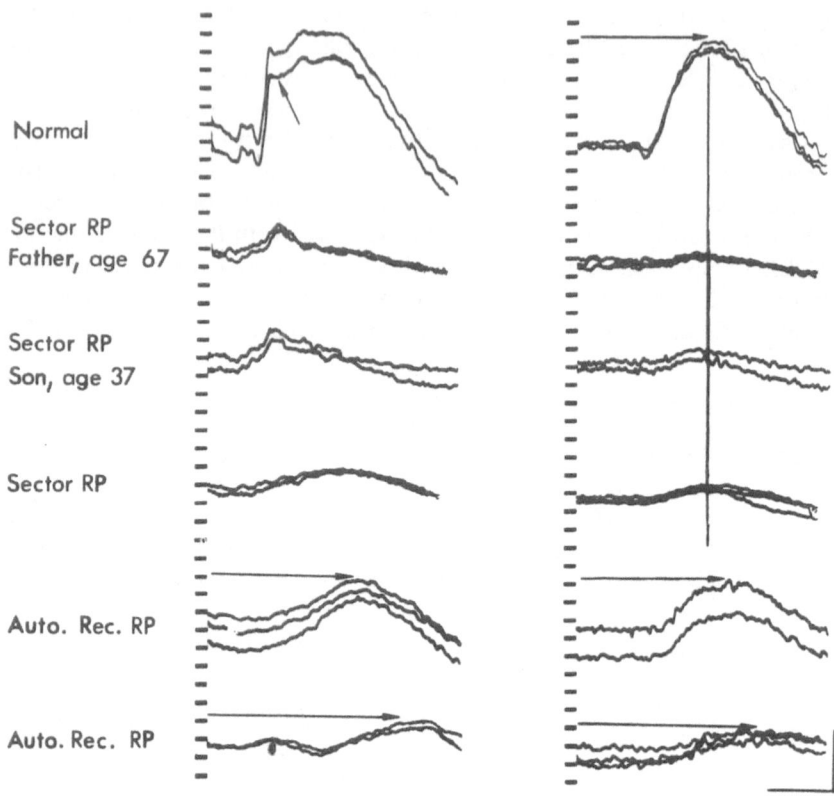

Fig. 5. ERGs to scotopically balanced light stimuli successively from top to bottom for normal subject, three patients with sector retinitis pigmentosa and two children with recessively inherited retinitis pigmentosa. Responses on left are obtained with red light stimuli ($\lambda > 600$ nm) and on right with scotopically matched blue light stimuli ($\lambda < 470$ nm). Calibration symbol (lower right corner) signifies 50 msec horizontally and 100 μV vertically. Vertical line and arrows (see text). (From Berson, E.L., and Howard, J.: Arch. Ophthalmol. 86 : 653, 1971.)

Following complete dark adaptation (after 12 hours), these patients have a normal rod b-wave amplitude and normal rod b-wave implicit time but only in response to one or two flashes of light (Gouras, 1970); the test flash used to elicit the ERG can be intense enough to light adapt the rod system. Rhodopsin kinetics measured by retinal densitometry are normal. The defect appears to be proximal to the rod photoreceptors in the neural mechanism of rod adaptation (Carr, Ripps, Siegel & Weale, 1966). These patients also have normal cone ERG implicit times (Berson, 1975) (Fig. 4).

From a practical view, the full-field ERG helps to establish that either the cone or rod system is essentially normal in patients included in this first group and that their long-term visual prognosis is good for maintaining large areas of functioning retina. Patients with complete cone deficiency suffer

154

from decrease in acuity, color blindness, and problems in adaptation; rod-deficient patients suffer from night blindness. With either the cone or rod system, these patients retain a full peripheral field with bright test lights. With either the cone or rod system and appropriate lenses, these patients can read 8-point (newspaper) print. With the aid of a night vision pocket-scope, night blind patients can use their cones to see under dim scotopic conditions (Berson, Mehaffey & Rabin, 1974). With protection afforded by dark sunglasses (with side shields) coated with metallic silver to reduce light transmission down to about 5%, rod monochromats or patients with cone degeneration can see under bright photopic conditions.

II. HEREDITARY RETINAL DISEASES THAT INVOLVE BOTH CONE AND ROD FUNCTION BUT ONLY IN LOCALIZED AREAS OF THE RETINA

A second category of hereditary retinal diseases are those that involve both the cone and rod system but only in localized regions of the retina. Previous studies have indicated that a close relationship exists between ERG amplitude and the area of functioning retina (Armington, Tepas, Kropfl & Hengst, 1961). Furthermore, focal and complete destruction of photoreceptors following photocoagulation (François & DeRouck, 1966) or secondary

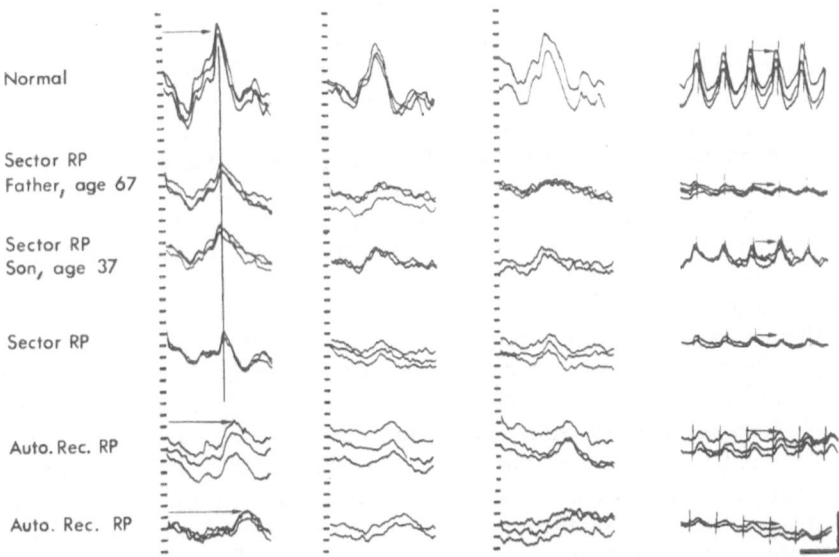

Fig. 6. Cone ERGs successively from top to bottom for normal subject, three patients with sector retinitis pigmentosa, and two children with widespread recessively inherited retinitis pigmentosa. Stimulus conditions same as those in figure legend 4. Calibration symbol (lower right corner) signifies horizontally 25 msec for columns 1 to 3 and 50 msec for column 4; calibration signifies vertically 40 μV for columns 1 to 3 and 100 μV for column 4. Vertical line and arrows (see text). (From Berson, E.L., and Howard, J.: Arch. Ophthalmol. 86 : 653, 1971.)

to old chorioretinitis (Berson, Gouras & Hoff, 1969) either in the periphery or in the macula of man has been associated with reduction in ERG b-wave amplitudes without delays in ERG b-wave implicit times. These findings are consistent with the observation that patients with localized hereditary retinal diseases such as dominant sector retinitis pigmentosa or hereditary macular degenerations have normal implicit times (Berson & Howard, 1971; Berson, 1974).

Studies of the ERG in dominant sector retinitis pigmentosa (which is minimally, if at all, progressive) have shown that this type of retinitis pigmentosa can be distinguished from the early stages of widespread types of recessive retinitis pigmentosa (which are clearly progressive). Patients with sector retinitis pigmentosa have bone spicule pigmentation and retinal arteriolar narrowing in one or more quadrants of the fundus and have abnormal final dark adapted rod thresholds in at least one area of the retina and normal thresholds in other areas.* In contrast, patients with widespread recessive retinitis pigmentosa characteristically have elevated final dark-adapted rod thresholds in all quadrants in the early stages and pigmentary changes in all quadrants in the more advanced stages.

Figure 5 illustrates dark-adapted ERGs for a normal subject, 3 patients with sector retinitis pigmentosa, and 2 children with autosomal recessive retinitis pigmentosa. The oblique arrow (top, left tracing) indicates the splitting of the earlier cone from the later rod component in a normal response to red light, and the horizontal arrow (top, right tracing) shows rod b-wave implicit time in a normal response to a scotopically matched blue light. Recordings from a father and son (ages 67 and 37, respectively), who have bone spicule pigmentation only in the nasal quadrants, are reduced in amplitude, but the rod implicit times are normal. The amplitudes of the father's responses (second row) are almost identical to those of his son (third row), supporting the idea that sector retinitis pigmentosa is minimally, if at all, progressive. Recordings from a 16-year-old girl with sector retinitis pigmentosa (fourth row) also show normal rod implicit times despite a marked reduction in ERG amplitude. A line has been extended vertically (right column) from the major cornea-positive component of the rod response of the normal through the ERG waveforms of these three patients with localized degenerations to emphasize that their rod implicit times are normal. Two children (ages 7 and 11) with autosomal recessive widespread retinitis pigmentosa (fifth and sixth rows) show delayed rod b-wave implicit times (horizontal arrows), even though the amplitudes of their rod responses are comparable to those of patients with sector retinitis pigmentosa. In some tracings, the early oscillation seen in response to red light, and not in response to blue light stimuli, are presumably from the cone system, and the reduced amplitudes of these early oscillations reflect varying amounts of loss of cone function (Berson & Howard, 1971).

Figure 6 shows cone ERG responses for a normal subject and the same group of patients. The three patients with sector retinitis pigmentosa have

---

* Dark adaptation testing was performed in the Goldmann-Weekers dark adaptometer with an 11° white test light.

reduced cone ERG amplitudes, but the implicit times are within the normal range. A line has been extended vertically in the left column from the major cornea-positive component of the normal cone response through the ERG waveforms of these patients to emphasize that their cone implicit times are normal. The two children with widespread recessively inherited retinitis pigmentosa have delayed cone implicit times (horizontal arrows) even though the amplitudes of their cone ERGs are comparable to those of patients with sector retinitis pigmentosa. The equality of the responses to long- and short-wavelength light stimuli in the second and third columns indicates that these ERGs must be due to cone function. The amplitudes are reduced, but the implicit times are normal in patients with sector retinitis pigmentosa; the amplitudes are comparably reduced, but the implicit times are markedly delayed in the two children with widespread recessive retinitis pigmentosa. Responses to flicker at 30 cps (fourth column) indicate similar results. The cone implicit times are within the normal range in all the patients with sector retinitis pigmentosa (Berson & Howard, 1971; Berson, 1974), but are so delayed in the children with widespread retinitis pigmentosa (Hill, Arbel & Berson, 1974; Berson, 1974; Berson & Kanters, 1970), that a shift occurs between the relationship of stimulus artifacts and response peaks, and an additional stimulus artifact can be seen before the flicker response to the previous light flash is completed (see arrows).

Patients with reduced central vision and hereditary degenerative changes localized in the macula** show findings similar to those from patients with focal macular scars secondary to old chorioretinitis; that is, the cone and rod b-wave implicit times are normal in the full-field ERG. If the abnormal central area includes the perimacula (i.e., 10-20°) as well as the macula (central 10°), full-field cone and rod ERGs can be slightly reduced (20-25% below normal) in amplitude, but implicit times remain normal (Berson, Gouras & Hoff, 1969; Berson, 1974). Final dark adapted rod thresholds in the Goldmann-Weekers adaptometer are normal when retinal areas outside the central scotoma are tested. These findings in patients with macular degenerations should be distinguished from those seen in patients with progressive cone-rod degeneration (Berson, Gouras & Gunkel, 1968); in progressive cone-rod degeneration, the patient has decreased central vision, elevated final dark adapted rod threshold across the retina, and very reduced cone and rod ERG amplitudes. Patients with macular degenerations and normal or nearly normal full-field ERG amplitudes with normal cone and rod implicit times appear to retain large areas of normal peripheral cone and rod retinal function for many years, while those with progressive cone-rod degeneration eventually lose macular and most peripheral retinal function (Berson, 1974; Berson, Gouras & Gunkel, 1968).

** The normal macula (central 10°) contains maximally only 7% of the entire retinal cone population and about as many rods as cones, while the normal peripheral retina has about fourteen rods for every cone (Wyszechi & Stiles, 1967; Osterberg, 1935). Patients with retinal scars confined to the macula apparently have a large percentage of the total number of photoreceptors and, therefore, show normal full-field ERGs.

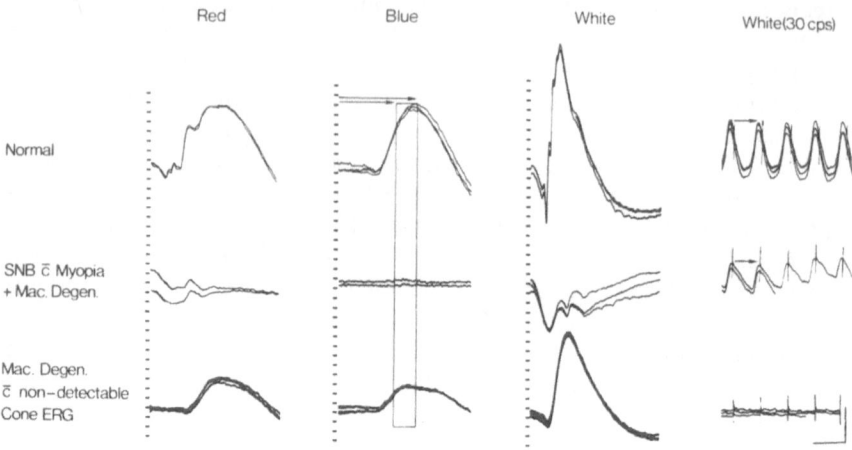

Fig. 7. ERG responses for a normal emmetropic subject (top row), a 67-year-old white male with congenital stationary night blindness with myopia and macular degeneration (second row), and a 62-year-old white male with macular degeneration and nondetectable cone function (third row). Responses were obtained to single flashes of scotopically matched red (column 1) and blue (column 2) light stimuli and white light (column 3) after 45 minutes dark adaptation. Responses (right column) were obtained to white flicker presented at 30 cps. Horizontal arrows (column 2) designate range of normal rod b-wave implicit times and a vertical bar defining this range (mean ± 2 S.D.) has been extended through the patients' responses. Horizontal arrows (right column) designate cone implicit times. Calibration symbol (lower right) signifies 50 msec horizontally and 100 μV vertically for all tracings.

III. HEREDITARY RETINAL DISEASES THAT INVOLVE EITHER CONE OR ROD FUNCTION ACROSS ALL OR NEARLY ALL THE RETINA WITH MACULAR DEGENERATION

Either loss of peripheral rod function with macular degeneration or loss of peripheral cone function with macular degeneration has been observed in a few patients. Figure 7 shows ERGs from an emmetropic normal subject (top row), a 67-year-old male with congenital stationary night blindness with myopia and macular degeneration (second row), and a 62-year-old male with nondetectable cone function and macular degeneration (bottom row). Both patients reported visual acuities of 10/400 and both also have some perimacular degeneration with 15-20° central scotomas. The patient with congenital stationary night blindness with myopia and macular and perimacular degeneration has a large cone ERG to 30 cps white stimuli with normal cone ERG implicit time (see arrow) in association with preserved peripheral cone function; peripheral dark-adapted rod thresholds are elevated when retinal areas outside his central scotoma are tested. The patient with macular and perimacular degeneration with absent cone function has reduced rod b-wave responses to scotopically matched red and blue light stimuli in association with loss of central rod function; however, the rod

158

b-wave implicit time is within the normal range (vertical bar, second column), and peripheral dark-adapted rod thresholds are normal when retinal areas outside his central scotomas are tested. The former can read 8-point print with high magnification with his peripheral cones, and the latter can read 8-point print with high magnification with his peripheral rods. Available evidence suggests that patients with macular degeneration and large areas of normal peripheral cone function with relatively large cone amplitudes (at least 50% of normal) and normal cone ERG implicit times retain their peripheral cone retinal function for many years; similarly, patients with macular degeneration and large areas of normal peripheral rod function with relatively large rod amplitudes (at least 50% of normal) and normal rod ERG implicit times retain their peripheral rod function for many years (Berson, unpubl. observations).

IV. HEREDITARY RETINAL DISEASES THAT INVOLVE BOTH CONE AND ROD FUNCTION OVER ALL OR NEARLY ALL THE RETINA

When focal areas of retina are destroyed, cone and rod ERG b-wave implicit times remain normal; in contrast, when the entire retina is abnormal, cone and rod ERG b-wave implicit times are delayed. Examples of generalized retinal disease come from laboratory studies of nutritionally induced retinal degenerations. Rats depleted of vitamin A and maintained in cyclic light show rod b-wave responses that are reduced in amplitude and delayed in implicit time (Noell, Delmelle & Albrecht, 1971; Berson & Rabin, Unpubl. observations). Cats fed a taurine-free casein diet show delayed cone b-wave responses (Rabin, Hayes & Berson, 1973) with the development of retinal taurine deficiency (Schmidt, Berson & Hayes, 1976; Berson, Hayes, Rabin & Schmidt, 1976). These delays in ERG b-waves reflect widespread impairment of photoreceptor function; if vitamin A or taurine deficiency continues, the ERGs become nondetectable and the photoreceptors degenerate. These laboratory studies have provided a basis for considering the ERG waveforms in hereditary retinal diseases that involve both the cone and rod system over all or nearly all the retina.

The original reports of ERGs in primary retinitis pigmentosa revealed that affected patients had nondetectable or small responses (Karpe, 1945; Bjork & Karpe, 1951; Henkes, Van der Tweel & Van der Gon, 1956), but these patients usually had advanced disease with extensive field loss, attenuation of the retinal arterioles, and widespread pigmentary changes in the retina. More recent studies have demonstrated that patients with the early stages of retinitis pigmentosa can have subnormal[***] ERGs (Goodman &

*** In the Ganzfeld system used in these studies, the normal amplitude (mean $\pm$ 2 S.D.) for 75 normal patients (age range 6 to 30 years) was $425 \pm 75 \mu V$ when these patients were fully dark-adapted and tested with single flashes of white light with brightness of 8 ft-L. The normal values were obtained from patients with no significant refractive error and no sedation prior to testing. The patients with subnormal ERGs discussed in this study had amplitudes less than $275 \mu V$ in response to the same white light flash.

Gunkel, 1958; Ruedemann & Noell, 1959; Gouras & Carr, 1964) that are still large enough to separate into cone and rod components. (Gouras & Carr, 1964; Berson, Gouras & Gunkel, 1968; Berson, Gouras, Gunkel & Myrianthopoulos, 1969) Many young patients with subnormal ERGs have minimal if any changes visible with the ophthalmoscope.

Representative subnormal ERGs (Fig. 8) from patients 9-14 years of age

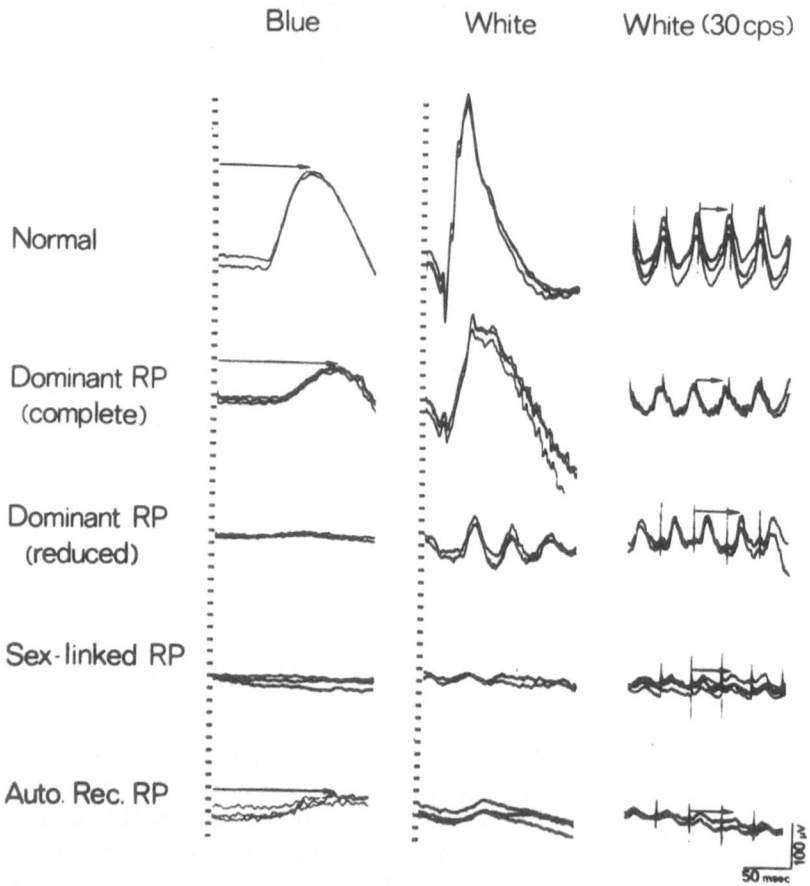

ERGs in EARLY RETINITIS PIGMENTOSA (RP)

Fig. 8. ERG responses for a normal subject and four patients with retinitis pigmentosa (ages 13, 14, 14 and 9). Responses were obtained after 45 minutes of dark adaptation to single flashes of blue light (left column) and white light (middle column). Responses (right column) were obtained to 30 cps white light. Calibration symbol (lower right corner) signifies 50 msec horizontally and 100 microvolts vertically. Rod b-wave implicit times in column 1 and cone implicit times in column 3 are designated with arrows. (From Berson, E.L.: Retinitis pigmentosa and allied retinal diseases: Electrophysiological findings. Trans. Acad. Ophthalmol. Otolaryngol., 81: 659, 1976).

with early retinitis pigmentosa show that two dominant forms can be separated from each other and from autosomal recessive and sex-linked forms. In dominant retinitis pigmentosa with complete penetrance, rod b-wave responses to blue light (left column) are reduced in amplitude and delayed in implicit time while the cone responses to 30 cps stimuli (right column) are normal or slightly reduced in amplitude with normal implicit times. In dominant retinitis pigmentosa with reduced penetrance, rod b-wave responses (left column) are usually nondetectable while the cone responses (right column) are normal or slightly reduced in amplitude and delayed in implicit time. In the autosomal recessive and sex-linked types, cone b-wave responses (right column) are reduced and delayed, and the rod b-waves, when detectable, are also delayed. Since the a-wave is generated by the photoreceptors, reduction of the a-wave amplitude in all cases (middle column) points to the involvement of the photoreceptors in the early stages of these diseases (Berson, 1976).

These recordings from patients of comparable age with early retinitis pigmentosa reveal that the more slowly progressive, dominantly inherited forms usually retain larger full-field cone ERG responses than the more rapidly progressive autosomal recessive and sex-linked forms. The rods are typically more severely affected than the cones, but it is important to note that both the cone and rod systems generate abnormal responses in the early stages.**** In most types, cone 30 cps responses (right column) are so delayed that a shift occurs between the stimulus artifacts and the response peaks. In one less common type of retinitis pigmentosa called progressive cone-rod degeneration (Berson, Gouras & Gunkel, 1968), cone function is lost first while rod function can be detected beyond age 30. Patients with progressive degenerations allied to retinitis pigmentosa, namely choroideremia and generalized choroidal sclerosis, also show reduced and delayed cone ERG responses (Berson, 1976). (Fig. 9).

Differences in cone implicit times can be seen not only in response to 30 cps stimuli but also in cone responses obtained with single flashes of white light in the presence of a steady white background light just sufficient to eliminate the rod contribution to the ERG. The cone implicit times of normal subjects or patients with focal or stationary retinal diseases fall into range A (Fig. 10) while the implicit times of progressive forms of retinitis pigmentosa (except the dominant with complete penetrance) fall into range B (Fig. 10) in a Ganzfeld test system (Berson, 1976).

Delays in the cone or rod b-wave implicit times or both, when measurable, have been demonstrated without exception in all patients with progres-

---

**** Some children with the early stages of dominant retinitis pigmentosa with complete penetrance have normal full-field cone ERGs with respect to amplitude and implicit time; however, cone function as measured by recovery rates of the early receptor potential (ERP) during dark adaptation has been found to be abnormal in these patients (see Fig. 14). Furthermore, psychophysical testing (2.5° stimulus) with Stiles' two-color increment threshold technique has shown that these children (under age 20) have normal cone thresholds in the central fovea but clearly elevated cone thresholds only 10° from the central fovea (Sandberg & Berson, Invest. Ophthal., 1977, in press).

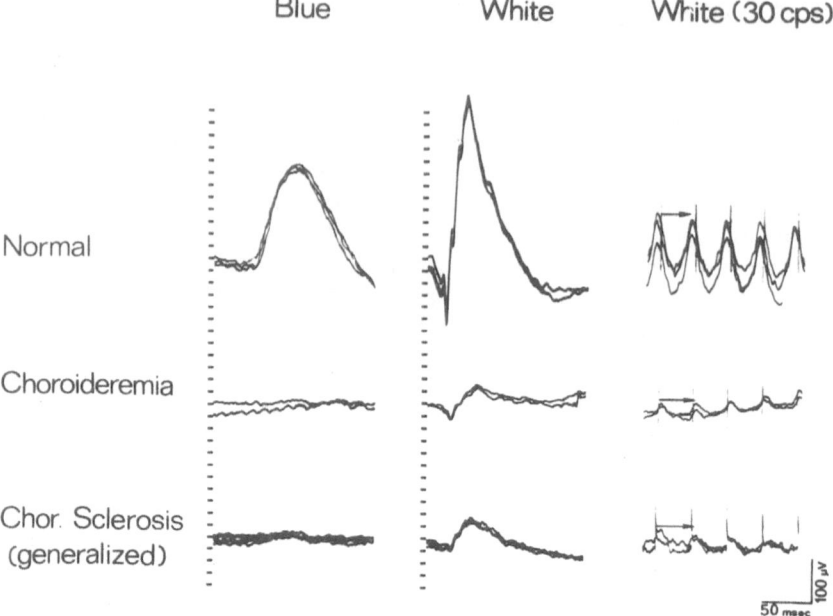

Fig. 9. ERGs for a normal subject (top row), a 25-year-old male with sex-linked choroideremia (second row), and a 17-year-old male with generalized choroidal sclerosis (third row). Stimulus conditions and calibration symbol same as figure legend 8. Cone implicit times in column 3 are designated by arrows. (From Berson, E.L.: Retinitis pigmentosa and allied retinal diseases: Electrophysiological findings. Trans. Am. Acad. Ophthalmol. Otolaryngol., 81: 659, 1976).

sive forms of retinitis pigmentosa (Berson, 1976) (Table 1). These delays in implicit times suggest widespread involvement of all or nearly all the photoreceptors across the retina in progressive forms even in the early stages (Berson, Gouras & Hoff, 1969; Berson, 1974; 1976). No patient with a subnormal and delayed cone ERG and elevated final dark adapted rod threshold in all quadrants has shown a spontaneous increase in ERG amplitude, and many followed over a 10-year period have developed further reduction in ERG amplitudes. Many of these patients have a parent, grandparent, uncle, or aunt with retinitis pigmentosa; in every instance, the older affected relative has had more extensive visual field loss and, when measured, further reduction in ERG amplitude compared with the younger affected relative (Berson, 1974). These findings contrast with the normal cone and rod implicit times (Table 2) and large areas of preserved visual field that are characteristically seen in patients with focal or stationary retinal diseases (Berson, 1976).

The percentages of normal and abnormal ERGs among siblings, 6-20 years of age, in families with autosomal recessive or autosomal dominant retinitis pigmentosa agree closely with percentages of normal and affected patients predicted from Mendelian laws describing these patterns of inheritance (Berson, 1974) (Table 3). These findings support the idea that, in these families, patients with subnormal and delayed ERGs have the early stages of retinitis pigmentosa even when changes visible with the ophthalmoscope are minimal or absent and will develop the advanced stages; in contrast, patients with normal ERGs do not have these diseases and do not

Table. I.

ERGs* IN WIDESPREAD, PROGRESSIVE RETINITIS PIGMENTOSA (RP)

| TYPE OF DEGENERATION | CASES† | CONE ERG (b-wave) | | ROD ERG (b-wave)†† | |
		Amplitude	Implicit Time	Amplitude	Implicit Time
Dominant RP with complete penetrance	11	Normal or reduced	Normal	Reduced	Delayed
Dominant RP with reduced penetrance	8	Normal or reduced	Delayed	Reduced	Delayed
Autosomal recessive RP	75	Reduced	Delayed	Reduced	Delayed or normal
Sex-linked recessive RP	7	Reduced	Delayed	Reduced	Delayed

*Ganzfeld, clear media, dilated pupil, large enough responses to separate into cone and rod components.
†Patients under age 25.
††Nondetectable in most patients by age 25.

Table. II

ERGs* IN SECTOR OR STATIONARY RETINAL DISEASE

| TYPE OF DISEASE | CASES | CONE ERG (b-wave) | | ROD ERG (b-wave) | |
		Amplitude	Implicit Time	Amplitude	Implicit Time
Sector retinitis pigmentosa	11	Reduced	Normal	Reduced	Normal
Stationary night blindness	20	Normal or reduced	Normal	Absent or normal for one flash	Normal if present
Macular degenerations	40	Reduced	Normal	Reduced	Normal
Chorioretinal scars	50	Reduced	Normal	Reduced	Normal

*Ganzfeld, clear media, dilated pupil.

Table. III.

RETINITIS PIGMENTOSA (RP), THE ELECTRORETINOGRAM AND MENDEL'S LAWS

	Dominant RP		Recessive RP	
Number of families	6		18	
Number of siblings	11		49	
	Normal	Affected	Normal	Affected
Predicted	50%	50%	75%	25%
Observed	54.5%	45.5%	74.4%	25.6%

appear to have the genetic defects that lead to these diseases. Subnormal and delayed ERGs have been recorded in children between ages 1 and 6 representing all genetic types. High risk relatives under age 20 with normal cone and rod ERG amplitudes and implicit times have not been seen to develop primary retinitis pigmentosa at a later time.

WHITE (SINGLE FLASHES)
c̄ BACKGROUND

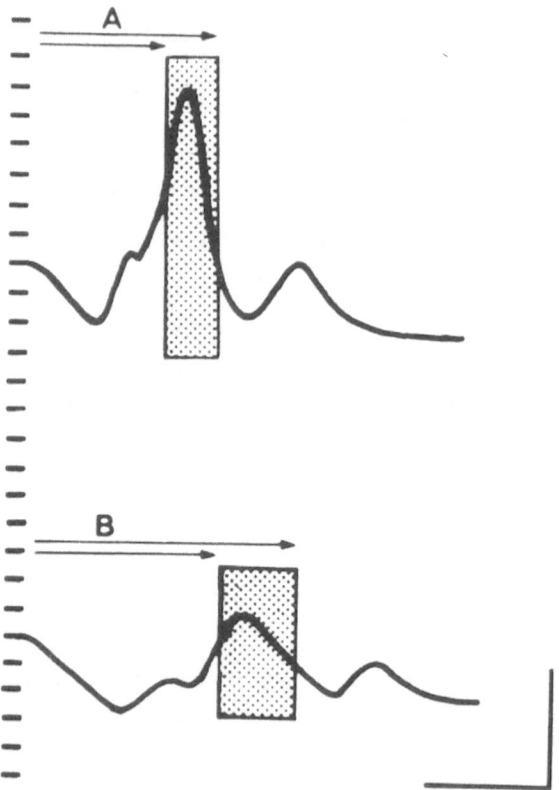

Fig. 10. Diagrammatic tracings to illustrate the temporal aspects of the cone ERG in reponse to single flashes of white light presented in the presence of a 10 ft-L, full-field background light sufficient to eliminate the rod contribution to the ERG. Horizontal arrows (A) designate the range (mean ± 2 S.D.) of the cone b-wave implicit times observed in normal subjects and patients with sector or stationary retinal diseases and horizontal arrows (B) the range for patients with most types of progressive retinitis pigmentosa. Calibration symbol (lower right) signifies horizontally 25 msec for all tracings and vertically 50 microvolts or less depending on the type of retinal disease (see text). (From Berson, E.L.: Retinitis pigmentosa and allied retinal diseases: Electrophysiological findings. Trans. Am. Acad. Ophthalmol. Otolaryngol., 81: 659, 1976).

164

The early involvement of the cone system in retinitis pigmentosa is seen not only in full-field ERG responses but also in early receptor potential (ERP) responses to high intensity flashes of light. The ERP is a rapid biphasic response that precedes the leading edge of the a-wave of the ERG (Fig. 11); the ERP is generated primarily by the cones in man (Goldstein & Berson, 1969; Carr & Siegel, 1970). In all patients with early widespread retinitis pigmentosa who have been tested (Fig. 12), ERP amplitudes have been reduced well below normal (Berson, 1976). Possible explanations for a decrease in ERP amplitude include decreased concentration of visual pigment in the photoreceptors, disorientation of the photoreceptor outer segment membranes, abnormal orientation of the visual pigment molecules within the membranes, changes in the chemical environment of the photoreceptors, a decrease in the number of photoreceptors, or any combination. Reduced ERP amplitudes without delays in response peaks have been observed in patients with delayed cone and rod ERG b-wave implicit times (Berson & Goldstein, 1970) (Fig. 13).

In addition to the reduction in ERP amplitudes, patients with early retinitis pigmentosa have shown faster-than-normal ERP recovery rates during dark adaptation after a bleaching flash (Fig. 14). Measurements of ERP amplitudes obtained during recovery yielded data that closely approximated curves describing first order exponential functions, and the half times of regeneration were about twice as fast as the half times of regeneration recorded from normal subjects tested under the same bleaching conditions. The half times of regeneration have appeared to be characteristic for a given family. Comparison was made between the rates of ERP recovery of normals ($t_{1/2}$ = 1.6 min), patients with early retinitis pigmentosa ($t_{1/2}$ = 0.6 to

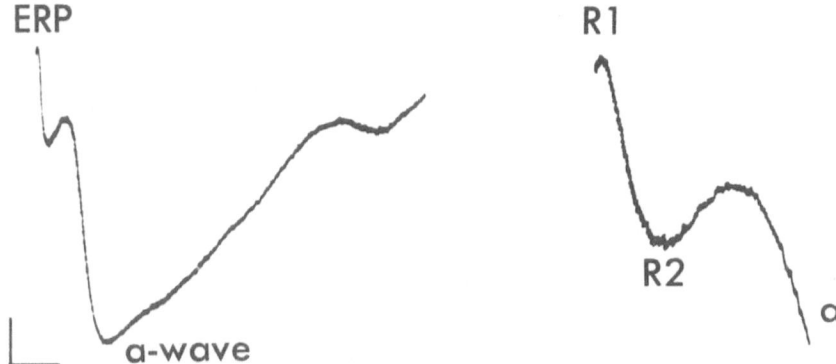

Fig. 11. Normal human early receptor potential (ERP) followed by the a-wave of the electroretinogram (ERG) in the left tracing and the normal ERP with higher sweep speed and amplification in the right tracing. The cornea positive peak (R1) and later cornea negative peak (R2) of the ERP are designated. Stimulus onset is at the beginning of each trace. Calibration (lower left) signifies 2 msec horizontally and 100 microvolts vertically for the left tracing and 0.5 msec horizontally and 50 microvolts vertically for the right tracing. (From Berson, E.L. & Goldstein, E.B.: Early receptor potential in dominantly inherited retinitis pigmentosa. Arch. Ophthalmol. 83 : 412, 1970.)

165

1.0 min), and patients with minimal or absent cone function and normal rod function ($t_{1/2}$ = 3 to 5.6 min). Although loss of rod function may contribute to the acceleration of ERP recovery rates in patients with retinitis pigmentosa, it is difficult to explain the faster-than-normal recovery rates of patients with retinitis pigmentosa on the basis of loss of rod function alone (Berson & Goldstein, 1970). Since the human ERP has been shown to be generated primarily by the cones and since ERP recovery rates have been correlated with regeneration rates of visual pigments, the faster-than-normal ERP recovery rates in patients with early retinitis pigmentosa suggested as

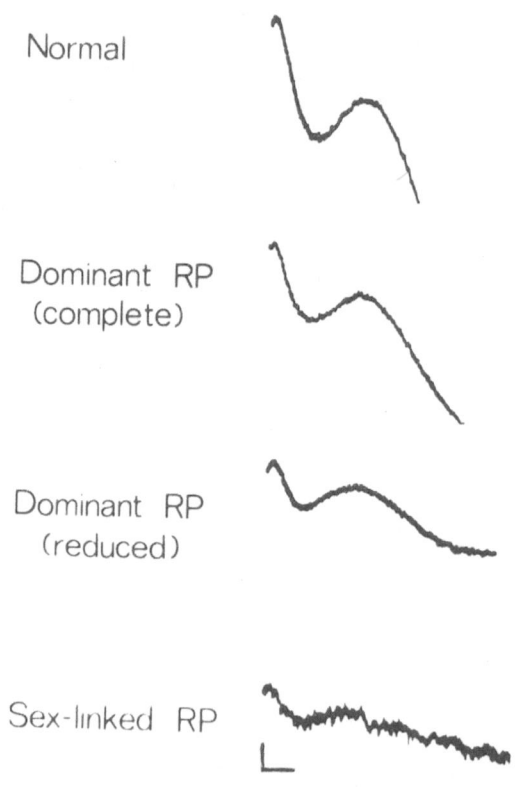

ERPs in EARLY RETINITIS PIGMENTOSA (RP)

Normal

Dominant RP (complete)

Dominant RP (reduced)

Sex-linked RP

Fig. 12. ERPs recorded from a normal subject and three patients (ages 18, 6, and 14) with retinitis pigmentosa. Calibration symbol (lower left corner) signifies 0.5 msec horizontally and 50 microvolts vertically for the upper three tracings and 20 microvolts vertically for the bottom tracing. (From Berson, E.L.: Retinitis pigmentosa and allied retinal diseases: Electrophysiological findings. Trans. Am. Acad. Ophthalmol. Otolaryngol., 81: 659, 1976).

one possibility that some abnormality in the cone pigment regeneration process had occurred in these diseased retinas. These faster-than-normal recovery rates were measured in both the dominant and sex-linked types of retinitis pigmentosa (Berson & Goldstein, 1970). Retinal densitometry measurements in some patients with retinal dystrophy have also demonstrated that pigment regeneration is faster than normal (Alpern, Holland & Ohba, 1972).

The close relationship of the photoreceptors to adjacent cells makes it impossible at present to decide from ERG or ERP responses whether the primary defects in the different types of hereditary retinitis pigmentosa are in the photoreceptors, pigment epithelial cells, or Müller cells or any combination. No histopathologic specimens of the early stages of retinitis pigmentosa have been reported. In a postmortem specimen from a 68-year-old woman with advanced dominant retinitis pigmentosa with complete penetrance, disorientation and disruption of outer segment membranes was ob-

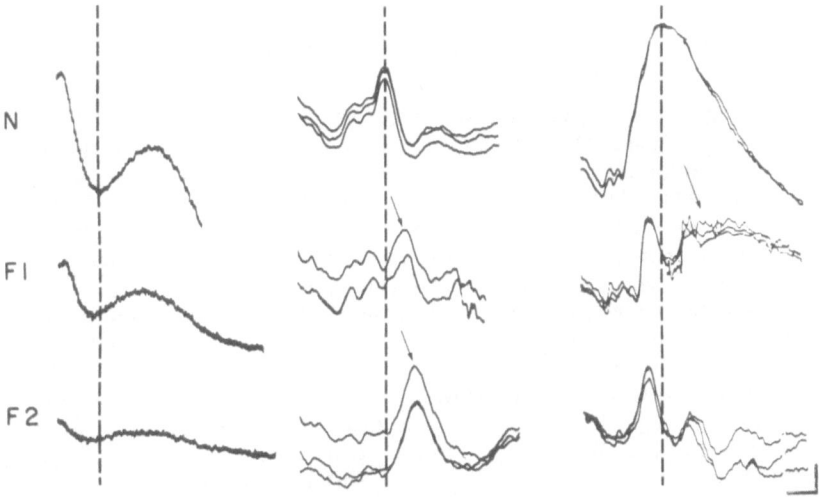

Fig. 13. ERPs (column 1) and ERGs (columns 2 and 3) for normal subject (N) and two children with dominant retinitis pigmentosa with reduced penetrance (F1 and F2). Responses in column 2 are cone responses to 8 ft-L white light flash in presence of steady white background light of 10 ft-L. Responses in column 3 are dark-adapted ERGs to single flashes of long-wavelength light ($\lambda > 550$ nm) of sufficient intensity to elicit both cone and rod components in response. Arrows point to delayed cone (column 2) and rod (column 3) b-waves. Rod component in column 3 is so delayed in F1 compared with normal that clear splitting of rod and cone components can be seen. Stimulus onset is at beginning of each trace. Two or three consecutive responses are superimposed for responses in columns 2 and 3. Dashed line has been vertically extended from peak of R2 of normal subject through responses of F1 and F2. Calibration symbol (lower right corner) is 50 μV vertically and 0.5 msec horizontally for column 1, 12.5 msec horizontally and 50 μV vertically for column 2, and 25 msec horizontally and 30 μV vertically for column 3. (From Berson, E.L., and Goldstein, E.B.: Arch. Ophthalmol. 83 : 412, 1970).

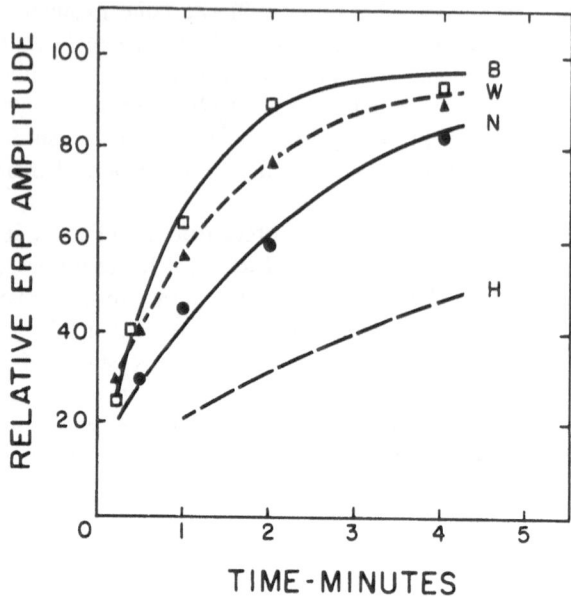

TIME-MINUTES

Fig. 14. Average ERP recovery curves for four normal subjects (•) and for two siblings (B1, age 16; and B2, age 14) in family B (□) and three siblings (W1, age 18; W2, age 13; and W3, age 11) in family W (▲) with dominantly inherited pigmentosa, after yellow (λ > 500 nm) bleaching flash at time zero. ERP amplitudes (peak of R1 to peak of R2) for each subject are responses to white light flashes and are expressed as percentage of response of dark-adapted eye. Curve N is based on average of four normal subjects, curve B on average of B1 and B2, and curve W on average of W1, W2, and W3. Data for each patient are based on average of two to four responses at 30 sec, 1 min, 2 min, and 4 min after bleaching flash. Only one white light test flash was presented after bleaching flash in each sequence of recordings, and patient was dark adapted for minimum of 1 hour between each sequence. Average variation from the mean for each determination for each patient and normal subject was ± 5%. Recovery curves could be described by exponential functions (normal subjects, $t_{1/2}$ = 1.6 min; family B, $t_{1/2}$ = 35 sec; family W, $t_{1/2}$ = 1.0 min). Because final level of recovery for normal subjects was about 97%, all exponential curves were calculated to asymptote at this level. Patient H (long dashed line) is 16-year-old congenital rod monochromat; his recovery curve is described by slower exponential ($t_{1/2}$ = 5.6 min) curve. (From Berson, E.L., and Goldstein, E.B.: Arch. Ophthalmol. 83 : 412, 1970).

served in remaining foveal cones (Kolb & Gouras, 1974). This woman was the paternal grandmother of the 18-year-old male with a reduced ERP illustrated in Figure 12. The mechanism that leads to abnormal ERPs and delayed ERG b-wave implicit times in the early stages and to disoriented and disrupted outer segments and photoreceptor cell death in advanced stages is not known.

Patients in group IV with abnormal cone and rod function across all or nearly all the retina, even in the early stages, have worse long-term visual prognoses than patients in groups I-III. Patients in group IV can have minimal if any changes visible with the ophthalmoscope at a time when amplitudes and implicit times of the ERG are clearly abnormal. Although no treatments are known at present for patients with primary retinitis pigmentosa and allied diseases, early diagnosis and definition of visual prognosis aid in genetic counseling, vocational guidance, and selection of patients for possible therapeutic trials such as light deprivation of one eye with an opaque scleral contact lens (Berson, 1973).

SUMMARY AND CONCLUSIONS

Full-field ERGs, separated into cone and rod components, have been presented to show that hereditary retinal diseases can be classified into four major groups:

I. Diseases that involve either cone or rod function across all or nearly all the retina (i.e., stationary night blindness, congenital rod monochromacy, etc.)

II. Diseases that involve cone and rod function but only in localized areas of the retina (i.e., sector retinitis pigmentosa, macular degeneration)

III. Diseases that involve cone or rod function across all or nearly all the retina with macular degeneration

IV. Diseases that involve both cone and rod function across all or nearly all the retina (i.e., widespread retinitis pigmentosa, choroideremia, etc.)

The full-field ERGs not only help to define the extent and type of hereditary retinal disease but also provide an aid in determining long-term visual prognoses of affected patients. Patients with sector or self-limited hereditary retinal diseases (groups I to III) characteristically have reduced ERG amplitudes and normal ERG b-wave implicit times, while those with progressive widespread forms of hereditary retinal disease (group IV) characteristically have reduced ERG amplitudes and delayed ERG b-wave implicit times. The full-field ERG can be used in early life to establish the diagnosis of different types of primary retinitis pigmentosa and allied diseases and to determine visual prognoses even when changes visible with the ophthalmoscope are minimal or absent.

REFERENCES

Alpern, M., Lee, G.B. & Spivey, B.E.: π_1 monochromatism. *Arch. Ophthalmol.* 74, *334*, (1965).

Alpern, M., Holland, M.G. & Ohba, N.: Rhodopsin bleaching signals in essential night blindness. *J. Physiol. (London)* 225, *457*, (1972).

Armington, J.C., Tepas, D.I., Kropfl, W.J. & Hengst, W.H.: Summation of retinal potentials. *J. Opt. Soc. Am.* 51, *877*, (1961).

Auerbach, E., Godel, V. & Rowe, H.: An electrophysiological and psychophysical study of two forms of congenital night blindness. *Invest. Ophthalmol.* 8, *332-345*, (1969).

Berson, E.L., Gouras, P. & Gunkel, R.D.: Progressive cone degeneration, dominantly inherited. *Arch. Ophthalmol.* 80, 77, (1968).

Berson, E.L., Gouras, P. & Gunkel, R.D.: Progressive cone-rod degeneration. *Arch. Ophthalmol.* 80, *68*, (1968).

Berson, E.L., Gouras, P. & Gunkel, R.D.: Rod responses in retinitis pigmentosa, dominantly inherited. *Arch. Ophthalmol.* 80, *58* (1968).

Berson, E.L., Gouras, P., Gunkel, R.D. & Myrianthopoulos, N.C.: Rod and cone responses in sex-linked retinitis pigmentosa. *Arch. Ophthalmol.* 81, *215*, (1969).

Berson, E.L., Gouras, P., Gunkel, R.D. & Myrianthopoulos, N.C.: Dominant retinitis pigmentosa with reduced penetrance. *Arch. Ophthalmol.* 81, *226*, (1969).

Berson, E.L., Gouras, P. & Hoff, M.: Temporal aspects of the electroretinogram. *Arch. Ophthalmol.* 81, *207*, (1969).

Berson, E.L. & Kanters, L.: Cone and rod responses in a family with recessively inherited retinitis pigmentosa. *Arch. Ophthalmol.* 84, *288*, (1970).

Berson, E.L. & Goldstein, E.B.: The early receptor potential in dominantly inherited retinitis pigmentosa. *Arch. Ophthalmol.* 83, *412*, (1970).

Berson, E.L. & Goldstein, E.B.: The early receptor potential in sex-linked retinitis pigmentosa. *Invest. Ophthalmol.* 9, *58*, (1970).

Berson, E.L. & Howard, J.: Temporal aspects of the electroretinogram in sector retinitis pigmentosa. *Arch. Ophthalmol.* 86, *653*, (1971).

Berson, E.L.: Experimental and therapeutic aspects of photic damage to the retina. *Invest. Ophthalmol.* 12, *35*, (1973).

Berson, E.L.: Electroretinographic testing as an aid in determining visual prognosis in families with hereditary retinal degenerations. In Pruett, R.C., & Regan, C.D.J., eds. *Retina Congress*, New York, 1974, Appleton-Century-Crofts, pp. *41-53*.

Berson, E.L., Mehaffey, L. & Rabin, A.R.: A night vision pocketscope for patients with retinitis pigmentosa: Design considerations. *Arch. Ophthalmol.* 91, *495* (1974).

Berson, E.L.: Electrical phenomena in the retina. In: *Adler's Physiology of the Eye*, 6th edition, R.A. Moses (ed.), C.V. Mosby, St. Louis, 1975, pp. 453-499.

Berson, E.L., Hayes, K.C., Rabin, A.R., Schmidt, S.Y. & Watson, G.: Retinal degeneration in cats fed casein: II. Supplementation with methionine, cysteine or taurine. *Invest. Ophthalmol.* 15, *52*, (1976).

Berson, E.L.: Retinitis pigmentosa and allied retinal diseases: Electrophysiological findings. *Trans. Am. Acad. Ophthalmol. Otolaryngol.*, 81, *659* (1976).

Berson, E.L.: Unpublished observations.

Berson, E.L., and Rabin, A.R.: Unpublished observations.

Bjork, A. & Karpe, G.: The electroretinogram in retinitis pigmentosa. *Acta Ophthalmol.* 29, *361*, (1951).

Carr, R.E., and Siegel, I.M.: Electrophysiologic aspects of several retinal diseases. *Am. J. Opthalmol.* 58, *95*, (1964).

Carr, R.E. & Gouras, P.: Oguchi's disease. *Arch. Ophthalmol.* 73, *646*, (1965).

Carr, R.E., Ripps, H., Siegel, I.M. & Weale, R.A.: Rhodopsin and the electrical activity of the retina in congenital night blindness. *Invest. Ophthalmol.* 5, *497*, (1966).

Carr, R.E. & Siegel, I.M.: Action spectrum of the human early receptor potential. *Nature* 225, *88*, (1970).

Dhanda, R.P.: ERG in myopic retinal degenerations. In Nakajima, A., ed.: *Jap. J. Ophthal.* 10 (suppl.), *325*, (1966).

François, J., Verriest, G., De Rouck, A. & Dejean, C.: Les fonctions visuelles dans l'héméralopie essentielle nougarienne. *Ophthalmologica (Basel)* 132, *244-257*, (1956).

François, J. & DeRouck, A.: Behavior of ERG and EOG in localized retinal destruction by photocoagulation. In Burian, H.M. & Jacobson, J.H., eds.: Clinical electroretinography; Proceedings of the Third International Symposium 1964, Oxford, 1966, Pergamon Press, Inc. pp. 191-202.

Goldstein, E.B. & Berson, E.L.: Cone dominance of the human early receptor potential. *Nature* 222, *1272*, (1969).

Goodman, G. & Gunkel, R.D.: Familial electroretinographic and adaptometric studies in retinitis pigmentosa. *Am. J. Ophthalmol.* 46, *142*, (1958).

Gouras, P. & Carr, R.E.: Electrophysiological studies in early retinitis pigmentosa. *Arch. Ophthalmol.* 72, *104*, (1964).

Gouras, P.: Electroretinography: Some basic principles. *Invest. Ophthalmol.* 9, *557*, (1970).

Gunkel, R.D., Bergsma, D.R. & Gouras, P.: A ganzfeld stimulator for electroretinography. *Arch. Ophthalmol.* 94, *669*, (1976).

Henkes, H.E., van der Tweel, L.H. & van der Gon, J.J.D.: Selective amplification of the electroretinogram. *Ophthalmologica (Basel)* 132, *140*, (1956).

Hill, D.A., Arbel, K. & Berson, E.L.: Cone electroretinograms in congenital nyctalopia with myopia. *Am. J. Ophthalmol.* 78, *127*, (1974).

Karpe, G.: Basis of clinical electroretinography. *Arch. Ophthalmol.* 24 (suppl.), *84*, (1945).

Kolb, H. & Gouras, P.: Electron microscopic observations of human retinitis pigmentosa, dominantly inherited. *Invest. Ophthalmol.* 13, *487*, (1974).

Krill, A.E.: Hereditary retinal and choroidal diseases, New York, 1972, Harper & Row, Publishers, pp. 248-249.

Mehaffey, L. & Berson, E.L.: Cone mechanisms in the electroretinogram of the cynomolgus monkey. *Invest. Ophthalmol.* 13, *266*, (1974).

Noell, W.K., Delmelle, M.C. & Albrecht, R.: Vitamin A deficiency effect on the retina: Dependency on light. *Science* 172, *72*, (1971).

Norren, D.V. & Padmos, P.: Human and macaque blue cones studied with electroretinography. *Vision Res.* 13, *1241*, (1973).

Osterberg, G.: Topography of the layer of rods and cones in the human retina. *Acta Ophthalmol. (Suppl.)* 6, *1*, (1935).

Rabin, A.R., Hayes, K.C. & Berson, E.L.: Cone and rod responses in nutritionally induced retinal degeneration in the cat. *Invest. Ophthalmol.* 12, *694*, (1973).

Rabin, A.R. & Berson, E.L.: A full-field system for clinical electroretinography. *Arch. Ophthalmol.* 92, *59*, (1974).

Ruedemann, A.D., Jr. & Noell, W.K.: A contribution to the electroretinogram of retinitis pigmentosa. *Am. J. Ophthalmol.* 47, *564*, (1959).

Sandberg, M. & Berson, E.L.: Blue and green cone mechanisms in retinitis pigmentosa. *Invest. Ophthal.* (1977, in press).

Schmidt, S.Y., Berson, E.L. & Hayes, K.C.: Retinal degeneration in cats fed casein: I. Taurine deficiency. *Invest. Ophthalmol.* 15, *47*, (1976).

Schubert, G. & Bornschein, H.: Beitrag zur Analyse des Menschlichen Electroretinograms. *Ophthalmologica* 123, *396*, (1952).

Völker-Dieben, H.G., Van Lith, G.H.M., West, L.N. & De Vries-De Mol, E.C.: Electroophthalmology of a family with x-chromosomal recessive nyctalopia and myopia. In Dodt, E. & Pearlman, J.T., eds: Documenta Ophthalmologica Proceedings, Series 4. Eleventh ISCERG Symposium. Bad Nauheim,. May 1973, Dr. W. Junk, B.V., The Hague, The Netherlands, pp. 169-177.

Wyszechi, G. & Stiles, W.S.: *Color Science*, New York, 1967, John Wiley & Sons, Inc., p. 206.

Author's address:
Berman-Gund Laboratory for the
Study of Retinal Degenerations
Harvard Medical School
Massachusetts Eye and Ear Infirmary
243 Charles Street
Boston, Mass. 02114
USA

ELECTROPHYSIOLOGICAL AND PSYCHOPHYSICAL STUDIES IN CONGENITAL RETINOSCHISIS OF X-LINKED RECESSIVE INHERITANCE

TATSUO HIROSE, ERNST WOLF & AKIRA HARA

(Boston)

SUMMARY

Twenty-eight eyes of 14 males affected with congenital retinoschisis were studied. The amplitude ratio of b- over a-wave (b/a ratio) of the ERG was lower than normal in all cases including those in which the clinically visible abnormality in the fundus was limited to the macula. This characteristic pattern of the ERG could even be recognized in an advanced stage when the responses became extremely small. VER obtained by focal stimulation of the macula showed delayed peak times in all cases suggesting abnormal macular function. The light rise of the EOG was normal in all cases except one of advanced stage. Kinetic perimetry showed depression in the center and in the upper fields corresponding to the locations of the fundus abnormalities visible ophthalmoscopically. Flicker perimetry showed diffuse impairment of the cone function in the entire field. Dark adaptation curves showed in most patients elevation of the tresholds of both cones and rods. In advanced stages, the rod portion of the dark adaptation curve was entirely missing, indicating complete night blindness. The results of these studies demonstrate that there is much more profound and widespread functional abnormality in congenital retinoschisis than one would suspect from the fundus appearance. The macula as well as the area outside the macula is involved. Pathology in this disease probably starts in the inner and middle layers of the retina, and initiates later the degeneration of the receptors.

Congenital retinoschisis should be noted as a disease leading to complete night blindness. In late stages, the fundus appearance, psychophysical and electrophysiological findings may resemble those found in retinitis pigmentosa.

INTRODUCTION

Retinoschisis is a splitting of the sensory retina. It can be classified into three groups: congenital (Kraushar, Schepens & Kaplan, 1972), acquired (Shea, Schepens & Pirquet, 1960), and secondary. Congenital retinoschisis is usually manifested by x-linked recessive transmission (Kraushar, Schepens & Kaplan, 1972). It is characterized ophthalmoscopically by a ballooning elevation of the retina, large oval holes in the inner layer of the retinoschisis and microcystic elevation of the macula with radiating folds from the fovea (Kraushar, Schepens & Kaplan, 1972). The vitreous, often degenerated, forms membranes which are partly attached to the retina or the optic disc and causes traction on the macula or the disc. Congenital retinoschisis usually appears almost stationary, but in some cases slow progression alternates with spontaneous remission. In late stages, chorioretinal atrophy and diffuse pigmentation are seen in the area underneath the retinoschisis. Histopathological studies in congenital retinoschisis show a splitting of the nerve fiber layer (Yanoff, Rahn & Zimmerman, 1968; Manschot, 1972).

The ERG response in congenital retinoschisis is subnormal to absent (Ricci, 1961; Sarin, Green & Dailey, 1964; Bengtsson & Linder, 1967; Vainio-Mattila, Eriksson & Forsius, 1969; Constantaras, Dobbie, Choromakis & Frankel, 1972; Denden, 1975; Boman, Heilig, Kolber, Giblett & Failkow, 1976), normal or subnormal a-wave with a much reduced b-wave amplitude (Guyot-Sionnest, 1969; Deutman, 0000; Forsius, Eriksson & Vainio-Mattila, 1963; Carr & Siegel, 1970; Thaler, Heilig & Slezak, 1973; Van Lith, 1977; Fishman, 1975), or scotopic ERG more affected than photopic ERG (Deutman, 1971; Harris & Yeung, 1976) and subnormal or loss of oscillatory potential (Deutman, 1971; Thaler, Heilig & Slezak, 1973). EOG was reported normal (Harris & Yeung, 1976) or abnormal (Constantaras, Dobbie, Choromakis & Frenkel, 1972; Carr & Siegel, 1970) or both (Denden, 1975; Deutman, 1971; Thaler, Heilig & Slezak, 1973). Local ERG and VER of the fovea was abnormal (Deutman, 1971). VER (Visual Evoked Response) to patterned stimuli shows reduced amplitude and delayed latency only in late stages of the disease (Harris & Yeung, 1976).

Central vision is impaired early (Kraushar, Schepens & Kaplan, 1972) and may become worse with advancing age (Forsius, Krause, Helve, et al., 1973). Color vision may be normal, (Ricci, 1961; Bengtsson & Linder, 1967; Constantaras, Dobbie, Choromakis & Frenkel, 1972; Levy, 1952) or abnormal to various degrees (Vainio-Mattila, Erikson & Forsius, 1969; Deutman, 1971; Forsius, Eriksson & Vainio-Mattila, 1963; Harris & Yeung, 1976; Forsius, Krause, Helve, et al., 1973; Levy, 1952) or severely impaired (Helve, 1972).

Dark adaptation is reported to be anywhere from normal (Ricci, 1961) at the lower limit of the normal range, to slightly impaired (Sarin, Green & Dailey, 1964; Bengtsson & Linder, 1967; Vainio-Mattilla, Eriksson & Forsius, 1969; Deutman, 1971; Forsius, Eriksson & Vainio-Mattila, 1963; Gieser & Falls, 1961) or with final rod thresholds significantly or severely elevated (Boman, Heilig, Kolder, Giblett & Fialkow, 1976; Carr & Siegel, 1970).

Static perimetry showed reduced sensitivity in the macula. (Harris & Yeung, 1976).

The fundus appearance in congenital retinoschisis is quite characteristic. Differentiation of the condition from retinal detachment may be of historical interest. (Levy, 1952; Sorsby, Klein, Gann, et al., 1951). However, because of its polymorphous manifestations in each patient and in each stage of the disease, it is still often misdiagnosed as nonspecific macular degenerations or retinitis pigmentosa. A variety of retinal function test results reported thus far appears to reflect the polymorphous clinical manifestations of the disease at different ages and in different individuals.

The purpose of the present paper is to correlate morphological changes with abnormalities of function, both electrophysiological and psychophysical, in order to shed some light upon the natural course and diagnosis of the disease.

METHODS

Twenty-eight eyes of 14 males aged from 7 to 59 years (Table 1) afflicted with X-linked recessive congenital retinoschisis comprise the material. Ophthalmic examination consisted of routine examinations, binocular indirect ophthalmoscopy with scleral depression, and biomicroscopy of the vitreous and fundus by slit-lamp microscopy with the aid of a Goldmann three-mirror lens.

Electrophysiological Tests

ERG: A contact lens electrode of the Jacobson type was used. A reference electrode was placed on the ipsilateral cheek. Potentials produced by photic stimulation were fed into an amplifier and displayed on a cathod ray oscilloscope. The frequency responses were lowered 50% at 0.3 and 3,000 Hz.

The light source was a Grass model PS-1 stroboscopic light which illuminated a translucent circular screen subtending a visual angle of 53°. Four different stimuli were used to isolate the specific components of the *ERG:* A contact lens electrode of the Jacobson type was used. A reference Wratten Filter No. 92, >610 nm) at stimulus intensity 16. The scotopic b-wave was recorded with dim blue light (Kodak Wratten No. 47B) at intensity 1. Photopic flicker responses were obtained with white light setting No. 8 and 30 Hz. The a-wave and the oscillatory potential were obtained with white light with intensity 16. The patient's eye was fully dilated with 1% cyclopentolate hydrochloride and 10% phenylephrine hydrochloride. A period of dark adaptation of 30 minutes or more preceded the recordings. *VER:* Visual evoked responses (VER) were recorded with 8-mm silver disc electrodes pasted on the scalp 3 cm lateral to and 2 cm above the inion and reference electrode was on the joined earlobes. The electrodes were connected to a Grass EEG machine through which the responses were amplified and further fed into a PDP 8 computer. The computer summed 150 responses which were displayed on the oscilloscope resulting in an upward

Table I. Age of Patients

Years	No.
Less than 10	1
11-20	6
21-30	2
31-40	4
51-60	1
Total	14

deflection with the negativity of the occipital electrodes. The frequency responses of the amplifier were down 50% at 1 and 500 Hz.

The light source was a glow modulator tube (Sylvania R1131C) driven by square wave generator. The light intensity produced by the tube was 14,290 millilamberts measured with a McBeth illuminometer. By interposition of neutral density filters, the stimulus was reduced to eliminate the effects of scattered light (Hirose & Larson, 1976).

A rectangular stimulus pulsating at 1.7 Hz with a fixed flash duration of 50 msec was delivered to the macula. The stimulus spot subtended a visual angle of 4.5° (Hirose & Larson, 1976) The patient was asked to see the center of the stimulus spot. Four dim red dots located about 7 degrees from the center helped to maintain the fixation in patients with relatively poor central vision.

EOG: The electrooculogram (EOG) was recorded as described by Arden and others (Arden, Barrada & Kelsey, 1962). Patients spent at least half an hour in complete darkness while their pupils were being dilated with topical 1% cyclopentolate hydrochloride and 10% phenylephrine hydrochloride. When the ERG was recorded prior to the EOG we waited 10 to 15 minutes in the dark before recording the EOG. Under very dim ambient light, two silver disc electrodes were pasted near the outer and inner canthi of each eye and the ground electrode on the center of the forehead. The patients sat 1 meter from the center of the adaptation screen of 90 cm x 90 cm, upon which two small red fixation lights were presented on the horizontal of the visual field, separated by a visual angle of 30°. The screen consisted of translucent plexiglass, transilluminated by four 40-watt daylight fluorescent tubes. Patients placed their chins on a chin rest and their foreheads flush against the bar and were asked to move their eyes rhythmically from one fixation light to the other to a metronome click at a frequency of about 1.2 Hz. The potentials recorded from the electrodes were led to the Grass EEG machine and registered with a penwriter on paper. The time constant of the amplifier was set at 0.45 seconds.

The EOG was recorded in darkness for about 15 seconds every two minutes. After five recording sessions the screen was illuminated, and the responses were recorded again in the same manner every two minutes for an additional 15 minutes. Amplitudes of several responses recorded in each session were measured and averaged. The ratio between the largest averaged amplitude in the light and the smallest averaged amplitude in the darkness (Light Peak/Dark Trough: LP/DT ratio) was measured. Several normal subjects were tested. As their amplitudes fell within the range found by Arden and others (Arden, Barrada & Kelsey, 1962) their criterion for abnormality was used. LP/DT ratio smaller than 1.85 was considered abnormal.

Psychophysical Tests

Kinetic perimetry was performed with a Goldmann perimeter under photopic background illumination. Two isopters were plotted, one with a target of 64 mm² and maximum intensity, the other with a 16 mm² spot with the intensity reduced to one-tenth that of the large target. Flicker perimetry was performed by the method of Wolf et al. (1968). Critical flicker frequencies (CFF) were determined monocularly by lowering the frequency from fusion to the point at which flicker became noticeable. CFF values were obtained along the horizontal and vertical meridians, from the center out to 60°. The results were plotted as flicker profiles and compared with those obtained from normal individuals.

Dark adaptation was tested with a Tübinger perimeter. Preadaptation consisted of exposure for three minutes to white light of 385 foot-lamberts reflected from the evenly illuminated hemisphere of the perimeter. A white test field subtending an angle of 2° was presented 10° nasal on the horizontal meridian in single flashes of 0.1 second. The patient was asked to respond to each presentation simply by indicating whether he saw the stimulus. The examiner adjusted the luminance of each flash until the threshold was determined. A dark adaptation curve was obtained by plotting log threshold luminance against time in darkness. After the termination of the test, light thresholds were measured at different locations along the horizontal meridian. Thus a sensivity profile from 30° nasal to 30° temporal was obtained.

RESULTS

I. OPHTHALMOSCOPIC FINDINGS

Group I – Macular abnormality without peripheral retinoschisis

Eleven eyes of six patients showed characteristic macular abnormalities (Kraushar, Schepens & Kaplan, 1972) without obvious elevation of the peripheral retina. Among them, six eyes of three patients showed a metallic reflex in the inferotemporal quadrant of the fundus, and two eyes of one patient revealed a beaten metal appearance deep in the retina with the surface of the retina appearing very slightly elevated when viewed in profile with a binocular indirect ophthalmoscope and scleral depression. Five eyes out of three patients showed extensive white-with-pressure in the inferotemporal quadrant. The ages of patients in thsi group were 13, 17, 31, 33, 34, and 38 years.

Group II – Macular abnormality plus typical ballooning peripheral retinoschisis with large inner layer holes

Thirteen eyes of seven patients belong to this group. The ages of patients in this group range from 7 to 29.

Group III – Macular abnormality plus extensive peripheral retinoschisis with multiple inner layer holes, loss of blood vessels, or extensive pigmentation

Two eyes of one patient showed extensive retinoschisis with multiple inner layer holes located not only in the inferotemporal quadrant but also superiorly and temporally. In addition typical macular abnormalities were present. Two eyes of another patient showed no elevation of the inner layer but relatively dense extensive pigmentation, mainly in the inferior half of the fundus where no retinal vessels are visible ophthalmoscopically. The superior half of the fundus appeared ophthalmoscopically normal. The macula of this patient showed elevation and a typical star-shaped pattern of folds radiating from the fovea (Kraushar, Schepens & Kaplan, 1972). The ages of the two patients are 18 and 59 years.

II. ERG

A. Photopic b-wave recorded with red stimulus

ERGs on twenty eyes of 14 patients were recorded.Among them 15 eyes showed a significant decrease in amplitude and 3 eyes showed nonrecordable photopic b-waves. Recordings of two eyes showed an artifact due to blinking and were not suitable for evaluation. None showed a normal photopic b-wave. Of three eyes which showed nonrecordable photopic b-waves, one eye was from Group II and two eyes from Group III.

B. Scotopic b-wave recorded with red and blue stimuli

Seventeen eyes showed a decrease in amplitude of the scotopic b-wave. Three eyes which showed nonrecordable photopic b-waves had nonrecordable scotopic b-wave also. None showed a normal scotopic b-wave.

C. Photopic flicker responses

Seventeen eyes showed reduced amplitudes. Three eyes which had nonrecordable photopic and scotopic b-waves showed barely noticeable photopic flicker responses. All 20 eyes showed a significant delay in peak after the onset of each flicker stimulus. None showed normal responses.

D. A-wave

The a-wave was recorded in 27 eyes. Decrease of the amplitude of the a-wave appeared proportional to the extent or severity of the fundus lesion revealed by ophthalmoscopy. Two eyes of two patients in Group I showed normal amplitudes (Fig. 1B). Seven eyes of five patients in Group I revealed very slight but significant decrease in amplitude. One eye in Group I and 14 eyes of 7 patients in Group II showed moderately decreased amplitudes (Fig. 1C). Three eyes of two patients in Group III showed marked decrease in amplitude (Fig. 1D).

E. b/a ratio

The amplitude ratio of the b-wave to the a-wave in ERG recorded with bright white light was studied. Twenty-two eyes of 11 patients showed b/a ratios of less than 1. In other words, the b-wave was smaller than the a-wave. Five eyes of three patients (two patients in Group II, one in Group I) showed a b/a ratio larger than 1, but smaller than normal. None showed a normal or higher than normal b/a ratio. A low b/a ratio seems to be characteristic for congenital retinoschisis.

F. Oscillatory potential

Twenty-five eyes of 13 patients showed no oscillatory potential. Only two eyes of one patient in Group I showed a trace of it. A normal oscillatory potential was never observed.

III. EOG

Twenty-two eyes of 11 patients were tested. Two eyes of one patient in Group III showed lower than normal light peak vs dark trough ratio (LP/DT ratio). The ratio was above 1.85 in 14 eyes of 8 patients and above 3.5 in 6 eyes of 4 patients.

IV. VER

VER recorded by focal stimulation (central 4.5°) of the macula showed three major deflections which form a W-shaped configuration with negativity of the occipital electrode taken as an upward deflection (Hirose, Wolf & Malin, 1974).

Twenty-four eyes of 12 patients with congenital retinoschisis were tested. Nine eyes of five patients showed the VERs whose peaks of the Wave II (Hirose, Wolf & Malin, 1974) were delayed more than 50 msec as compared with the normal mean. From thirteen eyes of seven patients no VER could be recorded. The recordings of two eyes of one patient could not be interpreted because of the huge spontaneous EEG which was not cancelled out by the computer averaging.

V. KINETIC PERIMETRY

Results correspond relatively well to the extent of peripheral retinoschisis. Cases which showed retinoschisis inferiorly showed field defect superiorly. Cases without peripheral retinoschisis showed normal peripheral fields.

VI. FLICKER PERIMETRY

Twenty-eight eyes of 14 patients were tested. All showed significant decrease of critical flicker frequency (CFF) in the center and periphery not only in the area corresponding to the retinoschisis but often in the area where there was no obvious retinoschisis visible ophthalmoscopically. In some cases which showed only macular lesion ophthalmoscopically, depressed CFF were observed in the upper and nasal fields.

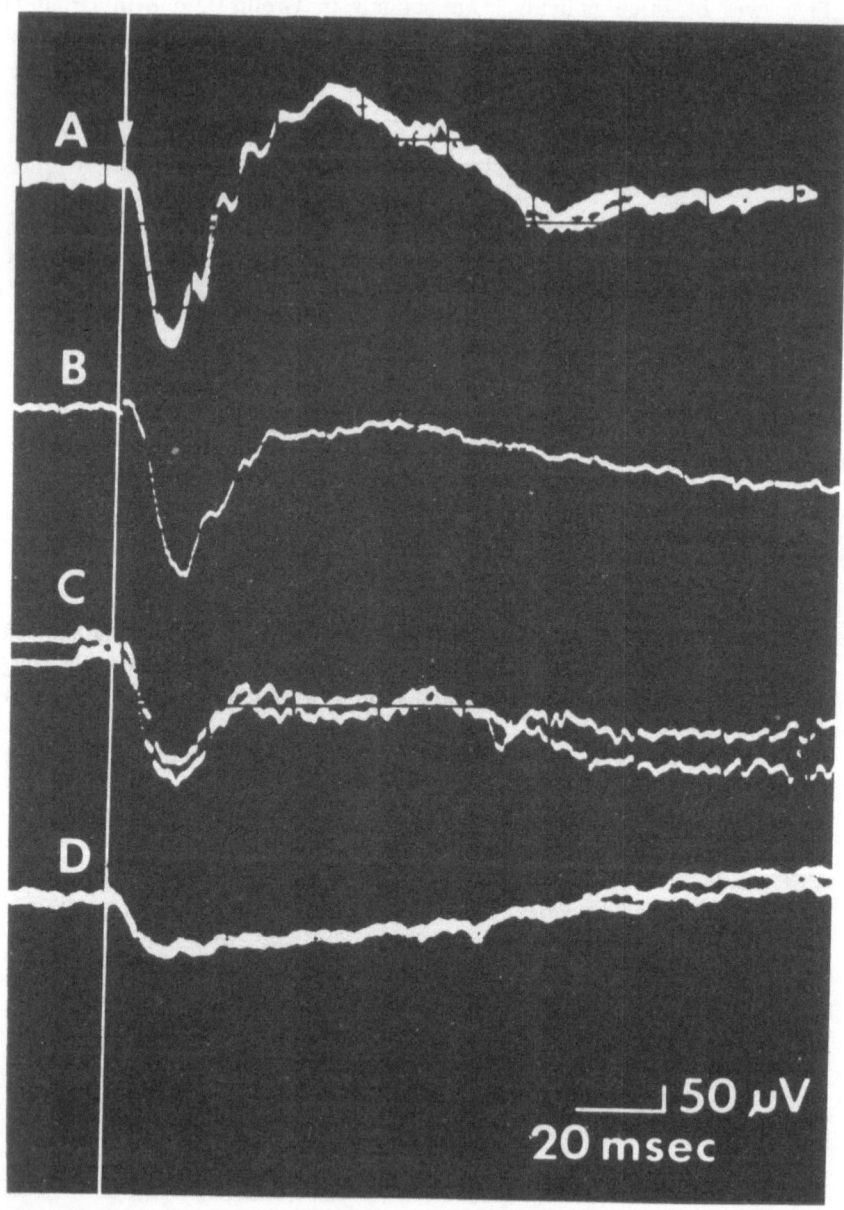

Fig. 1. ERG in congenital retinoschisis recorded white bright white stimulus. A: Normal ERG. B: ERG in patient with macular lesion without peripheral retinoschisis. C: ERG in patient with macular lesion and ballooning peripheral retinoschisis. D: ERG in patient with late stage of the disease. Note that b- and a-waves become small with more extensive lesions of the fundus and that b/a amplitude ratio is lower than normal in all cases.

VII. DARK ADAPTATION AND SENSITIVITY PROFILES

Nine eyes of nine patients were tested. Thresholds of cones and rods are elevated including all cases with macular abnormality only (Fig. 2A). The thresholds tend to be higher in the eyes with extensive fundus lesions. The curve in Fig. 2B was obtained from an eye in Group II. One eye in Group III showed that the rod portion of the curve was entirely missing indicating complete night blindness (Fig. 2C). When thresholds are measured at various locations from the center along the horizontal meridian at the end of dark adaptation testing (Sensitivity profile) it is significantly elevated not only in the area corresponding to the retinoschisis but in the areas where no retinoschisis was found indicating that the rod function is extensively impaired.

COMMENTS

ERG and VER findings in patients in the present study are quite uniform and diagnostically characteristic. Most characteristic is the reduced b/a amplitude ratio. This ERG finding is seen regardless of the extent, severity of the fundus appearance and the age of patients; even in cases which show only macular lesion without peripheral retinoschisis as well as in cases which are advanced showing extensive fundus pigmentation. It also can be used in

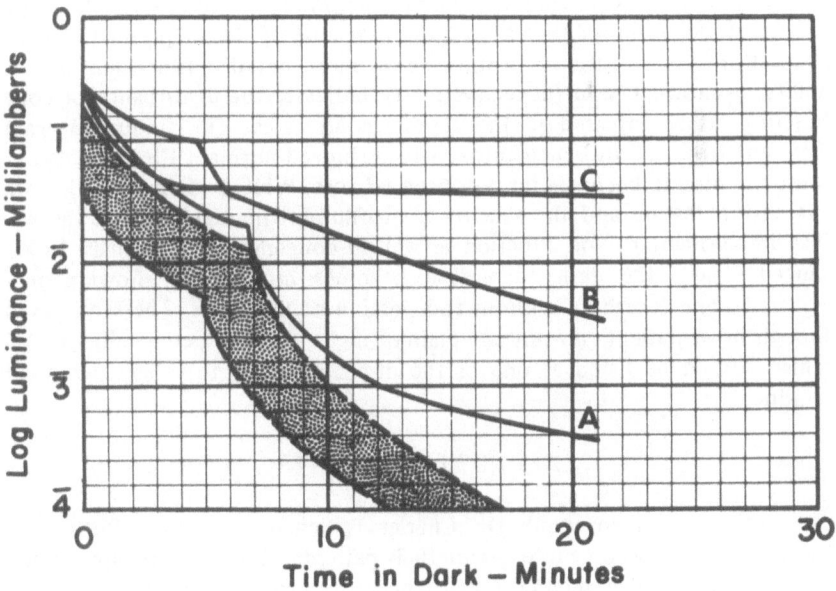

Fig. 2. Dark adaptation curve in congenital retinoschisis. A: Patient with macular lesion without visible peripheral retinoschisis. B: Patient with macular lesion and ballooning peripheral retinoschisis. C: Patient in late stage of the disease. Area between dashed lines represents normal range of dark adaptation curve.

differentiating congenital retinoschisis from retinal detachment which shows decrease of amplitude of both b- and a-wave proportional to the extent of detachment (Guyot-Sionnest, 1969). Decrease in amplitude of the a-wave appears somewhat parallel with the extent of visible lesions in the fundus in retinoschisis. As the b-wave is considered to be generated in the middle layer of the retina (Brown, 1968) including the Müller cells (Dowling, 1970) and the a-wave in the outer layer, (Brown, 1968) the reduced ERG b/a amplitude ratio in congenital retinoschisis suggests that the diffuse involvement of the middle layer of the retina precedes that of the receptors. Loss of oscillatory potential combined with a normal a-wave in some cases, and normal EOG light rise in most cases seem to support this view. Although all our cases showed recordable ERGs, the ERG may become non-recordable in far advanced stages as others reported (Constantaras, Dobbie, Choromakis & Frenkel, 1972; Denden, 1975; Deutman, 1971; Thaler, Heilig & Slezak, 1973). Abnormal VER to stimulation of the macula suggests the impairment of macular function present in all cases studied. These electrophysiological results in congenital retinoschisis are quite different from those in retinitis pigmentosa although the former at its late stage is sometimes mistaken as retinitis pigmentosa. In retinitis pigmentosa, the b-wave does not usually become smaller than the a-wave (Berson, Gouras, Gunkel & Myrianthopoulos, 1969) and the EOG light rise becomes abnormal (Arden, Barrada & Kelsey, 1962) while the VER is normal in early stage (Hirose & Jacobson, 1968).

Visual field defects found in kinetic perimetry correspond well to the extent of the retinoschisis, however, the results of flicker perimetry, dark adaptation and sensitivity profiles show more detailed functional abnormality. Abnormality in flicker perimetry indicates the disturbance of cone function. It is impaired in the center in all cases. The finding is again different from retinitis pigmentosa which showed normal CFF in the center until the disease becomes far advanced (Hirose, Wolf & Malin, 1974). Dark adaptation testing and the sensitivity profile plotting demonstrate the diffuse impairment of rod function as well in congenital retinoschisis. In advanced stages, the dark adaptation becomes monophasic showing only elevated cone threshold without rod portion of the curve. Therefore, even though most patients do not complain of night blindness, congenital retinoschisis should be listed as one of the diseases leading to progressive night blindness.

ACKNOWLEDGEMENTS

The authors wish to thank Dr. Charles L. Schepens and the Retina Associates who allowed us to examine their patients, and for their support and encouragement. The technical assistance was provided by Mrs. Elizabeth Larson. The artwork was done by Mr. David Tilden. This work was supported by Public Health Service Research Grant EY 01259 from the National Eye Institute, National Institutes of Health.

REFERENCES

Arden, G.B., Barrada, A. & Kelsey, J.H.: New clinical test of retinal function based upon the standing potential of the eye. *Brit. J. Ophthal.* 46, *449*, (1962).

Bengtsson, B., Linder, B.: Sex-linked hereditary juvenile retinoschisis. *Acta Ophthal.* 45, *411* (1967).

Berson, E.L., Gouras, P., Gunkel, R.D. & Myrianthopoulos, N.C.: Rod and cone responses and sex-linked retinitis pigmentosa. *Arch. Ophthal.* 81, *215*, (1969).

Boman, H., Heilig, P., Kolder, H.E., Giblett, E.R. & Fialkow, P.J.: Hereditary retinoschisis: linkage studies in a family and considerations in genetic counselling. *Canad. J. Ophthal.* 11, *11*, (1976).

Brown, K.T.: The electroretinogram: Its components and their origin. *Vision Res.* 8. *633*, (1968).

Burns, R.P., Lovrien, E.W. & Cibis, A.B.: Juvenile sex-linked retinoschisis. Clinical and genetic studies. *Trans. Amer. Acad. Ophthal. Otolaryn.* 72, *1011*, (1971).

Carr, R.E. & Siegel, I.M.: The vitreo-tapeto-retinal degenerations. *Arch. Ophthal.* 84, *436*, (1970).

Constantaras, A.A., Dobbie, J.G., Choromakis, E.A. & Frenkel, M.: Juvenile sex-linked recessive retinoschisis in a black family. *Amer. J. Ophthal.* 74, *1166*, (1972).

Denden, A.: X-chromosomale vitreo-retinale Degeneration. ERG- und EOG-Untersuchungsergebnisse. *Klin. Mbl. Augenheilk.* 166, *35*, (1975).

Deutman, A.F.: Hereditary Dystrophies of the Posterior Pole of the Eye. Springfield, Charles Thomas, 1971, p. 48.

Dowling, J.E.: Organization of vertebrate retinas. *Invest. Ophthal.* 9, *655*, (1970).

Fishman, G.A.: The electroretinogram and electro-oculogram in retinal and choroidal disease. Rochester, Minn., *Amer. Acad. Ophthal. Otolaryn.* 1975, p. 28.

Forsius, H., Eriksson, A. & Vainio-Mattila, B.: Geschlechtsgebundene erbliche Retinoschisis in zwei Familien in Finland. *Klin. Mbl. Augenheilk.* 143, *806*, (1963).

Forsius, H., Krause, U. & Helve, J., et al: Visual acuity in 183 cases of x-chromosomal retinoschisis. *Canad. J. Ophthal.* 8, *385*, (1973).

Gieser, E.P. & Falls, H.F.: Hereditary retinoschisis. *Amer. J. Ophthal.* 51, *1193*, (1961).

Guyot-Sionnest: A propos d'une famille atteinte de retinoschisis idiopathique recessif lie au sexe. *Ann. Ocul. (Paris)* 202, *573*, (1969).

Harris, G.S. & Yeung, J.W.-S.: Maculopathy of sex-linked juvenile retinoschisis. *Canad. J. Ophthal.* 10, *1*, (1976).

Helve, J.: Colour vision in x-chromosomal juvenile retinoschisis. *Mod. Probl. Ophthal.* 11, *122* (1972).

Hirose, T. & Jacobson, J.H.: Combined recording of the electroretinogram (ERG) and visual evoked occipital response (VER) in lesions of the visual pathways. In Schmöger, E., (ed): Advances in Electrophysiology and Pathology of the Visual System. Leipzig, Thieme, 1968, p. 125.

Hirose, T., Wolf, E. & Malin, S.: Human visual evoked responses to focal stimulation of the retina. Clinical applications. In Pruett, R.C. & Regan, C.D. (eds): Retina Congress. New York, Appleton-Century-Croft, 1974, p. 55.

Hirose, T. & Larson, E.: Photostimulator for local VER. *Jap. J. Ophthal.* 20, *347*, 1976.

Kraushar, M.F., Schepens, C.L. & Kaplan, J.: Congenital retinoschisis. In Bellows, J.G. (ed): Contemporary Ophthalmology. Honoring Sir Stewart Duke-Elder. Baltimore, Williams and Wilkins Co., 1972, p. 265.

Levy, J.: Inherited retinal detachment. *Brit. J. Ophthal.* 36, *626* (1952).

van Lith, G.H.M.: Familile fovealen Dystrophien. *Ber. Deutsch. Ophthal. Ges.* (in press).

Manschot, W.A.: Pathology of hereditary juvenile retinoschisis. *Arch. Ophthal.* 88, *131*, (1972).

Ricci, A.: Clinique et transmission héréditaire des dégénérescences vitreo-rétiniennes. *Bull. Soc. Ophtal. Franc.* 61, *618*, (1961).

Sarin, L.K., Green, W.R. & Dailey, E.G.: Juvenile retinoschisis: Congenital vascular veils and hereditary retinoschisis. *Amer. J. Ophthal.* 57, *793*, (1964).

Shea, M., Schepens, C.L. & von Pirquet, S.R.: Retinoschisis. 1. Senile type: A clinical report of one hundred seven cases. *Arch. Ophthal.* 63, *1*, (1960).

Sorsby, A., Klein, M. & Gann, J.H., et al: Unusual retinal detachment possibly sex-linked. *Brit. J. Ophthal.* 35, *1*, (1951).

Thaler, A., Heilig, P. & Slezak, H.: Elektroretinogramm und Elektrookulogramm bei juveniler Retinoschisis. *Klin. Mbl. Augenheilk.* 163, *699*, (1973).

Vainio-Mattila, B., Eriksson, A.W. & Forsius, H.: X-chromosomal recessive retinoschisis in the Region of Pori. An ophthalmogenetical analysis of 103 cases. *Acta Ophthal.* 47, *1135*, (1969).

Wolf, E., Gaeta, A.M. & Geer, S.E.: Critical flicker frequencies in flicker perimetry: Standard and confidence limits. *Arch. Ophthal.* 80, *347*, (1968).

Yanoff, M., Rahn, E.K. & Zimmerman, L.E.: Histopathology of juvenile retinoschisis. *Arch. Ophthal.* 79, *49*, (1968).

Author's address:
Dept of Retina Research
Retina Foundation
20 Staniford Street
Boston, Mass. 02114
USA

THE SIGNIFICANCE OF THE DC-ERG IN HEREDITARY RETINAL DISEASE

M.H. FOERSTER

(Tübingen)

The DC-ERG of the human was first described by SACHS who, recorded it as early as 1928 with a cotton wick electrode and a string galvanometer attached to an amplifier. This caused severe technical problems of drift compensation. In order to bypass these difficulties the technique of the RC-coupled ERG with Ag/AgCl electrodes was developed for use in clinical practice. Since that time the ERP, A-, B- and C-wave, together with the OFF-response have been described experimentally and clinically. Most of the experiments were conducted with flash stimuli some with stimuli of longer duration.

The response to a flash stimulus is oscillatory in nature; the response to a longer stimulus is more in the direction of a steady-state.

Up to the ganglion cell level, every retinal cell reacts with slow intracellular potential changes. These are integrated and finally transformed at the axon hillock of the ganglion cell into an impulse code. The medium membrane potential controls the transmission in a given cell. This may be equally valid in a summed response.

If we use a square wave stimulus instead of a flash we are able to record the DC-component in the ERG. This was first described by Brown & Wiesel (1961) in the cat. Laters studies tried to link the OFF-response to the rod and conesystem, where rod dominated answers showed a negative and cone dominated answers showed a positive OFF-response.

The DC-Component depends on the level of adaptation. Kawasaki et al. (1972) saw a positive DC-component in the dark whereas, in light, no positive plateau was noted. In 1973, Knave & Nilsson described their method of DC-recording of the ERG. They used matched kalomel halfcells attached to electrolytebridges and a contact-glass receiving the potential. We use a similar setup with standardized electrodes to record the clinical ERG. The kalomel electrodes exhibit minimal drift and develop no polarization current. The light-stimulus is projected onto a 100 Dpt. Medical Workshop Contact Lens from which the Ag/AgCl-electrode has been removed and replaced by an electrolyte-bridge which is coupled to the recording kalomel-electrode. The indifferent electrode is on the forhead. The stimulus of 1 sec. duration could be varied by neutral density filters, 0 intensity being equal to about $14000 \, cd/m^2$. We have recorded the averages of 5 sweeps by means of a Mnemotron Cat 400 computer. The analysis time was 4 sec. A calibration signal is placed on the starting sweep. One eye was used to fixate on a dim red light.

Fig. 1a and 1b show a normal human DC-ERG at different lightintensities with dark and light background illumination (10 cd/m²). With dark backgrounds we see a positive plateau which increases with increasing light intensity. By further increasing the light intensity the DC-component returns to the base line and becomes negative. With a light background we only see a negative DC-potential. The C-wave which is fairly small because of the brevity of the light stimulus increases with increasing light intensity too. Note in fig. 1b that the intensity function of the DC-component and the OFF-response exhibit a different slope.

In fig. 2 we see the adaptation of the B-wave, the DC-potential and the OFF-response after preadaptation to 1400 cd/m² with a stimulus of 2 log. units above B-wave threshold in the dark. B-wave and DC-potential adaptation are running a somewhat similar course whereas the slope of the OFF-response is different again.

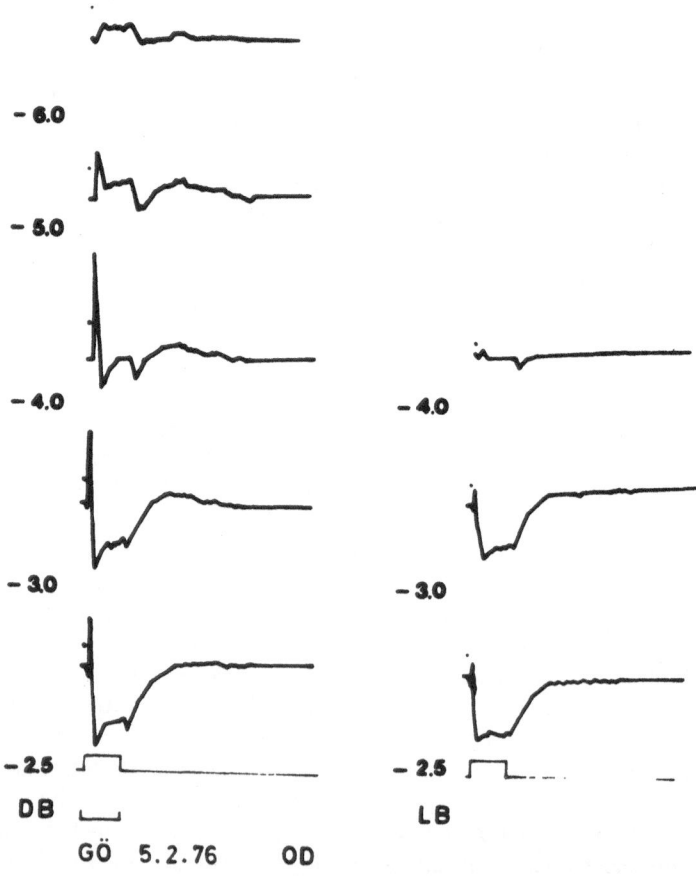

Fig. 1a. ERG of a normal human subject at different stimulus intensities with dark background left and light background right. Calibration signal at the beginning of each sweep 100 μv. Stimulus time 1 sec.

If one applies these data to the patients suffering from retinal disease one might be able to gain further information about retinal changes, since now we have A and B-waves including their latencies and implicit times, the DC-potential and the C-wave for judgement of the objective functional state.

Fig. 3 shows the ERG of a 52 year old patient with dominantly inherited retinopathia pigmentosa. The visual acuity is 0,6 OD, 0,7 OS. After dark adaptation for 1 hour we notice a positive DC-potential and an increasing B-wave. They are nevertheless decreased by 1/3. At intensity −2,6 there is no negative DC-potential as one would expect, but a positive waveform which further increases with light adaptaion. At intensity −2,0 with light background the most prominent feature is a negative DC-shift, which does not outlast the stimulus. An OFF-response is present only in the dark at low luminances. No C-wave is seen.

In summary in this case we find all waves decreased. The OFF-response is present only in the dark. In the light the DC-potential shift is markedly reduced and does not outlast the stimulus.

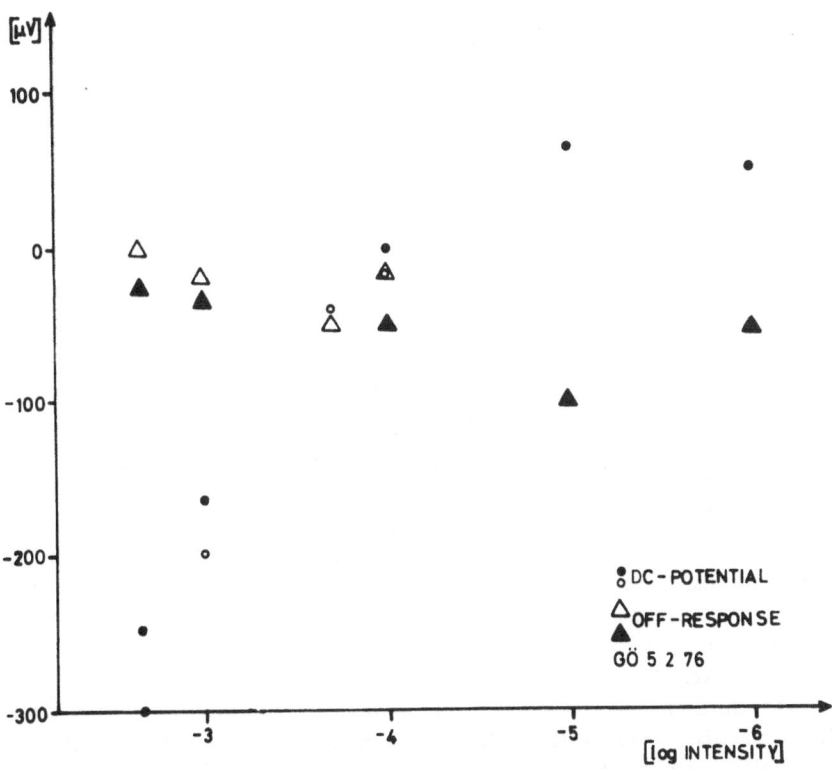

Fig. 1b. Intensity function of the DC-component and the OFF-response. Filled symbols at dark background illumination open symbols at light background illumination.

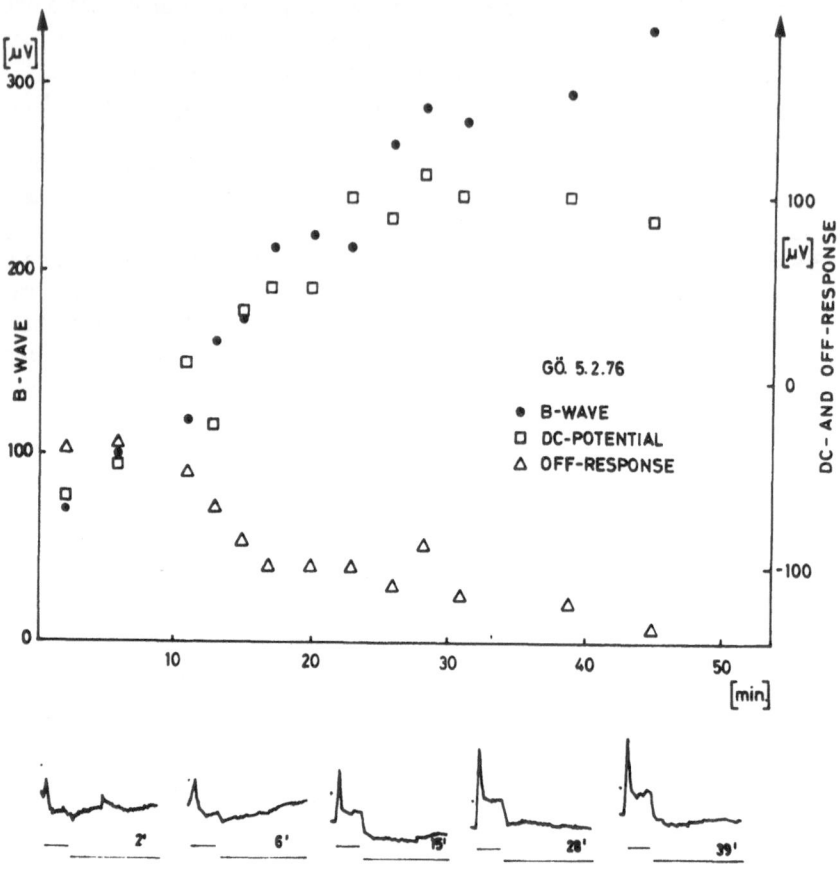

Fig. 2. Time course of the readaptation of the B-wave, the DC-component and the OFF-response after preadaptation to 1400 cd/m^2 in response to light stimuli of 1 sec. duration 2 log. units above B-wave threshold. Note the difference in the slope of the DC-component and the OFF-response.

In fig. 4 we see the ERG of a 9 year old boy with X-linked hereditary retinoschisis with macular involvement. Because of fixation problems there are lid and movement artefacts, in the last 3 sec. of the recording. The A-waves are normal in amplitude and the B-waves are reduced, especially with light backgrounds. The DC-potential reveals diminished values in the entire intensity range. In contrast to the former patient we see over the whole intensity range an OFF-response, which is negative at first and becomes positive at intensity −3,0. In intensities −3,6 and 3,0 we even recognize a C-wave.

The third case in fig. 5 is recorded from a 21 year old patient suffering from macular degeneration with large central scotomata together with peripheral tapetoretinal degeneration. Here again, A and B-waves are diminished at least 75% in light and dark background illumination. The DC-potential which is negative except for the uppermost record exhibits a photopic behaviour with no signs of adaptation. An OFF-response is present in all of

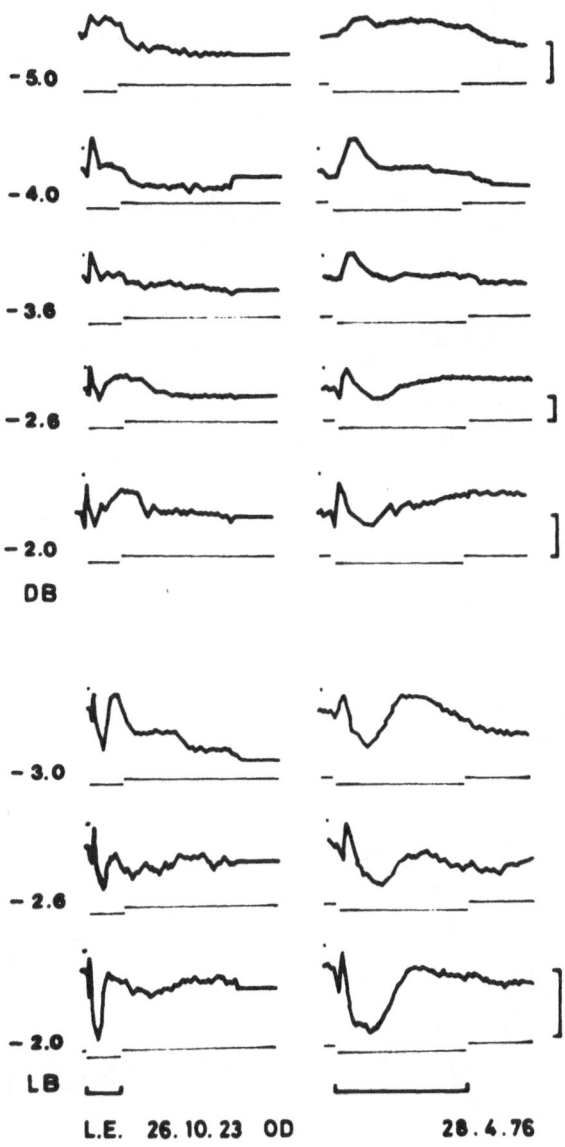

Fig. 3 ERG of 52 y. old patient with dominantly inherited retinopathia pigmentosa. On the right is the same recording as on the left at an enlarged scale. Vertical calibration 100 μv horizontal calibration 1 sec. Upper part with dark background, lower part with light background.

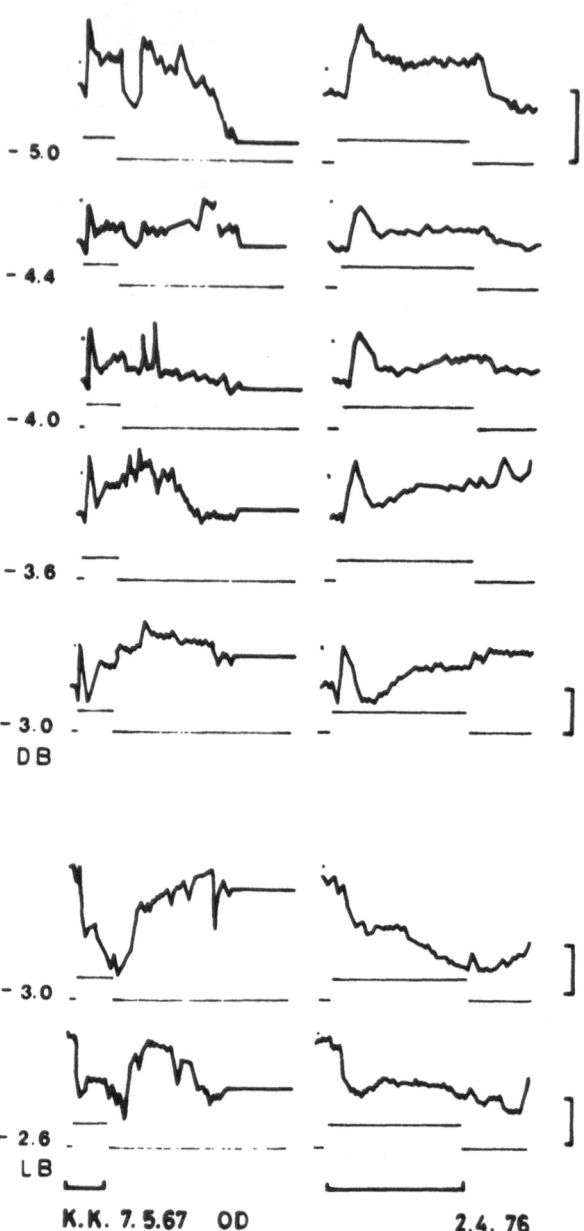

Fig. 4. DC-ERG of a 9 y. old boy with X-linked retinoschisis. Calibration same as in fig. 3. Because of fixation difficulties, there are blink and movement artefacts in the last 3 seconds of some traces.

190

the recordings. The C-wave is difficult to judge because of the fixation problems.

The recordings from a 22 year old patient with fundus flavimaculatus and macular dystrophy (fig. 6) showed normal A- and B-waves in the dark. The DC-potential increases and becomes negative. With light background A- and B-waves together with the C-potential are decreased. No C-wave could be recorded.

Fig. 7 shows the ERG of a 28 year old patient who complained of eye strain and dazzling. Ophtalmoscopy revealed defects in the pigment epi-

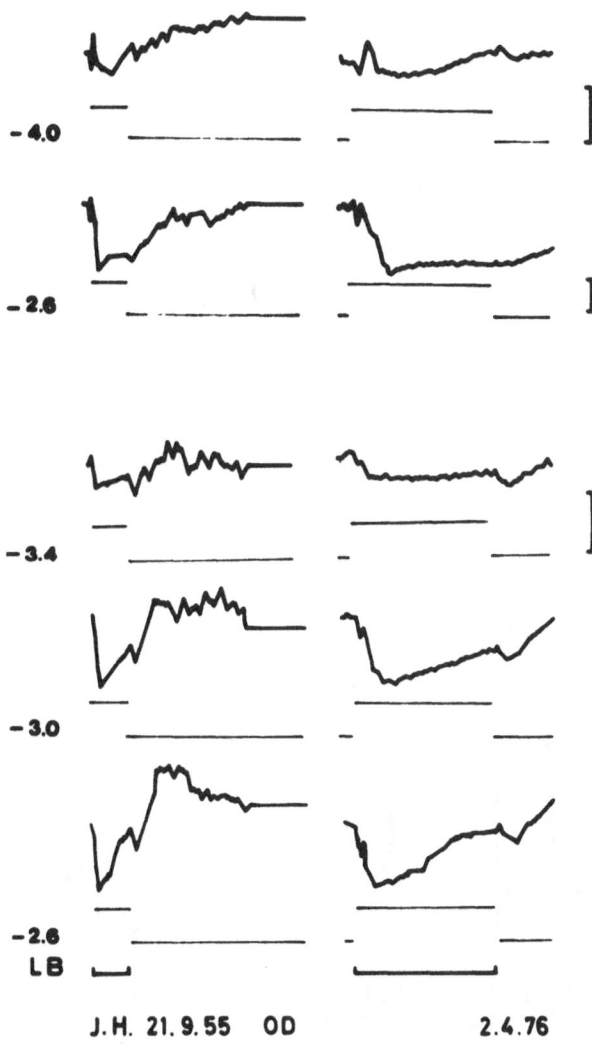

J. H. 21. 9. 55   OD   2.4.76

Fig. 5. DC-ERG of a 21 y. old male with tapetoretinal degeneration with macular involvement.

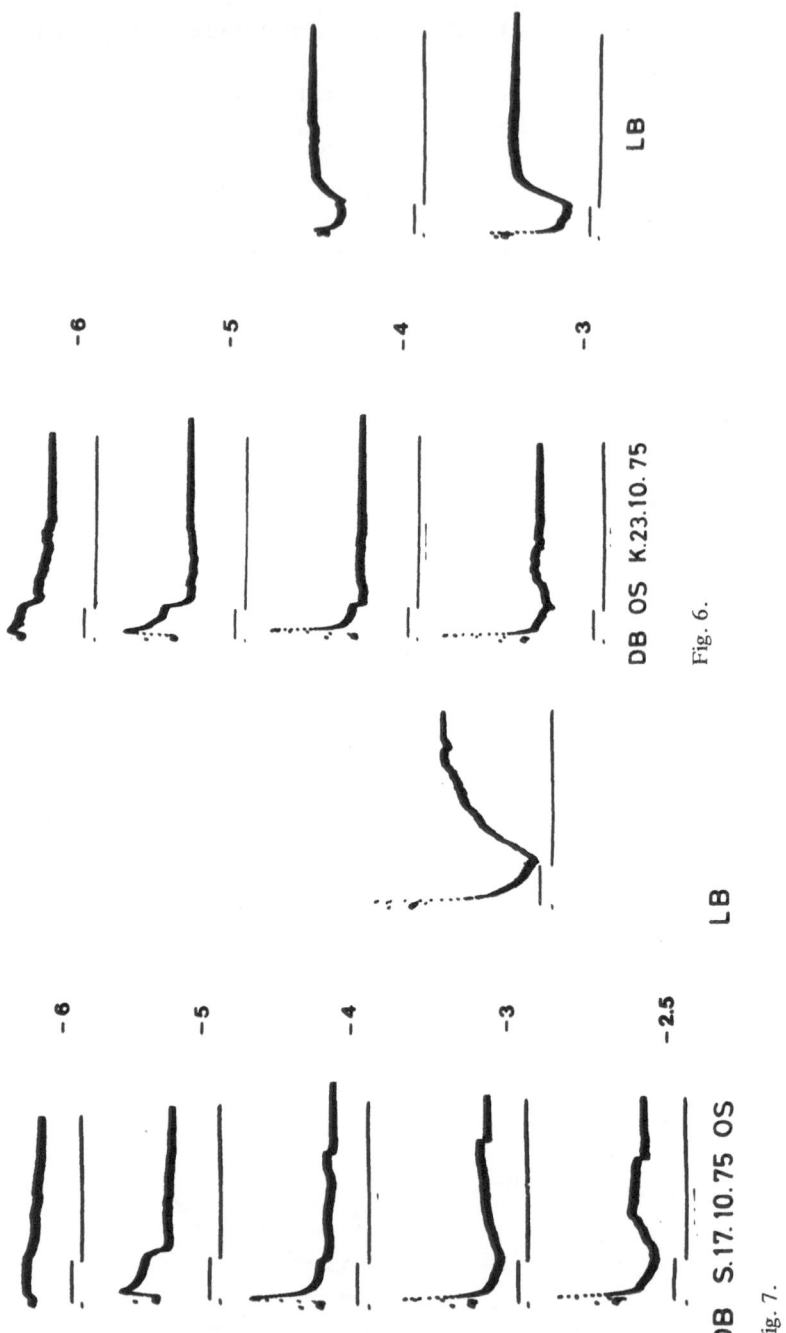

Fig. 6. DC-ERG of a 22 y. old male with fundus flavimaculatus. Note the missing of the C-wave even with the brightest light stimuli. Vertical calibration at left 100 μv and at right 30 μv at each starting sweep. Light stimuli of 1 sec. duration.

Fig. 7. DC-ERG of a 28 y. old male with pigment epitheliopathy. Vertical calibration 100 μv; light stimuli 1 sec.

thelium with intact choriocapillaris and relatively narrow retinal vessels. In darkness A- and B-waves and even the DC-potential are normal, but there is no C-wave at all. In the light adapted state A-wave, B-wave and the DC-potential are decreased. No C-wave can be noted.

These clinical cases allow one to draw the following conclusions: The DC-ERG provides an opportunity to record the known ERG components. With the DC-method we can simultaneously record the DC-component, the OFF-effect and the C-wave. These can all be recorded without undesirable polarization and driftpotentials. The DC-potential follows an intensity function from positive to negative with increasing light stimuli. The time course of adaptation with low luminance stimuli shows a parallel behaviour between B-wave and DC-potential over a fairly large range.

Up to date we have only qualitative experience with this method and no quantitative data are yet available. Nevertheless we hope that clinical application of this method might be judged useful for the following reasons: 1. It enables a steady state examination. 2. We can describe the adaptive behaviour of the retina. 3. We can record the intensity function of the DC-potential which reveals the dynamic range of the adaptation.

This might provide further clues regarding pathogenesis of retinal disease.

LITERATURE

Brown, K.T. Wiesel, T.N.: Analysis of the intraretinal electroretinogram in the intact cat eye. *J. Physiol.* 158, *229-256* (1961).

Kawasaki, K., Tsuchida, Y. & J.H. Jacobson: The direct current component of the electroretinogram in man. *Amer. J. Ophthalmol.* 73, *243-249* (1972).

Knave, B., Nilsson, S.E.G. & T. Lunt: The human electroretinogram: d.c. recordings at low and conventional stimulus intensities. Description of a new method for clinical use. *Acta ophthal.* (Kbh) 51, *716-726* (1973).

Sachs, E.: Die Aktionsströme des menschlichen Auges. *Klin. Wochenschrift* 8, *136*, (1929).

Author's address:
Universitäts-Augenklinik
Abt. für Pathophysiologie des Sehens
74 Tübingen
FR 9

STATISTICAL ANALYSIS OF ERG AMPLITUDE AND WAVEFORM ABNORMALITIES IN MACULAR DEGENERATION

RICHARD SREBRO

(Buffalo, N.Y.)

Several previous studies have suggested that the dark adapted electroretino-gram (ERG) may be abnormal in patients with macular degeneration (Krill, 1966; Merin & Auerbach, 1970; Orpin, Orpin & McCulloch, 1974; Ruede-mann, 1966; Jacobson, Najae, Stephens, Kara & Gideon, 1960; Jayle, Boyer & Dubert, 1959; Niemeyer, 1969; Ruedemann & Noell, 1961; Henkes, 1956). Two types of abnormality have been reported: a reduction in the overall amplitude of all ERG components, and (Merin & Auerbach, 1970) a 'slowing' of the a-wave. However, a critical examination of these reports raises some questions concerning the validity and interpretation of the findings. First, many of the reports are based on a more or less casual or 'by eye' comparison between relatively small numbers of ERG records from patients with macular degeneration and normals and lack adequate statistical tests. Second, the effect of age on the ERG has often been ignored in making comparisons. Third, the extent of the lesion observed ophthalmoscopically has not been carefully correlated to ERG findings. Since, it appears that ophthalmoloscopically visible abnormalities less than 3 disc diameters in extent usually do not produce ERG abnormalities (Jacobson, Najae, Stephens, Kara & Gideon, 1960; François & DeRouck, 1966; Ponte, 1961) this correlation is important. Finally, the considerable variability in ERG waveform from patient to patient has not received adequate attention.

The purpose of this study is to compare dark adapted ERGs from patients with macular degeneration with ERGs from normals in a quantitive way which considers the factors listed above and which allows statistical testing. The study was done in the hope that such a comparison may help to develop an understanding of the pathophysiology of macular degeneration. Although the study is limited to the dark adapted ERG, it is appreciated that several other types of ERG tests (such as light adaptation, flicker responses, and spectral analysis) may also be useful. The restriction to dark adapted ERGs reflects the data currently available to me.

METHODS

The data is based on ERG records taken from over 750 patients at E.J. Meyer Memorial Hospital, Buffalo, N.Y. during the period 1967-1975. The testing facility was established by Prof. W.K. Noell, and patients

195

were examined by virtually the same technique and by one technician during this period. The recording technique follows that of Ruedemann and Noell (1968) exactly. It includes full cycloplegia and dilitation, a clear modified Karpe contact lens, a wide (0.1 to 2000 Hz) bandpass for pre-amplification, and photographic recording of the ERGs from an oscilloscope trace. Both eyes are done simultaneously. A Grass photic stimulator provides a brief white light flash. The records analyzed in this study were those taken after 15 minutes of dark adaptation.

All ERG records were converted to digital form from photographic records using a laboratory computer and a specially developed device that permitted semiautomatic analog to digital conversion. The effective analog to digital conversion rate was 500 Hz. Each ERG record consisted of the first 100 msecs following the flash and was stored on digital magnetic tapes along with identifying information (age, diagnosis etc.). The tape 'library' could be scanned by the computer to select those particular records needed for the analysis.

In order to be designated as a 'normal' a best corrected vision of 20/25 (Snellen) or better was required and no significant anterior segment, lens, or fundus abnormalities were permitted. Modest lens changes occasional drusen in older patient, and 'bear track' markings were not considered significant abnormalities. A total of 285 eyes met the criteria for normal and were derived from the following sources: volunteers, patients being evaluated for 'dyslexia', and the fellow eye of a patient with unilateral disease, usually trauma or strabismic amblyopia.

These eyes classified as having macular degeneration had a best corrected visual acuity no better than 20/30, and the vast majority had much worse visual acuity. The macular degeneration group was subdivided into several sub-catagories: (1) probable macular degeneration (irregularity of pigment epithelium confined to the macular region, 74 eyes), (2) dry macular degeneration less than 3 disc diameters in extent (definite pigment clumping, atrophy, macular holes or cysts confined to the macular region, 112 eyes). (3) dry macular degeneration greater than 3 disc diameters in extent (as in 2 but larger area of visible lesions, or macular lesions associated with more widespread changes such as extensive drusen, patchy chorioretinal atrophy, extensive choroidal sclerosis, or angoid streaks, 50 eyes), (4) disciform macular degeneration less than 3 disc diameters in extent (presence of a localized sub-retinal or sub-pigment epithelial hemorrhage or detachment, 14 eyes). (There were too few eyes with disciform macular degeneration and associated widespread retinal abnormalities to analyze).

Measurements of ERG records were done by computer. The a-wave amplitude was measured from the baseline to the a-wave minimum voltage. The b-wave amplitude was measured from the a-wave minimum to the b-wave maximum. ERG waveforms were analyzed in two ways. The first method, a qualitative one, was to construct an average waveform for each diagnostic category. To avoid bias due to ERG amplitude, each ERG record was first area normalized, and then all ERGs within a single diagnostic category were averaged across patients. The second method was quantitative and consisted of a 3 factor analysis of variance. The 3 factors used were time after onset of light flash, diagnostic category, and age. The analysis of variance technique is well described in several texts (Lindquist, 1953; Brunnig & Kintz, 1968) and permitted a quantitive comparison of waveform. An F test was used to decide if there was an effect of diagnostic category on ERG waveform.

RESULTS

ERGs from normal subjects had a mean a-wave amplitude of 250 uvolts (250×10^{-6} volts) and a standard deviation of 61 uvolts, and a mean b-wave

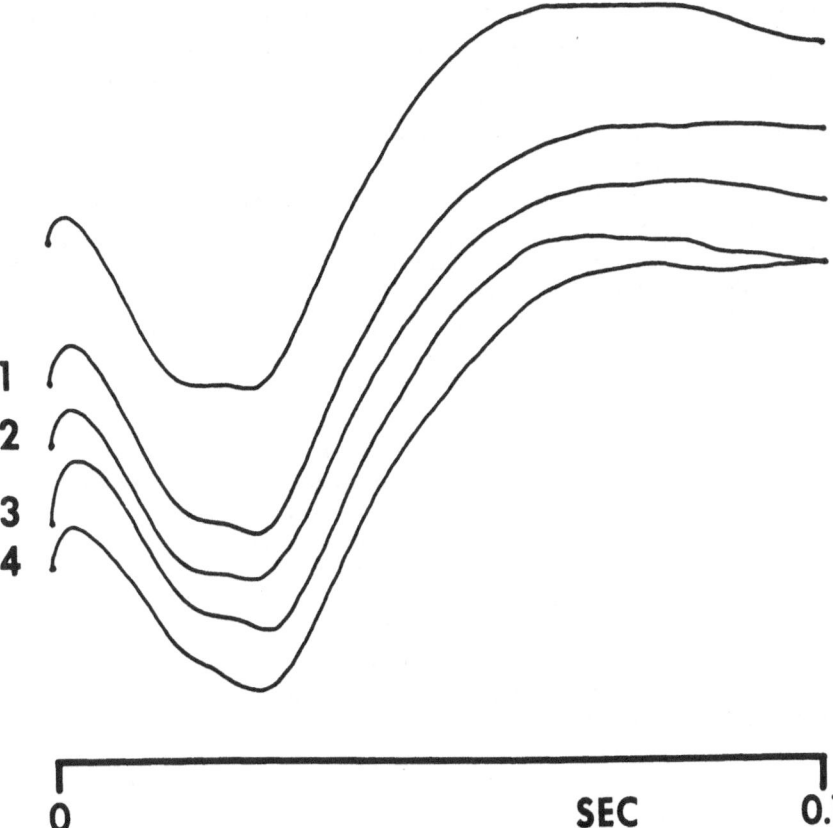

Fig. 1. Average normalized dark adapted ERGs for normal subjects and for 4 sub-categories of macular degeneration. Each record shows 100 msecs following a 10 usec flash of white light synchronous with the start of the record. The top most record is for a population of 285 normals. The number to the left of each record desingnates the sub-categories: (1) probable macular degeneration, (2) dry macular degeneration less than 3 disc diameters in extent, (3) dry macular degeneration greater than 3 disc diameters in extent, (4) disciform macular degeneration less than 3 disc diameters in extent. (See text for further description of the sub-categories). Averaging was done across patients in each sub-category. The initial sharp downward deflection and subsequent recovery (lating 4-5 msecs) is a flash artifact.

197

amplitude of 527 uvolts and a standard deviation of 112 uvolts. However, there was a significant effect of age on ERG component amplitude. The mean a-wave amplitude fell from 266 uvolts in subjects under 10 years of age to 225 uvolts in subjects 60 or more years old. The mean b-wave amplitude fell from 560 uvolts to 461 uvolts in the same age span. This confirms a previous report (Peterson, 1968).

A two factor (time after flash and age) analysis of variance of area normalized ERGs showed a significant age dependent affect on waveform within the normal category ($F = 3.6$ degrees of freedom 210 by 10,080). An examination of average ERG waveforms in normals taken seperately by age in decades suggested that the systematic waveform change consists of a decrease in the slope of both the initial phase of the a-wave and b-wave rise, and a delay in the minimum of the a-wave potential with increasing age.

When appropriate corrections for the generally unequal age distributions of the normal subjects and each diagnostic sub-category of macular degeneration was made, only one sub-category of the macular degeneration group showed significant abnormalities in either the a-wave or b-wave amplitude. This was the sub-category of dry macular degeneration greater than 3 disc diameters in extent. The mean a-wave amplitude for this group was 179 uvolts (age corrected expected normal 245 uvolts) and the mean b-wave amplitude was 376 uvolts (age corrected expected normal 517 uvolts). These differences from the normal age corrected expected values were significant at the 1% level of the t test.

A three factor (time after flash, age, diagnostic category), analysis of variance of area normalized ERGs, however, showed a significant waveform difference between every sub-category of macular degeneration and normal at the 1% level of the F test. (In contrast, no significant waveform differences were found between normals and either strabismic amblyopia, or visual acuity loss of unknown eitiology using the same technique).

Fig. 1 shows the average ERG waveforms for the normals and for each sub-category of macular degeneration. Note particularly the progressive decrease in slope of the initial portion of the a-wave and delay in the time to reach the minimum a-wave voltage (a-wave implicit time) in sub-categories 1, 2, and 3 which represent increasing severity of dry macular degeneration.

DISCUSSION

The results presented here suggest that there is no significant reduction in the component amplitudes of the dark adapted ERG in macular degeneration unless the ophthalmoloscopically visible lesion is larger than 3 disc diameters in extent or is associated with widespread retinal abnormalities visible on ophthalmoscopy. This finding argues against the hypothesis that macular degeneration is the 'tip of an iceberg', that is that even though lesions may appear to be localized to the macula region, a much wider retinal degeneration may be present. It does *not*, however, disprove the hypothesis, since more sensitive tests than the ERG may disclose a more widespread retinal disease, nor does it preclude the possibility that the natural history of the disease involves a spread of the degeneration, initially confined to the macula, to more perpheral retinal regions.

In striking contrast to the results concerning the ERG component amplitude, the data presented here confirm an ERG waveform change in all sub-categories of macular degeneration similar to those reported by Ruedemann and Noell (1961). As Fig. 1 shows these waveform changes are subtle and further analysis shows that any attempt to diagnose macular degeneration entirely on the basis of a single dark adapted ERG record is unreliable. However, the nature of the ERG waveform changes are intriguing because they imply a selective loss of faster components. Such a loss could come about in several ways. (1) There may be a selective loss of cones in the retina. (2) The non-uniform light distribution produced by stroboscopic stimulation thru a clear contact lens may selectively stimulate the central retinal, cone rich, region of the retina and exaggerate its contribution to the ERG. A degeneration of central retinal receptors would then produce waveform changes that simulate a selective loss of cones even though *no* selection between rods and cones occurred at a biological level. (3) Macular degeneration may represent a widespread retinal disease which although not completely destroying retinal cells (except perhaps at the macula) affects the time-course of their individual responses. Clearly further work and the development of more discriminating tests will be required to decide the issue.

ACKNOWLEDGEMENTS

I wish to thank Mrs. Dorothy Bechtold who accomplished all ERG recordings with meticulous care over the 8 year period of this study.

I also wish to thank Dr. Seymour Axelrod, Dept. of Psychiatry, S.U.N.Y. Buffalo, for his helpful suggestions concerning the statistical analysis of the data.

And, finally, I wish to thank Dr. W.K. Noell who developed the ERG testing facility, devised the protocol an directed the operation of the facility during the period in which the data was collected.

BIBLIOGRAPHY

Bruning, J.L. & Kintz, B.L.: Computational handbook of statistics. Scott, Foresman Company, Glenview, Ill. 1968.

Francois, J. & DeRouck, A.: Behavior of ERG and EOG in localized retinal destruction by photocoagulation. Proceedings of the Third I.S.C.E.R.G. Symposium, Supp. Vision Research (1966).

Henkes, H.F.: Electroretinography in circulatery disturbances of the retina. *Arch. Ophthal.* 51, *54* (1956).

Jacobson, J.H., Najae, H., Stephens, G., Kara, G.B. & Gideon, F.G.: The role of the macular in the electroretinogram of monkey and man. *Amer. J. Ophthal.* 50, *889* (1960).

Jayle, G.E., Boyer, R. & Dubert, L.: Etude de differents test functionnels electro-retinographiques dans la degenerescence maculaire senile grave. *Ann. D'Oculistique* 192, *36* (1959).

Krill, A.E.: The electroretinographic and electrooculographic findings in patients with macular lesions. *Trans. Amer. Acad. Ophthal. and Otol.* 70, *1063* (1966).

Lindquist, E.F.: Design and analysis of experiments in psycholgy and education. Houghton Mifflin Company, Boston, Mas. (1953).

Merin, S. & Auerbach, E.: The central and peripheral retina in macular degenerations. *Arch. Ophthal.* 48, *710* (1970).

Niemeyer, G.: Elektroretinographie bei maculadegenerationen. *Graefes Arch. klin. exp. Ophthal.* 177, *39*, (1969).

Orpin, J., Orpin, E. & McCulloch, C.: The electroretinogram in macular degeneration. *Canad. J. Ophthal.* 9, *214* (1974).

Peterson, H.: The normal 8-potential in the single-flash clinical electroretinogram. *Acta Ophthal. Supp.* 99, (1968).

Ponte, F.: Electroretinography in solar macular injury. *Acta Ophthal. Supp.* 70, *238* (1961).

Ruedemann, A.D. Jr. & Noell, W.K.: The electroretinogram in central retinal degeneration. *Tr. Amer. Acad. Ophthal. and Otol.* 65, *576* (1961).

Ruedemann, A.D, Jr.: The ERG in hereditary central retinal degeneration or heredo-macular disease. *Amer. J. Ophthal.* 61, *240* (1966).

Author's address:
2211 Main Street
Buffalo, N.Y. 14214
USA

SOME CHARACTERISTICS OF THE ELECTRORETINOGRAM
IN HEREDITARY RETINAL PIGMENTARY DYSTROPHY.
I. THE CORRELATION OF RECORDABILITY BY SINGLE STIMULUS
AND MODE OF INHERITANCE*

N. OHBA, T. TANINO & K. OMOTO

(Tokyo)

ABSTRACT

Single-stimulus electroretinograms were recorded in dark adapted condition from patients with heriditary retinal pigmentary dystrophy of diffuse type. Responses were recordable from 27.6% of 123 patients. The recordability was significantly dependent upon the mode of inheritance: 59.4% of 32 patients with autosomal dominant inheritance showed recordable responses, whereas only 16.4% of 91 patients with autosomal recessive inheritance revealed detectable responses. An hypothesis seems valid that progression in autosomal dominant form is much slower than autosomal recessive form.

INTRODUCTION

Single-stimulus electroretinogram (ERG) in primary retinal pigmentary dystrophy (i.e. retinitis pigmentosa) is conventionally classified into recordable and non recordable type, and it is well known that the majority of patients shows non-recordable responses and only small number of patients reveal detectable but reduced responses (Franceschetti, Prançois & Babel, 1974; Imaizumi, 1969). It is important to understand what clinical aspects are responsible for the recordability. According to the previous investigations, patients with recordable ERG responses are in a less advanced state of retinal dystrophy, and it has also been suggested that patients with autosomal dominant inheritance are more frequently recordable than those with autosomal recessive inheritance (Franceschetti et al., 1974). The purpose of this paper is to test the hypothesis that the detectability of the ERG responses in primary retinal pigmentary dystrophy is dependent upon its mode of inheritance.

METHOD

One hundred twenty three patients were used with the typical clinical picture of diffuse pigmentary dystrophy of the retina, and the diagnosis was made by integral studies with fundus examinations, functional examinations (visual fields, dark adaptation, color vision etc.) and family investigations.

* This work was supported by a research grant for retinitis pigmentosa from the Japanese Department of Health and Welfare.

Atypical forms of pigmentary dystrophy, e.g. sectorial, pericentral form, other clinical entities of tapetoretinal dystrophy and secondary retinal degeneration were carefully excluded from the study.

The mode of inheriance was determined by assessing the pattern of the pedgree chart obtained by detailed family studies in each patient. Of the 123 patients, 32 patients were from 12 families with autosomal dominant mode, and 91 patients were from 84 families with autosomal recessive mode.

Single-stimulus ERGs were recorded by a ganzfeld white test flash in a fully dark adapted condition. The stimulus was produced with a Xenon photoflash tube (Nihonkohde, Tokyo MSP-2, 80 joule). The flash was led through a combination of convexing lens and glass fiber optics into a small integrating sphere, which produced a uniform stimulation of the entire retina. The ERG responses were picked up by a lo-vac contact lens electrode (Medical Workshop, Holland) and were amplified by an AC coupled preamplifier with a time constant of 0.1 seconds and displayed on an oscilloscope (Nihonkohden VC-7, Tokyo). Attempts were made in each patient, in a fully dark adapted condition with a fully dilated pupil by two drops of tropicamide, to observe whether or not responses could be recorded by use of the strongest available flash stimulus. Several recordings were superimposed with suitable amplification on the oscilloscope in order to facilitate the determination of the responses.

Ten normal subjects participated for a control study.

RESULTS AND COMMENT

ERG responses elicited by single flash in the white ganzfeld under fully dark adapted condition were abnormal in all patients. With the brightest stimulus, in normal subjects, recorded responses were for the a-wave (310-410 μV, N = 10) and for the b-wave (445-560 μV) accompanied by oscillatory potentials. 27.6% of 123 patients revealed abnormally reduced but measurable responses, while 72.4% did not show any detectable responses (Table 1). This rate of detectability is similar to previous studies (Imaizumi, 1969; Franceschetti et al., 1974).

It was of interest in the present studies that the detectability varied significantly with the mode of inheritance: 59.4% of 32 patients belonging to 12 autosomal dominant families revealed responses, whereas only 16.4% of 91 patients with autosomal recessive form revealed responses. These findings confirm the previous suggestions (Krill et al., 1959; Botermans, 1972; Franceschetti et al., 1974) and lead to a view that ERG responses are in general more frequently recordable in autosomal dominant disease than in autosomal recessive disease.

How different is the dominant disease from the recessive disease? In our view, the two diseases are essentially different in that the dystrophy progresses more slowly in the dominant form as compared with the recessive form. This view is based on our recent observations of 50 patients with the dominant form and 150 patients with the recessive form that the disease onset as evaluated by recognition of night blindness showed a different

Table I. Electroretinograms in hereditary retinal pigmentary dystrophy*

Mode of inheritance		Recordable	Non-recordable	(total)
Autosomal dominant		19	13	32
Autosomal recessive		15	76	91
	(total)	34	89	123

* Cases with widespread dystrophy
Single white ganzfeld stimulus in dark

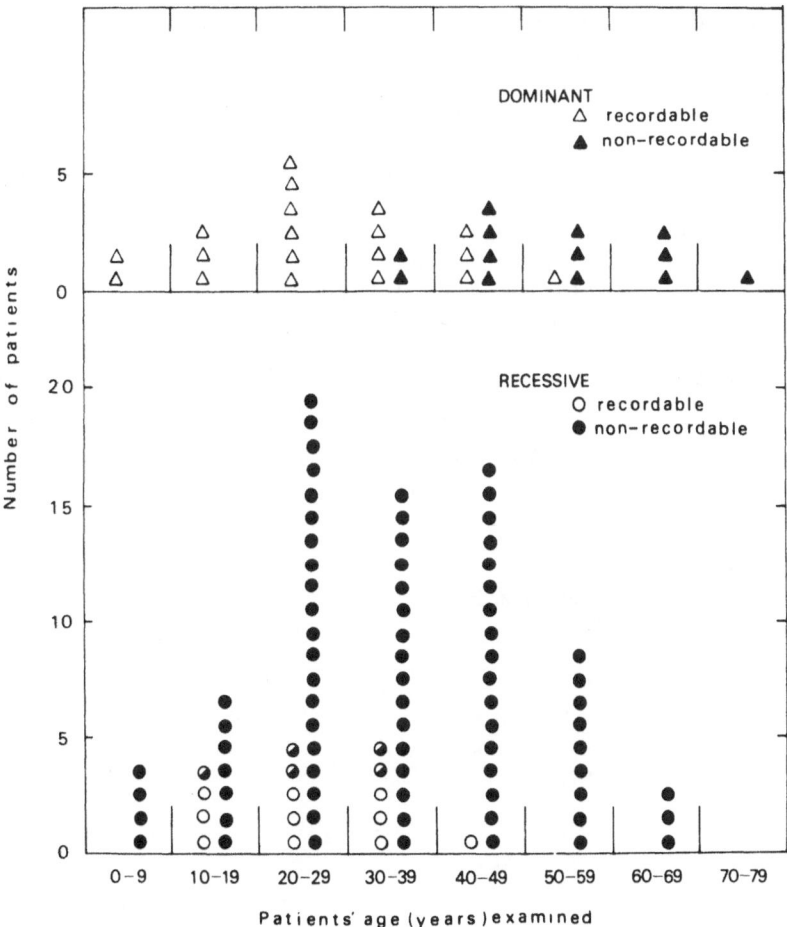

Fig. 1. Recordability of single-stimulus electroretinograms in fully dark adapted condition in patients with primary retinal pigmentary dystrophy. Upper part represents patients with autosomal dominant inheritance and lower part patients with autosomal recessive inheritance. Abscissa: patients' age at the time of examinations; Ordinate: number of patients. Open symbols: recordable cases; closed symbols: non-recordable cases. Semi-closed symbols: negative type responses.

203

distribution function in the two forms. And the degree of the disease, when compared each other of the same age group, revealed a more advanced state of retinal dystrophy in the recessive form (Tanino & Ohba, 1976). The present results showed that the detectability of ERG responses decreased with the age of the patients; but, as is seen in Figure 1, the time course was different in the two diseases. These findings support our view, since detectability of ERG responses no doubt indicates an earlier stage of retinal dystrophy (Ohba, Tanino & Omoto, 1976).

In conclusion, we believe in the validity of the hypothesis that autosomal dominant disease is relatively benign as compared with autosomal recessive disease. This view is of practical importance. It is, however, to be stressed that the view has been obtained from statistical observations: the speed of advancement of retinal dystrophy is variable among individual patients in each class of inheritance.

REFERENCES

Botermans, C.H.G.: Primary pigmentary retinal degeneration and its association with neurological diseases. In: Handbook of Clinical Neurology, vol. 13: 148-379. North-Holland Publ. Co., Amsterdam, (1972).

Franceschetti, A., François, J. & Babel, J.: Chorioretinal Heredodegenerations, pp. 176-180. Charles C. Thomas, Springfield, (1974).

Imaizumi, K.: Electrophysiological study of retinitis pigmentosa. *Acta Soc. Ophthalmol. Jap.*, 73, *2347-2487*, (1969).

Krill, A.E. & Iser, G.: The value of electroretinography in the diagnosis of pigmentary degenerations of the retina. *Amer. J. Ophthalmol.*, 47, *649-656*, (1959).

Ohba, N., Tanino, T. & Omoto, K.: this proceeding.

Tanino, T. & Ohba, N.: On the onset of hereditary retinal pigmentary dystrophy. *Jap. J. Ophthalmol.* in press, (1976).

Authors' address:
Dept of Opthalmology
University of Tokyo School of Medicine
Hongo 7-3-1, Bunkyo-ku
Tokyo 113
Japan

ONCE MORE: DOES UNILATERAL RETINITIS PIGMENTOSA REALLY EXIST?

HAROLD E. HENKES

(Rotterdam)

At the 3rd ISCERG-Symposium held in October 1964, I discussed 5 cases of unilateral retinitis pigmentosa, all fitting the criteria drawn up by France-schetti, François & Babel in 1963, viz.

1. Exclusion of inflammatory origin of the affection, in particular of syphilis or viral diseases.

2. Presence in the affected eye of symptoms typical for primary pigmentary degeneration - including the sine pigmento-type.

3. Absence in the fellow eye of symptoms of tapetoretinal dystrophy with the presence of a normal electroretinographic response.

However, in three of the patients the EOG-lightrise of the fellow eye was subnormal suggesting the probability of an abortive bilateral retinitis pigmentosa.

For this reason I added a fourth criterion, viz. a normal EOG-lightrise in the fellow eye. Based upon these criteria, only one case of the five cases described, was to be accepted as a genuine unilateral retinitis pigmentosa. I suggested at that time, that a genuine unilateral retinitis pigmentosa was probably extreemly rare, as opposed to the more common abortive bilateral retinitis pigmentosa. Four of the 5 patients could be reexamined after a period of 11 years. One patient (case number 4) had died.

Case 1: Mr. C. de J., born 1925, at the time (1964) diagnosed as suffering from a unilateral retinitis pigmentosa of the right eye. Based upon a deteriorating EOG-lightrise, the diagnosis in 1964 was changed into an abortive form of bilateral peripheral tapetoretinal dystrophy.

In 1976, visual acuity and fundus picture of the left eye were found to be normal. The fundus picture of the affected right eye showed a 'classical' pigmentary degeneration, more pronounced than at the examinations reported earlier. Neither a dark adaptation test nor electro-diagnostic tests could be performed in 1976, but 5 years earlier, in 1971 the scotopic and photopic ERG of the fellow eye showed normal values. The EOG-lightrise however, showed in 1971 a higher value than was reported in 1964 when the light/dark-ratio was clearly subnormal. The EOG-lightrise in 1971 fell just outside the normal range (LP/DT-ratio: 1.78).

In 1964 we felt rather sure that we were dealing with an abortive form of pigmentary dystrophy - which conviction was largely based upon the subnormal lightrise of the fellow eye registered at that time. At this moment we

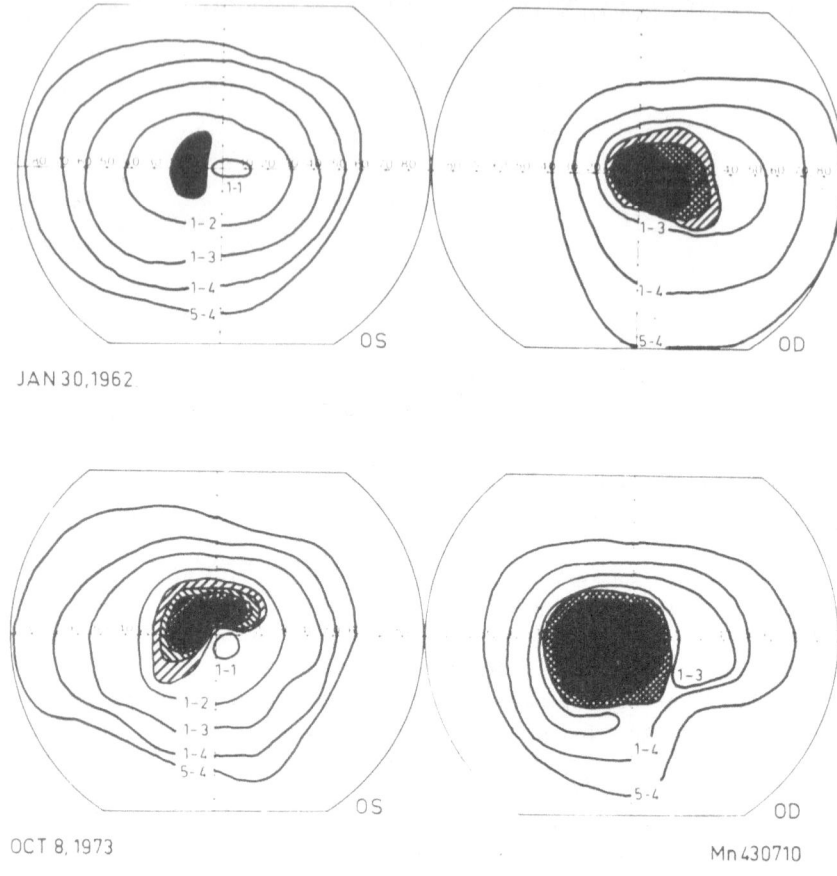

JAN 30, 1962

OCT 8, 1973

Mn 430710

Fig. 1. Case number 2. Abortive bilateral inverse retinitis pigmentosa. In 1962 a centrocoecal scotoma in the earlier affected right eye was found, together with a doubtful enlargement of the blind spot in the fellow eye. The latter had developed into a pericentral scotoma in 1973.

are not too sure this assumption was justified. As no further data are available, due to the patient's refusal to submit himself to electrodiagnostic tests, only time will tell whether we are indeed dealing with a genuine case of unilateral peripheral retinitis pigmentosa of the right eye.

Case 2: P.M., male, born 1943. Since the time of publication (1964), visual acuity of the so-called 'normal' left eye deteriorated from 1.0 to 0.2. The para-central and peripapillary retina of the fellow eye had clearly changed, showing the same atrophic aspect as was reported earlier in the first affected, right eye. The peripheral retina of both eyes, however, was still normal in 1976. A pericentral scotoma was found in both eyes (figure 1). In 1973, the scotoma in the fellow eye was still less outspoken than the massive centro-coecal scotoma recorded in the affected right eye.

206

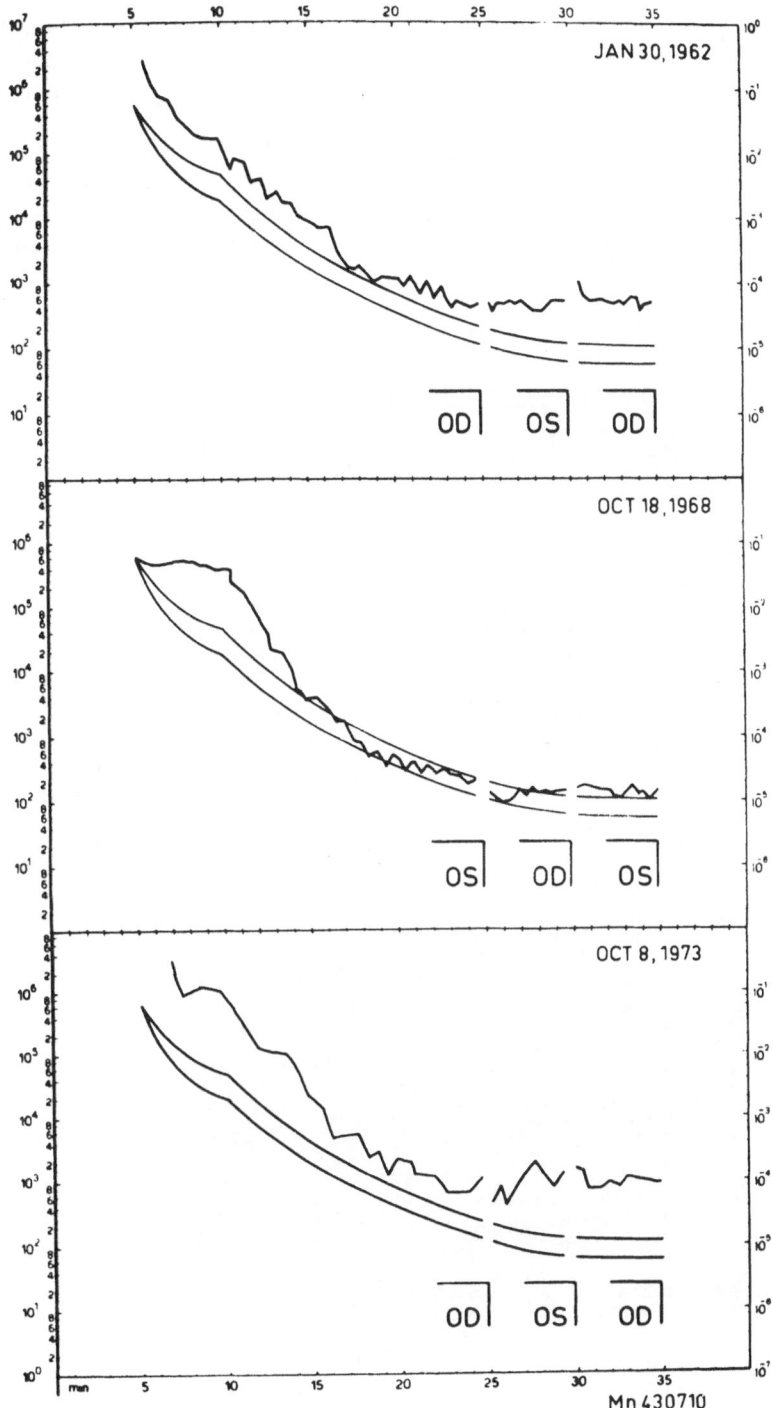

Fig. 2. Case number 2. Dark adaptation is only slightly affected due to still reasonable function of peripheral retina.

207

In comparison with the 1962-registration, the final rod threshold in the dark adaptation test of 1973 had not changed significantly. Due to the still reasonable function of the retinal periphery, the curve deviated not too much from the standard curve (figure 2).

Electrodiagnostic tests were repeated in 1973. Electroretinography revealed a marked deterioration of the electric responses of both retinae, though more outspoken in the grossly affected right eye. The EOG-lightrise as compared to the data found in 1964 had not changed significantly:

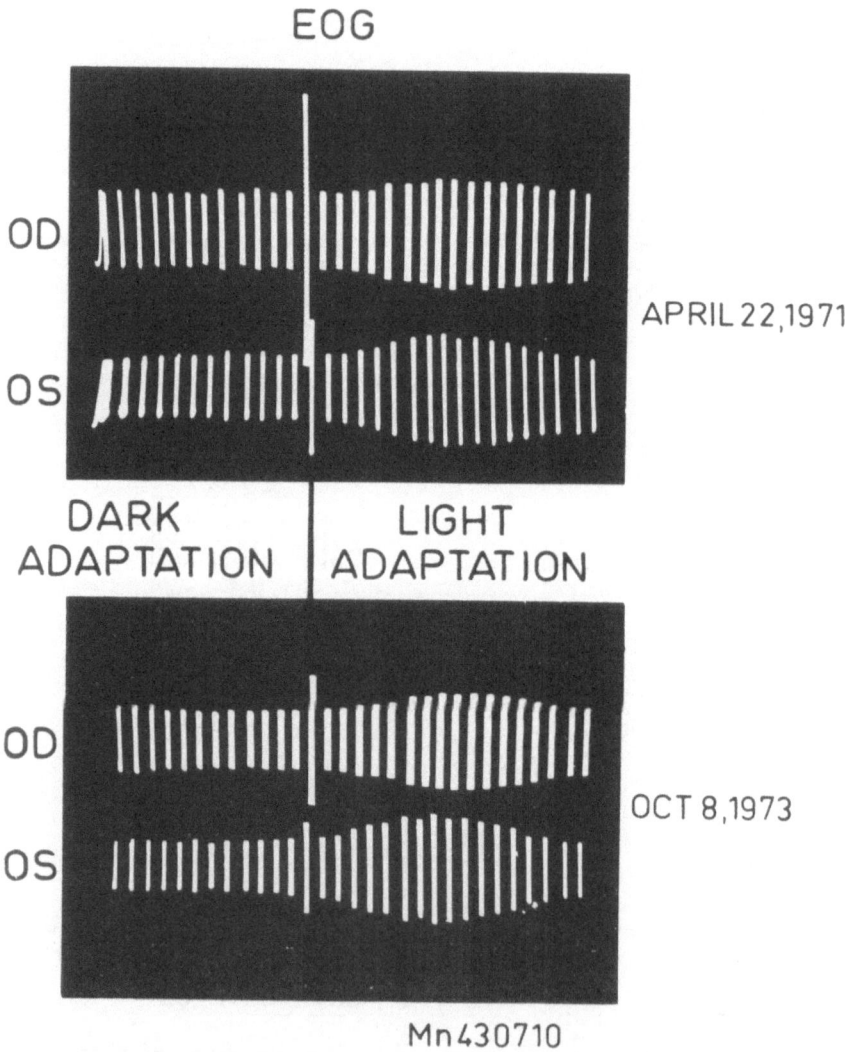

Fig. 3. Case number 2. EOG-lightrise is subnormal in the earlier affected right eye and still normal in the fellow eye.

subnormal in the right eye (1.65) and still normal in the left eye (2.11) (figure 3).

On account of the electroretinographic data and the fundus picture we can only corroborate the diagnosis of 1964, viz. bilateral pericentral (inverse) retinitis pigmentosa.

Case 3: L.L., male, born 1927. In 1964 a tentative diagnosis of unilateral peripheral tapetoretinal dystrophy of the left eye was considered doubtful on account of the subnormal EOG-lightrise of 1.57, found in the normal right eye, although the other retinal functions were at the time normal. Re-examination was done 5 years later; retinal functions were then normal,

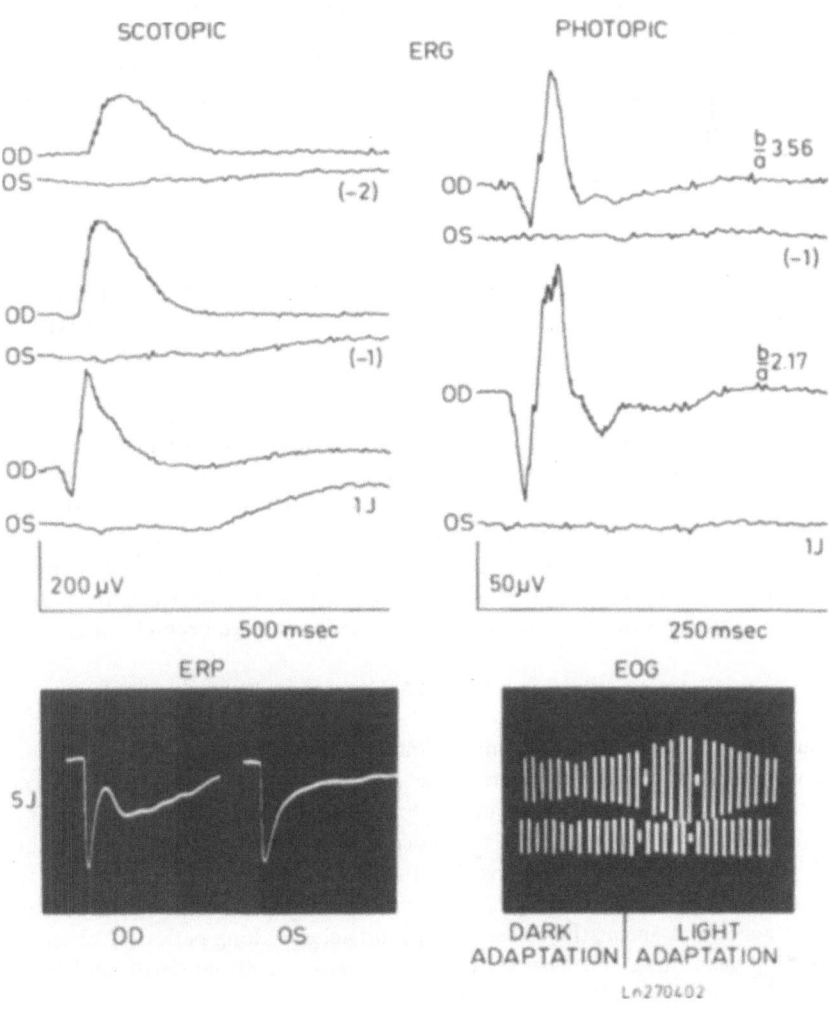

Fig. 4. Case number 3. Peripheral unilateral retinitis pigmentosa of the left eye. Normal electric responses of the right eye.

including a normal EOG-lightrise (1.82). In 1976 the patient was examined again; the findings of 1969 could be confirmed. The LP/DT-ratio was normal (2.05). A normal ERP was registered too (figure 4).

In conclusion: in this case we have to reject our previous assumption of an abortive bilateral retinitis pigmentosa. It is most probable that the case under consideration is one of unilateral retinitis pigmentosa of the peripheral type.

Case 5: J.v.O., male, born 1947, suffers from a unilateral pericentral retinitis pigmentosa of the right eye. In 1964 genuine unilateral retinitis pigmentosa, was the most likely diagnosis.

The patient was re-examined in 1976 but refused an electrodiagnostic test, which procedure was performed for the last time in 1969. At that time, retinal functions of the fellow eye, both subjective and objective, showed normal results. The EOG-lightrise in the fellow eye amounted to 2.32. In 1976 visual acuity, visual fields and fundus picture of the left eye were normal. We feel pretty sure that this case may be considered to represent a genuine case of unilateral pericentral retinitis pigmentosa.

DISCUSSION

Of the five unilateral cases of retinitis pigmentosa reported in 1964, the fellow eyes at that time fitted the criteria set by Franceschetti, François & Babel. However, in three the suggested additional fourth criterion, viz. a normal EOG-lightrise, was not fulfilled. Based upon this criterion, only one case (case nr. 5) was considered to represent a genuine unilateral retinitis pigmentosa. 4 of the 5 patients could be re-examined after a period of 11 years. In contradistinction to expectation, only in one of the 4 patients (case nr. 2) the diagnosis: abortive bilateral retinitis pigmentosa was established with a reasonable amount of certainty. Of the 3 patients left, the existence of a genuine unilateral retinitis pigmentosa is most likely in two subjects (nrs. 3 and 5) whereas this diagnosis in subject nr. 1 is highly probable. A safe period of observation however, necessary for a certified diagnosis of unilateral retinitis pigmentosa, may still not have been elapsed.

SUMMARY

Four out of 5 cases of presumed unilateral retinitis pigmentosa reported 11 years ago could be examined again. In 1964, all cases fitted the criteria for the normal fellow eye set up by Franceschetti, François & Babel. The fourth and added postulate, viz. a normal EOG-lightrise, seems not to be fully reliable, as in two, and possibly three cases the initial suggestion of an abortive bilateral retinitis pigmentosa has to be withdrawn. These findings stress again and again, the necessity of a sufficiently long period of observation between first and last examination, before a diagnosis of unilateral retinitis pigmentosa is to be certified.

REFERENCES

Franceschetti, A., François, J. & Babel, J.: Les hérédodégénérescences chorio-rétiniennes. Paris, Masson, (1963).

Henkes, H.E.: Does unilateral retinitis pigmentosa really exist? Proc. Third Int. Symposium, October 1964. In: Clinical electroretinography, p. 327-350. Oxford, Pergamon Press, (1966).

Author's address:
Eye Hospital
Erasmus University
180 Schiedamsevest
Rotterdam
The Netherlands

FUNDUS FLAVIMACULATUS: A CLINICAL CLASSIFICATION*

G.A. FISHMAN, G. BUCKMAN & T. VAN EVERY

(Chicago)

ABSTRACT

Various stages of fundus flavimaculatus seen ophthalmoscopically were correlated with findings on electrophysiologic and psychophysical tests. A new classification of fundus flavimaculatus into stages recognizes the nuances in genetic expression and their correlation with findings on retinal testing.

INTRODUCTION

Clinically recognizable patterns of expression of fundus flavimaculatus seemingly implicate a centrifugally advancing disease involving retinal pigment epithelium, photoreceptors, and choriocapillaris. Resultant from our investigation of 41 patients having fundus flecks is a classification into stages of the fundus changes that occur in fundus flavimaculatus. This classification considers both the area and severity of retinal pigment epithelium, photoreceptor, and choriocapillaris involvement. As the expression of this genetic disease may vary both within the same pedigree and among different pedigrees, these stages do not necessarily implicate the same sequence of evolution for all patients afflicted with this disease. With proper understanding of these stages, it is possible, however, to anticipate the severity and extent of retinal pigment epithelium, choriocapillaris, and photoreceptor involvement since fundus changes correlate well with results of electrophysiologic and psychophysical testing.

METHODS

EOG potentials were recorded from both eyes by silver-silver chloride contact skin electrodes attached with adhesive tape and electrode paste just below both medial and lateral canthi. A ground electrode was attached to the patient's forehead. The subjects were seated initially in a lighted room with head supported by a chin rest while facing a 180 degree diffusing sphere. For our recordings three small, dimly lit, red-fixation lights were placed 28 cm from the cornea in the patient's line of vision so that the

* Supported in part by training Grant No. EY 24-16 from the National Eye Institute, National Institutes of Health, and the Retinitis Pigmentosa Foundation.

213

center light served for center fixation while the peripheral lights allowed an excursion of 30 degrees as the patient looked from right to left at the approximate rate of 16 to 20 rotations per minute. The patients' pupils were maximally dilated with 10% NeoSynephrine and 1% Cyclogyl. After a standardized period of five minutes for room light adaptation (10 foot candles at the patient's eye), all lights are then turned off and the responses recorded for 15 minutes under dark-adapted conditions. After this time, the same room lights and four background lights (55 foot candles) were turned on, and responses recorded for another 15 minutes under light-adapted conditions. Sample recordings were obtained at approximately one minute intervals under both the light-adapted and dark-adapted conditions. The maximum amplitude in the light (LP) was then compared to the minimum amplitude in the dark (DT) to evaluate the normalcy of the responses. Normal patients under 50 years show ratios of 1.80 or greater. Ratios less than 1.70 are definitely subnormal in patients over 50 while values between 1.70 and 1.75 are borderline for this latter group.

The electroretinogram (ERG) was recorded from both eyes simultaneously while the patient was seated in an electrically shielded room. Pupils were maximally dilated with 10% NeoSynephrine and 1% Cyclogyl. Following the instillation of 5%proparacaine hydrochloride, as a topical anesthetic, Burian-Allen contact lenses were fixed to each eye. A 9 mm diameter silver-silver chloride disk fastened to the mid-forehead with recording electrode paste and adhesive tape served as an indifferent electrode. A similar disk fastened to the right ear, served as the ground electrode. For stimulation, a Xenon discharge lamp with a flash duration of approximately 10 microseconds and a peak luminance of about 1.5×10^6 candlepower was utilized. The lamp was activated by a Grass PS-2 photostimulator set at I-16. The Xenon lamp was placed above and behind the patient who was seated within a diffusing sphere so that the light stimulated the retina in a homogeneous (ganzfeld) manner. The elicited potentials were enhanced by a Grass P511E preamplifier having a ½ amplitude law frequency of 1 Hz. and a ½ Amp. high frequency of 1 kHz. Further amplification was achieved with a Tektronix 5A18N dual trace amplifier. All results were then displayed on a Tektronix 5103N oscilloscope and photographed with a Tektronix C-5 oscilloscope camera. Single flash photopic responses were recorded with the I-16 setting on the photostimulator after 5 minutes of adaptation to four 50 watt General Electric DC incandescent bulbs which provide 10 feet cd. of illumination at the patient's pupil. During dark adaptation, single flash recordings were obtained at 5, 10, 15 and 20 minutes, also at an I-16 intensity setting. The onset of the flash was delayed 40 milliseconds following the beam sweep to facilitate the measurement of implicit times. Following 20 minutes of adaptation, a Wratten 47 blue filter interposed between the light stimulus, coupled with an I_4 setting on the photostimulator, was used to measure predominantly rod responses. Subsequently, a Wratten 23-A orange-red filter was coupled with an I_{16} intensity to simultaneously record cone and rod components. The ERG determination was completed by measuring flicker fusion frequencies and amplitudes. One hundred responses at 30 cycles per second using an I_8 orange-red stimulus were averaged. Fifty

214

responses at 10 cycles per second with an I_4 blue stimulus coupled with a .5 Wratten neutral density filter were similarly recorded.

Dark adaptation testing was done on a Goldmann-Weekers dark adaptometer using standard techniques. Thresholds were obtained with 1 degree or 2 degree test targets 15 degrees above the fovea.

RESULTS

Fundus Flavimaculatus – Stage 1

(localized central retinal pigment epithelium, photoreceptor, and occasionally choriocapillaris disease)

The first evidence of disease is an insidiously progressive decrease in central vision generally with its onset between the ages of 8 and 16 years. In the majority of cases a ring of flecks surrounds a central, atrophic-appearing macular lesion (Fig. 1). The ring of flecks often circumscribes an area within 1 disk diameter of all sides of the fovea. The retinal vessels and optic disk are normal. Vision varies most frequently between 20/50 and 20/100. In my evaluation of 15 patients with stage 1 fundus flavimaculatus by ERG, EOG, and darkadaptation testing, the results were uniformly normal. Although the stages evolve very slowly, extending over several years, with time the central atrophic-appearing lesion extends in both width and depth. New flecks appear, often forming a broad garland around the posterior pole including the portion nasal to the optic disk.

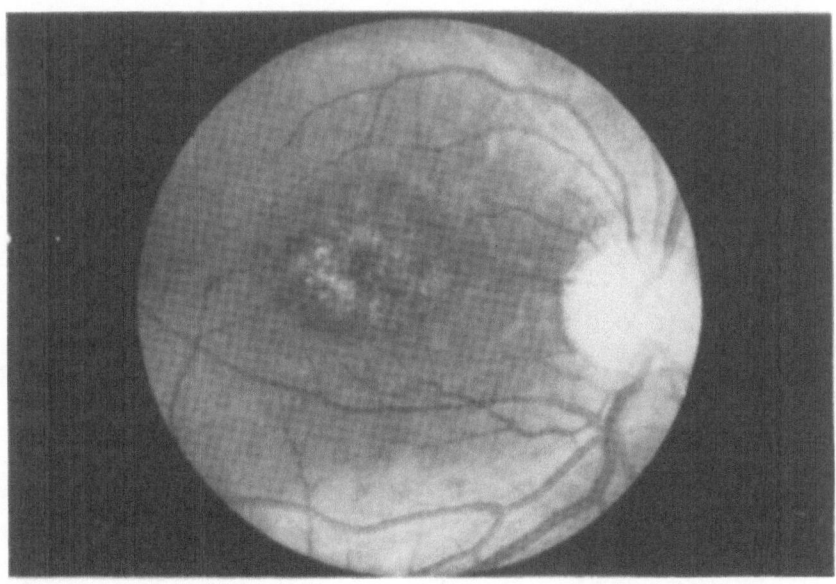

Fig. 1. Central atrophic lesion seen in stage 1 fundus flavimaculatus.

215

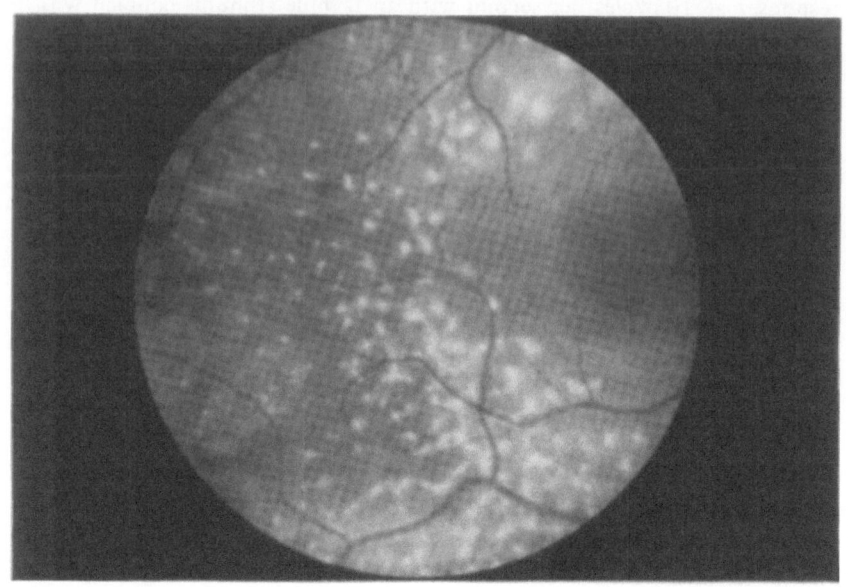

Fig. 2. Diffuse fishtail-like lesions of stage 2 fundus flavimaculatus.

Table I. Patients (16) with stage 2 fundus flavimaculatus

Patient,	Age (yr.),	Sex	EOG Ratios	
			OD	OS
1,	27	F	2.08	1.92
2,	19	M	2.67	2.04
3,	22	F	2.35	1.94
4,	21	F	2.00	1.94
5,	71	M	2.05	1.93
6,	31	F	1.85	1.82
7,	26	M	2.04	2.11
8,	49	F	2.00	2.17
9,	46	F	2.00	2.18
10,	48	F	2.14	2.28
11,	35	M	1.83	1.82
12,	54	M	2.45	2.55
13,	24	F	3.42	3.12
14,	37	F	2.14	2.33
15,	27	F	1.91	–
16,	49	F	2.11	2.38

(more diffuse, opaque, partially and totally resorbed flecks)

The yellowish-white flecks of stage 2 fundus flavimaculatus vary in size, shape (round, linear, fish-tail), and opacity and may extend to the equator (Fig. 2). In our series, there was a 90% incidence of atrophic-appearing macular lesions. The optic disk and retinal vessels are normal. Cases within stage 2, probably the stage most frequently seen by ophthalmologists, maintain normal ERG amplitudes and EOG ratios. Twenty three percent (patients 6, 12, and 13, Table 1) of our patients in this stage took a longer time (greater than the upper normal limit of 25 minutes in our lab) to reach normal scotopic ERG amplitudes. This finding may be missed if patients are not exposed to an intense enough preadaptation light. Both cone and rod implicit times are normal. Krill (1966) reported similar abnormal findings in ERG scotopic b-wave development, although he did not correlate the presence of these findings with ophthalmoscopic changes. These same three cases within stage 2 took a longer time (greater than 30 minutes) to reach normal final rod thresholds on dark-adaptation testing. Krill & Klien (1967) reported similar abnormalities on dark adaptation in some cases. In most stage 2 cases the flecks progressively resorb, leaving hypopigmented and presumably atrophic retinal pigment epithelium. The extent of the hypopigmentation is apparent by the numerous hyperfluorescent "window" defects on fluorescein angiography.

Fundus Flavimaculatus – Stage 3

(diffuse, totally resorbed flecks)

With progressive and extensive atrophy of the retinal pigment epithelium, the diagnosis of fundus flavimaculatus becomes more difficult. The retinal pigment epithelial defects become so widespread and confluent that unless specifically sought, residual, partially resorbed flecks will be missed and the diagnosis of fundus flavimaculatus will be in doubt (Fig. 3). In addition to the prevalence of diffusely resorbed flecks, stage 3 cases virtually always show choriocapillaris atrophy within the macula. During this stage, EOG ratios are first noted to be consistently abnormal (Table 2). This latter findings is contrary to some previous reports (Deutman, 1974; Krill & Klien, 1965).

In stage 3, ERG, amplitudes may be normal. In our series 57% of the cases showed normal cone and rod amplitudes while three of seven cases (43%) showed subnormal cone and rod ERG responses (Table 2). Of the 57% (4 Cases) with normal amplitudes, 50% (patients 1 and 2, Table 2) showed a longer time to reach normal amplitudes. As in stage 2, dark-adaptation testing showed a prolonged period to reach normal rod final thresholds in those cases showing similar prolonged time sequences on ERG testing. Some of the patients specifically complained of a mild decrease in their ability to see at night.

(diffuse, totally resorbed flecks and extensive choriocapillaris atrophy)

In addition to diffusely resorbed flecks, patients with stage 4 show extensive choriocapillaris atrophy throughout the fundus (Fig. 4). The patients in this study showed moderately or occasionally markedly reduced cone and rod ERG amplitudes (Table 2). Dark-adaptation findings on the three pa-

Table II. Patients (10) stages 3 or 4 fundus flavimaculatus

Patient,	Age (yr.),	Sex	ERG (Cone)*		ERG (Rod)*		EOG Ratios		Stage
			OD	OS	OD	OS	OD	OS	
1,	32	F	+	+	+	+	1.62	1.64	3
2,	47	F	+	+	+	+	1.56	1.50	3
3,	45	M	–	–	–	–	2.11	2.11	3
4,	35	M	+	+	+	+	1.64	1.60	3
5,	39	M	–	–	–	–	1.61	1.54	3
6,	21	F	+	+	+	+	1.50	1.46	3
7,	55	M	–	–	–	–	1.66	1.64	3
8,	56	F	–	–	–	–	1.43	1.31	4
9,	41	F	–	–	–	–	1.40	1.23	4
10,	74	M	–	–	–	–	1.33	1.37	4

* + indicates normal, – indicates subnormal.

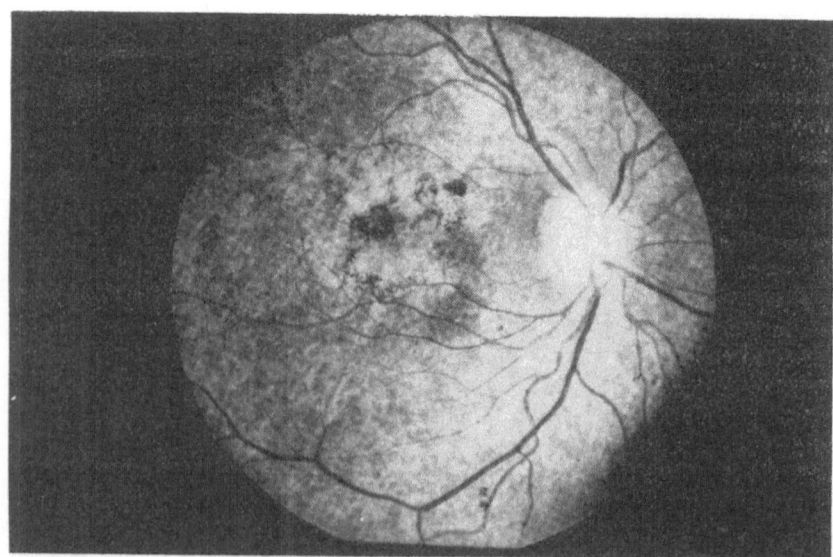

Fig. 3. Extensive retinal pigment epithelial atrophy as seen in stage 3 fundus flavimaculatus.

tients in this study classified in stage 4 showed elevated cone and rod thresholds which generally paralleled in degree the extent of abnormal cone and rod function measured by the ERG. Peripheral fields were either moderately or occasionally markedly constricted. The optic disks were normal while retinal vessels showed mild or moderate constriction. Nonspecific pigment clumping was sparse.

DISCUSSION

Fundus flavimaculatus is a progressive dystrophic disease initially involving the retinal pigment epithelium. This idea is consistent with electrophysiologic and psychophysical data. In our experience involvement of the macula with an atrophic-appearing lesion is the rule. The fact that a minority of cases with fundus flecks do not show an atrophic-appearing macular lesion probably reflects a variable expressivity and does not presently necessitate separate classification into Stargardt's macular dystrophy and fundus flavimaculatus.

This system of stages as proposed assists the examiner in quantitating by ophthalmoscopy the extent of retinal and choroidal disease since ophthalmoscopic changes correlate well with ERG amplitudes, EOG ratios, and dark adaptation thresholds.

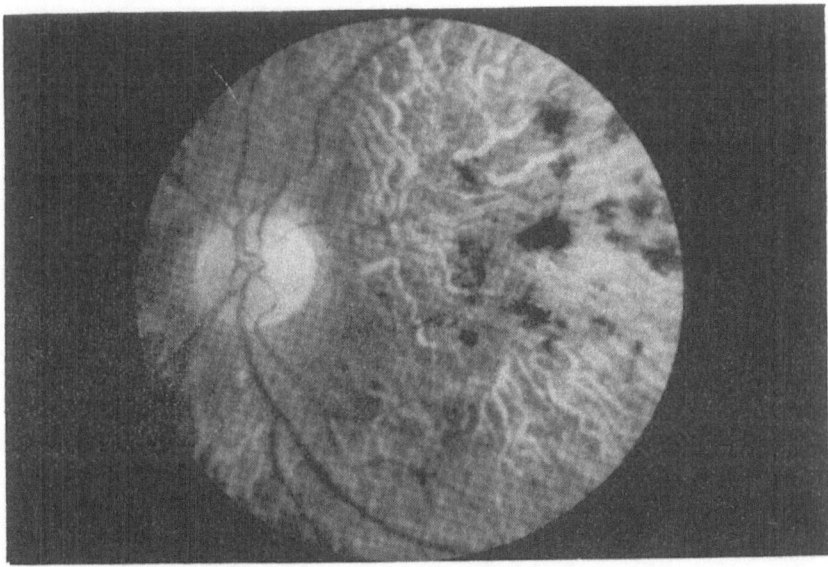

Fig. 4. Marked pigment epithelial and choriocapillaris atrophy seen in stage 4 fundus flavimaculatus.

REFERENCES

Deutman, A.F.: Macular dystrophies, in Goldberg MF: Genetic and Metabolic Eye Disease. Boston, Little, Brown and Co., 1974, pp. 380-385.

Krill, A.E.: ERG in fundus flavimaculatus. Proceedings of the 4th ISCERG Symposium. *Jap. J. Ophthalmol.* 10, *293-300,* (1966).

Klien, B.A. & Krill, A.E.: Fundus flavimaculatus: Clinical, functional and histopathologic observations. *Am. J. Ophthalmol.* 64, *3-23*, (1967).

Krill, A.E. & Klien, B.A.: Flecked retina syndrome. *Arch. Ophthalmol.* 74, *496-508*, (1965).

Authors' address:
Eye & Ear Infirmary
1855 W. Taylor
Chicago, Ill. 60612
USA

FUNDUS FLAVIMACULATUS ASSOCIATED WITH POLYCYSTIC
KIDNEY DISEASE: ANOTHER OCULO-RENAL DISORDER?

JEROME T. PEARLMAN

(Los Angeles, California)

A 47 year old woman was referred by her internist because of progressive bilateral visual loss. The patient's family history was significant in that her father died in his 40s of kidney disease, and the patient had one male and two female cousins who died of kidney disease. Her own long-standing renal disease was first clinically recognized in 1950, when she underwent a right nephrectomy for polycystic disease. She did reasonably well until 1967, when she developed progressive renal failure. In November, 1970, she underwent a cadaveric renal transplant, which was subsequently rejected, and had to be surgically removed later that same month. In March, 1971, the patient received her second cadaveric renal transplant, which functioned well until early 1973. From the time of her second kidney transplant, she had received a variety of medications, including azathioprine (150 mg/day), prednisone (20-80 mg/day), INH (300 mg/day), cycloheptadine hydrochloride (60 mg/day), chlorpheniramine maleate, and ascorbic acid. The patient was hypertensive both before and after her kidney transplant. She was maintained on varying doses of furosemide and methyldopa.

Her ophthalmic problems began in 1972, with the complaint of slowly progressive decreasing central vision in each eye. Visual acuity at that time was 20/40 on the right, and 16/100 on the left. In 1968, her ophthalmologist had recorded acuities of 20/25 on both sides. The same examiner found a ring scotoma on the left side. Intraocular pressures were normal by Schiotz tonometry. Examination in 1972 showed early bilateral posterior subcapsular cataracts. The ocular fundi revealed clear media, marked arteriolar sclerotic and hypertensive vascular changes, and pigmentary changes thought to be secondary to choroidal and retinal edema in each eye.

In May, 1973, her best visual acuity was 20/80 on the right, and 20/200 on the left. Her external examination was not remarkable. The posterior subcapsular cataracts were more advanced. She was sent for evaluation, because the referring physician wondered whether cataract extraction would significantly improve vision, particularly in view of concurrent macular pathology.

Inspection of the fundus through dilated pupils showed bilateral maculopathy with central 'cherry-red spots', surrounded by macular halos of diseased retinal pigment epithelium. In addition, a peculiar reticular pattern was noted peripheral to the macula. This suggested deposition of

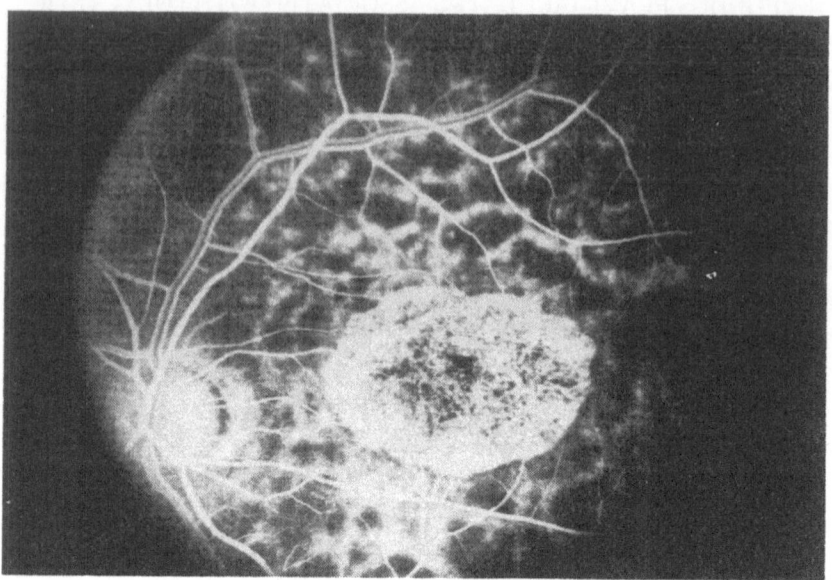

material at the level of the pigment epithelium. The retinas were flat, with no evidence of abnormal pigmentary migration within the retina. There were neither hemorrhages nor exudates.

Goldmann fields showed bilateral central scotomas of moderate density. A dark adaptation test, using a one degree test spot on the Goldmann-Weekers adaptometer, showed an elevation of both rod and cone thresholds. There was a delay of rod onset to about 17 minutes, and an elevated final rod threshold of 0.4 log units above the normal for our laboratory. The electroretinographic b-wave was normal bilaterally.

Fluorescein angiography (Fig. 1) revealed a normal appearing disc. The macula was characterized by a horizontally oval, moderately well-marginated area of almost total retinal pigment epithelial 'drop-out', except for a central hypofluorescent spot suggesting the local preservation of retinal pigment epithelium. The microvascular pattern of the choriocapillaris appeared to be intact. Peripheral to the macula was a reticulated pattern of hyperfluorescence.

The patient was followed intermittently through 1974, until the time of her death in January, 1975, due to renal failure. The post mortem, unfortunately, did not include histologic studies of the eyes.

DISCUSSION

The diagnosis of fundus flavimaculatus with central retinal involvement and reticulated peripheral deposits was made retrospectively, after the patient's death. During the patient's lifetime, the specific type of tapetoretinal degeneration remained open to question, because of the unusual fundus

222

features. At one point, the disorder seemed to resemble Sjögren's reticular dystrophy of the pigment epithelium. The patient even had Swedish ancestors. However, fluorescein angiography showed that this was not the case, as the reticular pattern was the inverse of that seen Sjögren's dystrophy. The bilateral central 'cherry-red-spots' and an overall glazed tapetal reflex, with no intraretinal pigmentation, suggested the unlikely diagnosis of 'inverse retinitis pigmentosa without pigment'.

Because the fundus features bore a resemblance to an illustration in Gass' book (1970), the most reasonable clinical diagnosis seemed to be fundus flavimaculatus with central involvement of the Stargardt variety. In 1975, Passmore & Robertson (1975) published an article with an illustration that lent further support to the above impression.

While the patient was alive, it was not readily known whether the alteration in central visual acuity was primary within the retina, or secondary to medications she was receiving. Cataract surgery, at best, would have improved only the clarity of peripheral vision without increasing central acuity.

The case has further interest because of the preservation of the microchoroidal vasculature in the region of each macula, despite the significant destruction of the retinal pigment epithelium overlying it. The atypical deposition of intraretinal material is unlike the usual yellow spots associated with fundus flavimaculatus.

The chief point of interest pertains to the possible relationship of the ocular and renal diseases: Fundus flavimaculatus has been known, on occasion, to appear in family pedigrees, together with retinitis pigmentosa (Franceschetti & Francois, 1965).Retinitis pigmentosa, in turn, has been known to be associated with a variety of renal disorders. In one form, retinitis pigmentosa may be associated with hypophosphataemic glycosuric rickets (Fanconi syndrome), where there is primary tubular disease of the kidneys (Linder, Bull & Grace, 1949). Other types of hereditary or familial nephropathies with retinitis pigmentosa are known (Senior, Friedmann & Braudo, 1961; Antoine, Braun-Vallon, D'Anglejeau, & Perrin & Ryckewaert, 1963; Meier & Hess, 1965; Asmal, 1969; Schimke, 1969; Mainzer,Saldino, Ozonoff & Minagi, 1970; Saraux, Dhermy, Fontaine, Boulesteix, Lasfargue, Grenet, N'Ghiem & Laplane, 1970; Durand, Bugiani, Palladini, Borrone, Della Cella & Siliato, 1971; Reiss, Porath & Schreier, 1971; Saldino & Mainzer, 1971; Senior, 1973; Abraham, Yanko, Licht & Viskoper, 1974; Hauser, 1974; Avasthi, Erikson & Gardner, 1976). Of these, there is no known association of retinitis pigmentosa with polycystic renal disease, nor has there been any description of polycystic renal disease with the flecked retina syndromes. The pathogenesis of polycystic renal disease is totally different from that of primary renal tubular deficiency, or tubulo-interstitial nephropathy of the nephronophthisis type.

Moreover, polycystic renal disease is transmitted as an autosomal dominant trait with incomplete penetrance, while fundus flavimaculatus is autosomal recessive. Their genetic relationship as concurrent conditions, therefore, seems remote.

Resolution of the complex question relating to the possible relationship of the ocular and renal disorders in this particular instance is complicated by the fact that there are no other living relatives of the deceased with familial polycystic renal disease, and no other family members with eye disorders. The deceased had no natural children.

It is not the intent of the author to force an association between retinitis pigmentosa or fundus flavimaculatus and yet another type of renal disease: The two conditions may be only coincidentally related. The association, however, does seem to be unusual, and the report is made in the hope that it may atract the attention of clinicians who possibly have encountered other similar cases that have previously gone unrecognized.

REFERENCES

Abraham, F.A., Yanko, L., Licht, A. & Viskoper, R.J.: Electrophysiologic study of the visual system in a family of juvenile nephronophthisis and tapetoretinal dystrophy. *Am. J. Ophthalmol.* 78, *591-597*, (1974).

Antoine, M.B., Braun-Vallon, S., d'Anglejeau, M.G., Perrin,,D., Dunod, J.P. & Ryckewaert, A.: Néphropathie familiale avec atteintes ossense et chorio-rétinienne. *J. d'Urologie et de Nephrologie* 69:(No. 1-2), *81-89*, (1963).

Asmal, A.C.: Hereditary renal disease, retinitis pigmentosa and other anomalies. *So. African Med. Journal* 43, *1033-1036*, (1969).

Avasthi, P.S., Erickson, D.G. & Gardner, K.D.: Hereditary renalretinal dysplasia and the medullary cystic disease – nephronophthisis complex. *Ann. of Int. Medicine* 84, *157-161*, (1976).

Durand, P., Bugiani, O., Palladini, G., Borrone, C., Della Cella, G. & Siliato, F.: Néphropathie tubulo-interstitielle chronique, dégénérescence tapéto-rétinienne et lipidose généralisée. *Arch. Franc. Ped.* 28, *915-927*, (1971).

Franceschetti, A. & Francois, J.: Fundus flavimaculatus *Arch. Ophthalmol.* 25, *505-530*, (1965).

Gass, J.D.M.: Stereoscopic Atlas of Macular Diseases: A funduscopic and angiographic presentation. St. Louis, C.V. Mosby Co., 1970, p. 123

Hauser, J.: Néphropathie chronique héréditaire avec surdité et attiente oculaire *Schweiz. med. Wschr.* 104, *724-728*, (1974). (The fundus findings were those of fundus albipunctatus)

Jackson, W.P.V. & Linder, G.C.: Innate functional defects of the renal tubules, with particular reference to the Fanconi syndrome – Cases with retinitis pigmentosa *Quart. J. of Medicine*, New Series XXII, No. 86, April, (1953).

Linder, G.C., Bull, G.M. & Grace, I.: Hypophosphataemic glycosuric rickets (Fanconi syndrome) – Report of a case with retinitis pigmentosa *Clin. Proceed.* 8, *1-20*, March, (1949).

Mainzer, F., Saldino, R.M., Ozonoff, M.B. & Minagi, H.: Familial nephropathy associated with retinitis pigmentosa, cerebellar ataxia and skeletal abnormalities. *Am. J. Medicine* 49, *556-562*, (1970).

Meier, D.A. & Hess, J.W.: Familial nephropathy with retinitis pigmentosa: A new oculorenal syndrome in adults. *Am. J. Medicine,* 39, *58-69*, (1965).

Passmore, J.A. & Robertson, D.M.: Ring scotomata in fundus flavimaculatus. *Am. J. Ophthalmol.* 80, *907*, (1975).

Reiss, D., Porath, U. & Schreier, K.: Nephronophthise mit tapetoretinaler Degeneration und Glycinurie bei 2 Brüdern (eine weitere familiäre Nephropathie) *Arch. f. Kinderheilkd* 183, *23-29*, (1971).

Saldino, R.M. &Mainzer, F.: Cone-shaped epiphyses (CSE) in siblings with hereditary renal disease and retinitis pigmentosa *Radiology* 98, *39-45*, (1971).

Saraux, H., Dhermy, P., Fontaine, J.-L., Boulesteix, J., Lasfargue, G., Grenet, P., N'Ghiem, M. &Laplane, R.: La dégénérescence rétino-tubulaire de Senior et Löken *Arch. Opht (Paris)* 30, *683-696*, (1970).

Schimke, R.N.: Hereditary renal-retinal dysplasia. *Am. J. of Int. Medicine* 70, *735-744*, (1969).

Senior, B., Friedmann, A.I. & Braudo, J.L.: Juvenile familial nephropathy with tapetoretinal degeneration: A new oculorenal dystrophy *Am. J. Ophthalmol.* 52, *625-633*, (1961).

Senior, B: Familial renal-retinal dystrophy. *Am. J. Dis. Child.* 125, *442-447*, (1973).

Author's address:
Jules Stein Eye Institute
800 Westwood Plaza
Los Angeles, Cal. 90024
USA

DEFINING FUNDUS ALBIPUNCTATUS

MICHAEL F. MARMOR,

(Stanford, California)

ABSTRACT

The ophthalmic literature contains argument about the distinction between fundus albipunctatus and the tapeto-retinal dystrophies. In 1974 Carr, Ripps & Siegel demonstrated abnormally slow photopigment regeneration in a family with fundus albipunctatus, and a physiological definition of the disorder seemed possible.

I have studied two new families with fundus albipunctatus. Scotopic functions, including the ERG and EOG, were virtually absent under ordinary test conditions (e.g. 30 minutes dark adaptation). However, after 3-4 hours of dark adaptation all of these parameters (including the a-wave, b-wave and b-wave threshold) returned to normal. These findings are consistent with abnormal pigment regeneration. They support the concept that fundus albipunctatus is a well defined disorder separable from stationary night blindness and from the progressive dystrophies.

Additional observations include angiography, which showed widespread pigment epithelial damage, while the punctate lesions were invisible or blocked fluorescence. The punctate lesions in one case showed a striking radial organization. Serial photographs from another case showed that the lesions may change. Mild abnormalities of photopic function were also present.

INTRODUCTION

Lauber (1910) made the distinction between fundus albipunctatus, a non-progressive condition, and retinitis punctata albescens, a severe progressive dystrophy. Subsequent authors have disagreed about the validity of this distinction. For example, Franceschetti, Francois & Babel (1974) described a continuum of disorders while Carr, Ripps & Siegel (1974) considered fundus albipunctatus to be a discrete disorder involving photopigment regeneration.

I have examined two families (Marmor, 1977) with fundus albipunctatus in which the affected individuals show a marked prolongation of subjective and electrophysiologic dark adaptation. These findings support the concept that this is a disorder of visual pigment regeneration. Some new observations are also made regarding cone involvement, the pattern and progression of lesions, and the angiographic appearance.

METHODS

The methods are described in more detail elsewhere (Marmor, 1976, 1977). Dark adaptometry was performed on a Goldmann-Weekers adaptometer,

227

after 7 minutes pre-adaptation to an intensity of 425 foot-lamberts. ERG's were performed with a full-field stimulator and bipolar Burian-Allen electrodes, and were displayed on an oscilloscope. The recording protocol allowed separation of cone and rod responses. The same full-field stimulator contained EOG fixation lights subtending an angle of 30° from the eyes; an intensity of 125 foot-lamberts was used for the light phase. The pupils were dilated for all of these tests.

CASE REPORTS

Two families were studied, each with one affected member who was the product of a consanguineous marriage. Family A is from the Azores; Family B is from southern Italy.

Case A (male, age 33): He has been aware for years of slow dark adaptation on going from a bright to a dim environment. Corrected acuity was 20/20 in either eye with a minor refractive error. His fundi (Figure 1) showed normal discs and retinal vessels, and a dense concentration of tiny white dots throughout much of the posterior pole. These dots came quite close to the fovea, were sharply demarcated, and were deep to vessels. Near the vascular arcades they formed rows which radiated from the macula, following neither retinal nor choroidal vessels. Peripherally, they gave way to larger fleck-like lesions which coalesced near the equator to give a mottled appearance to the fundus. They were no peripheral pigmentary lesions, but there was some dispersion of pigment beneath the foveas and both foveas appeared dull.

Case B (female, age 8): Asymptomatic until two years ago when she complained of poor vision on coming indoors from the sunlight. Corrected acuity was 20/20 in either eye with a refractive error roughly +1.25 sph. +0.75 cyl. x 90°. The fundi showed normal discs and vessels and many tiny white dots throughout the region of the vascular arcades. These lesions became more diffuse and fleck-like at the outer reaches of the arcades. They did *not* show a pattern of radiation as those of Case A, and in general were more sparse. A comparison of fundus photographs, spanning 15 months of observation, shows that while most of the lesions have been stable, a few have clearly faded and some new ones have appeared.

RESULTS

Angiograms of the affected cases showed mottled transmission of fluorescence in both posterior pole and periphery, but this did not correlate with the white dots or flecks. The punctate dots did not show aotofluorescence and on close examination some of them blocked fluorescein. Many of them could not be localized in the angiogram.

Visual fields showed slight constriction to a small dim target (I_2), and Case A had small paracentral scotomas. Both cases confused adjacent colors on the Farnsworth D-15 panel and had high error scores (132-201) on the Farnsworth 100-hue test. Their errors showed a weak tritan pattern.

Dark adaptometry on both patients showed an extremely slow bipartite curve (Figures 3 and 4). The cone plateau was not reached until 40-70 minutes, the cone/rod break until 100-120 minutes, and a normal rod threshold until 200-240 minutes. The final configuration resembled a normal dark adaptation curve on a greatly expanded time scale.

An EOG was performed on Case A after the left eye had been patched for 24 hours, while the right eye had only about 90 minutes dark adaptation. The light/dark ratios were 2.13 in the fully dark-adapted left eye, but only 1.33 in the poorly adapted right eye.

Photopic ERG's from both cases were of borderline amplitude (100-120 μV), but showed normal configuration and normal b-wave implicit time. However, 15 minutes of dark adaptation had almost no affect so that ordinary scotopic ERG lacked any rod contribution (see Figure 2). Case B-5 showed no change from records made 15 months earlier.

Dark-adapting for 3½ hours eliminated these scotopic abnormalities in both patients. A weak flash now produced a 300 μV rod b-wave, and a strong flash produced the typical response of a large a-wave, oscillatory potentials, and a 400 μV b-wave (Figure 2). In addition, repetition of the

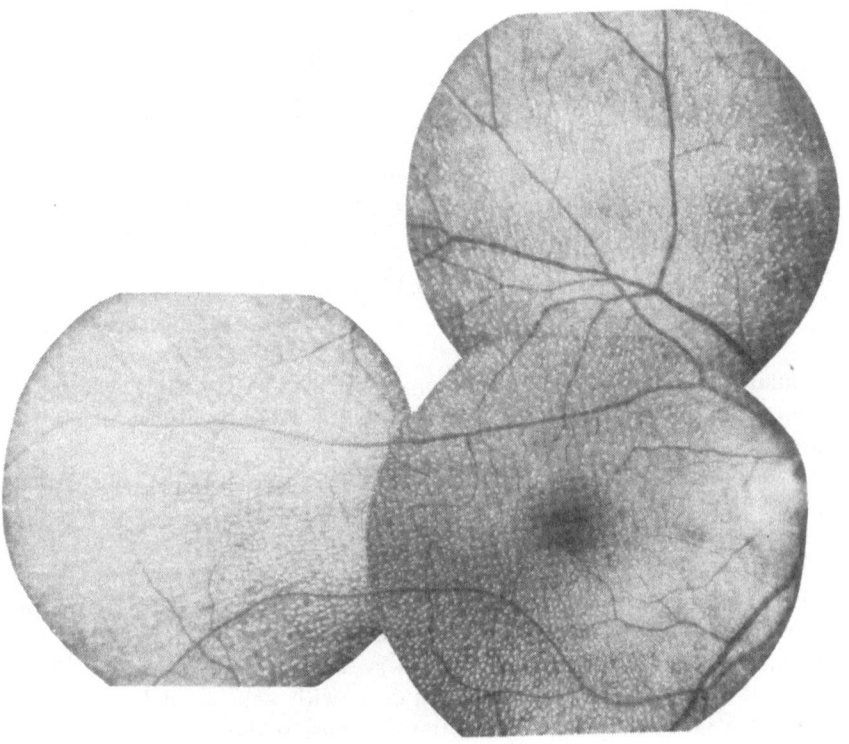

Fig. 1. Composite fundus photograph of Case A. The punctate lesions appear to radiate from the macula, but do not follow the visible retinal or choroidal vessels. The lesions change character beyond the arcades, becoming more fleck-like.

229

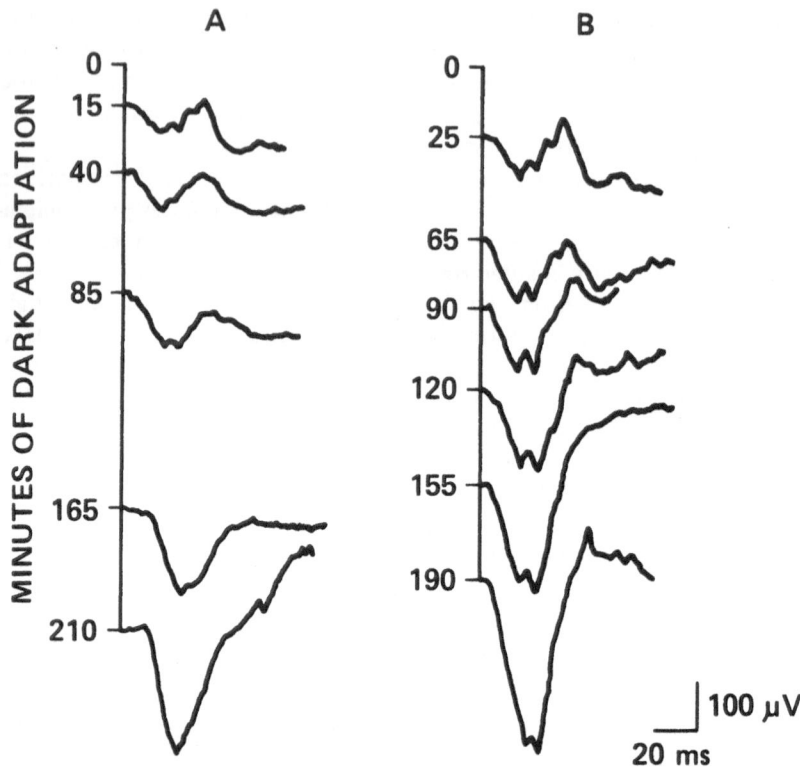

Fig. 2. ERG's from Cases A and B during dark adaptation. The time after pre-adaptation to light is shown on the ordinates. All responses are to a bright white (W-8) flash. For more than an hour, the signals resembled cone responses. Adaptation finally occurred, and after 3-4 hours the scotopic responses were within normal limits. The components of these responses are plotted in Figures 3 and 4.

stimulus flash after 10-15 seconds produced a superimposable waveform, demonstrating that the state of dark adaptation was not altered by a single flash.

ERG's were also performed at intervals during prolonged dark adaptation of both patients (Figures 3 and 4). Measurement of the a- and b-wave amplitudes showed good correlation between the timing of subjective dark adaptation and adaptation of the ERG components. The a-wave showed two phases of growth, consistent with the two portions of the dark adaptation curve. The cone b-wave was relatively stable during the initial period of dark adaptation, but both cone and rod b-waves increased after the cone/rod break. B-wave thresholds were also studied with Case A, and showed an initial plateau followed by descent after the cone/rod break.

DISCUSSION

In 1974, Carr, Ripps & Siegel studied two individuals with fundus albipunctatus who showed a marked prolongation of both cone and rod dark adaptation. Fundus reflectometry showed that the underlying problem was abnormal regeneration of visual pigment, in contrast to the normal pigment regeneration found in other forms of stationary night blindness (Carr, et al, 1966) and in Oguchi's disease (Carr & Ripps, 1967).

Both of my cases showed subjectively prolonged cone and rod dark adaptation, as well as slow adaptation of the EOG and the ERG (including the a-wave, b-wave, and b-wave threshold). These data suggest a defect which precedes generation of the a-wave. Appropriately, the dark-adapted ERG was unaffected by brief stimulus flashes that do not bleach a significant amount of rhodopsin (in contrast to Oguchi's disease – Gouras, 1970). These findings are consistent with the hypothesis that fundus albipunctatus involves abnormal pigment regeneration. The similarity between my patients and those of Carr, Ripps & Siegel suggests that a group of cases does exist

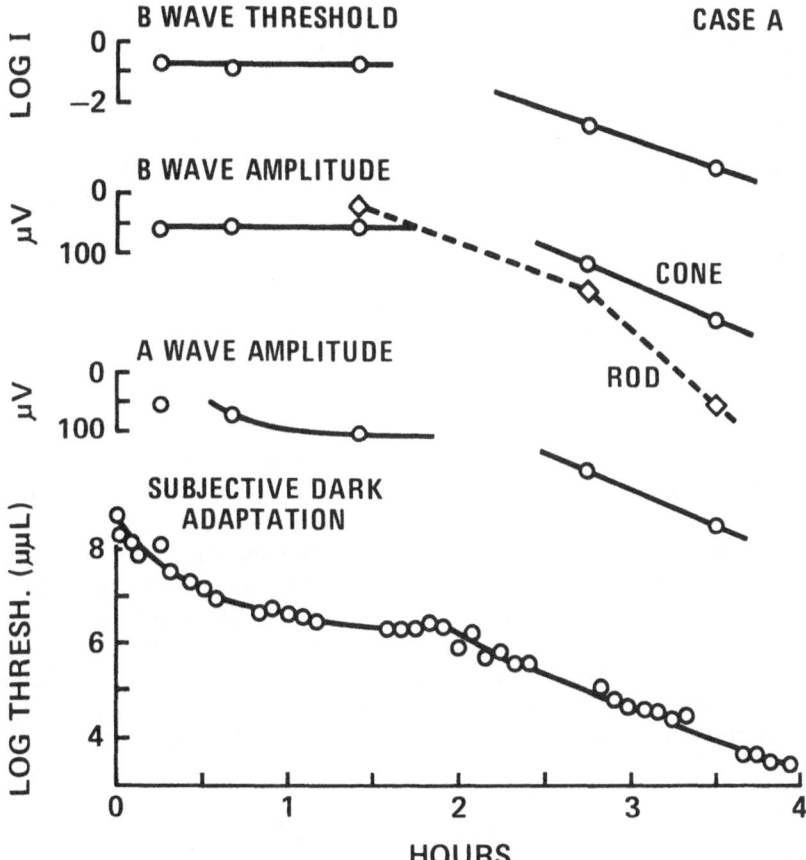

Fig. 3. Subjective and ERG dark adaptation in Case A. Note that the timescale reads in hours. The subjective dark adaptation curve is on the bottom; ERG components are shown above. Adaptation of the ERG components follows a timecourse similar to that of subjective adaptation.

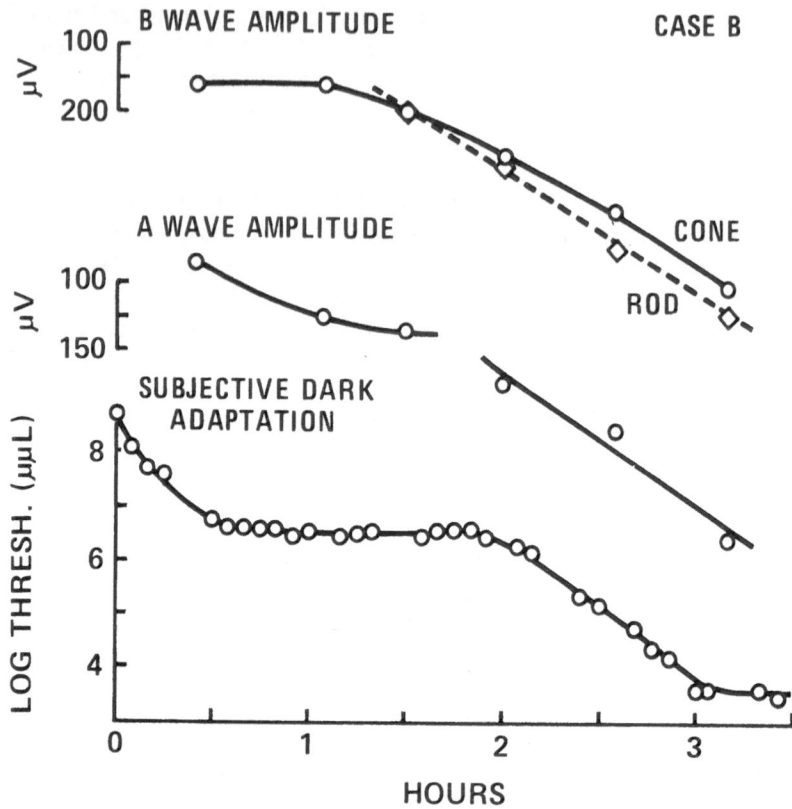

Fig. 4. Subjective and ERG adaptation in Case B. See legend for Figure 3.

for which fundus albipunctatus is a well defined disorder, physiologically distinct from the tapeto-retinal dystrophies and from other forms of stationary night blindness.

Among the case descriptions of fundus albipunctatus, dark adaptation has been markedly prolonged in some cases (Huber, Franceschetti & Dieterle, 1957; Franceschetti, et al, 1963), but only mildly affected in others (Smith, Ripps & Goodman, 1959; Krill & Folk, 1962). Thus, a spectrum of severity may exist. The ERG has been variously reported as normal (Franceschetti, et al, 1963; Franceschetti & Dieterle, 1954), subnormal (Franceschetti, et al, 1963; Franceschetti, Francois & Babel, 1974), and normal only after dark adaptation (Smith, Ripps & Goodman, 1959; Krill & Folk, 1962), but some of this variation may reflect different degrees of dark adaptation at the time of measurement. There should ordinarily be little problem with differentiation from retinitis punctata albescens. The latter will usually show, in addition to white dots, a diffuse retinal atrophy, attenuated vessels, disc pallor and frequently some black pigment spicules. There is permanent elevation of the dark adaptation threshold and depression of the ERG responses.

Although cone dark adaptation is abnormal, most reported cases of fundus albipunctatus have had no specific symptoms of photopic dysfunction. Subtle photopic abnormalities were evident in my two cases, including a mild tritan color defect, mild field constriction, borderline photopic b-wave amplitudes, and in Case A, abnormal-appearing foveas. The b-wave implicit times were not delayed, despite the diffuse nature of the disease.

The locus of the metabolic defect in fundus albipunctatus is unknown. The punctate lesions appear to be deep to the retinal vessels but they are not pigment epithelial defects. By angiography, the pigment epithelium seems to be diffusely involved by the disease. Perhaps some of the dots which appear to block fluorescein represent material within the pigment epithelial cell. The radial pattern of lesions in Case A (Figure 1) may be a clue to the disease, but its origin is obscure. The pattern does not follow the nerve fibres, or the visible retinal and choroidal vessels, or the segments of chorio-capillaris (Hayreh, 1975). The ciliary arteries radiate from the macula (Hayreh, 1975) but seem too distant.

The lesions in fundus albipunctatus have generally been described (without photographic comparison) as stable, including two cases followed for more than 35 years (Nettleship, 1914; Franceschetti & Chome-Bercioux, 1951). Case B has been followed for 15 months and her photographs (Marmor, 1977) show that some lesions have clearly changed. This flux of lesions is important because it may reflect a changing metabolic state that is amenable to analysis or therapy.

A similarity has been noted between fundus albipunctatus and 'fundus xerophthalmicus' (Uyemura, 1928; Teng Khoen Hing, 1965; Levy & Toskes, 1974), the latter being white spots in the fundus (generally reversible) as a result of vitamin A deficiency. White spots have also been observed in abetalipoproteinaemia (Gouras, Carr & Gunkel, 1971), a disease in which vitamin A is malabsorbed. Since fundus albipunctatus involves visual pigment regeneration, a relationship seems plausible between the fundus lesions and vitamin A metabolism. However, individuals with fundus albipunctatus have no signs of systemic vitamin A deficiency, and the dark adaptation curve in vitamin A deficiency may show elevated thresholds but is generally not prolonged (Russell, et al, 1973).

REFERENCES

Carr, R.E. & Ripps, H.: Rhodopsin kinetics and rod adaptation in Oguchi's disease. *Invest. Ophth.* 6, *426-436*, (1967).

Carr, R.E., Ripps, H. & Siegel, I.M.: Visual pigment kinetics and adaptation in fundus albipunctatus. In Documenta Ophthalmol. Proceedings Series, Vol. IV. The Hague, Dr. W. Junk B.V., 1974, pp. 193-204.

Carr, R.E., Ripps, H., Siegel, I.M. & Weale, R.A.: Rhodopsin and the electrical activity of the retina in congenital night blindness. *Invest. Ophthal.* 5, *497-507*, (1966).

Franceschetti, A. & Chome-Bercioux, N.: Fundus albipunctatus cum hemeralopia. *Ophthalmologica* 121, *185-193*, (1951).

Franceschetti, A. & Dieterle, P.: Importance diagnostique et pronostique de l'electro-retinogramme (ERG) dans les degenerescences tapeto-retiniennes avec retrecissement du champ visuel et hemeralopie. *Confin. Neurol.* 14, *184-186*, (1954).

Franceschetti, A., Francois, J. & Babel, J.: Chorioretinal Heredodegenerations. Springfield, Charles C. Thomas, (1974).

Franceschetti, A., Dieterle, P., Ammann, F. & Marty, F.: Une nouvelle forme de fundus albipunctatus cum hemeralopia. *Ophthalmologica* 145, *403-410*, (1963).

Gouras, P.: Electroretinography: some basic principles. *Invest. Ophthalmol.* 9, *557-569*, (1970).

Gouras, P., Carr, R.E. & Gunkel, R.D.: Retinitis pigmentosa in abetalipoproteinaemia: effects of vitamin A. *Invest. Ophthal.* 10, *784-793*, (1971).

Hayrch, S.S.: Segmental nature of the choroidal vasculature. *Brit. J. Ophthal.* 59, *631-648*, (1975).

Huber, V.O., Franceschetti, A. & Dieterle, P.: Zur differentialdiagnose zwischen fundus albipunctatus cum hemeralopia congenita und Oguchi's cher Krankheit. *Ophthalmologica* 133, *283-287*, (1957).

Krill, A.E. & Folk, M.R.: Retinitis punctata albescens. A functional evaluation of an unusual case. *Am. J. Ophth.* 53, *450-455*, (1962).

Lauber, H.: Die sogenannte retinitis punctata albescens. *Klin. Monatsbl. Augenh.* 48, *133-148*, (1910).

Levy, N.S. & Toskes, P.P.: Fundus albipunctatus and vitamin A deficiency. *Am. J. Ophth.* 78, *926-929*, (1974).

Marmor, M.F.: Corneal electroretinograms in children without sedation. *J. Ped. Ophth.* 13, *112-118*, (1976).

Marmor, M.F.: Fundus albipunctatus. In Press, 1977.

Nettleship, E.: A note on the progress of some cases of retinitis pigmentosa and of retinitis punctata albescens. *Roy. Long. Ophth. Hosp. Rep.* 19, *123-129*, (1914).

Russell, R.M., Smith, V.C., Multack, R., Krill, A.E. & Rosenberg, I.H.: Dark-adaptation testing for diagnosis of subclinical vitamin A deficiency and evaluation of therapy. *The Lancet, 1161-1164*, (1973).

Smith, B.F., Ripps, H. & Goodman, G.: Retinitis punctata albescens. *Arch. Ophthal.* 61, *93-101*, (1959).

Teng Khoen Hing: Further contributions to the fundus xerophthalmicus. *Ophthalmologica* 150, *219-238*, (1965).

Uyemura, M.: Ueber eine merkwurdige Augenhintergrundveränderung bei zwei Fällen von idiopathischer Hemeralopie. *Klin. Monatsbl. f. Augenh.* 81, *471-473*, (1928).

Author's address:
Ophthalmology Section (112 B1)
Veterans Administration Hospital
Palo Alto, Cal. 94304
USA

RETINITIS PIGMENTOSA: AN IMPROVED CLINICAL APPROACH

JEROME T. PEARLMAN

(Los Angeles, California)

Primary pigmentary degeneration of the retina, more commonly called 're-tinitis pigmentosa' has been recognized as a clinical entity since 1855. Its discovery came within a few years after the invention of the ophthal-moscope by Helmholtz in 1851. Since that time we have come to recognize RP as a group of similar-appearing clinical disorders characterized by night blindness, tunnel vision, retinal arteriolar narrowing, waxy pallor of the disc, and characteristic mid-peripheral and peripheral pigmentary deposits within the neurosensory retina. With the exception of one exceedingly rare form of the disease (Bassen-Kornzweig Syndrome), there is no known cure for any of the other forms of RP, although many different therapeutic approaches have been made, some of them bordering on the fantastic.

In terms of occurrence, RP is one of the most common of all genetically determined eye disorders, affecting about five in every one thousand of the world's population. That it represents not a single entity, but a group of clinically similar disorders, is borne out by the fact that all modes of genetic transmission and inheritance are known, including autosomal and X-chro-mosome linked varieties of the disease, together with both recessive and dominant forms. Diagnosis of the various forms of retinitis pigmentosa has been made considerably easier since different tests of retinal function have become available, including dark adaptometry, electroretinography, electro-oculography, and fluorescein angiography. When characteristic pigment deposition within the retina is present, there are relatively few disorders which need to be distinguished from RP.

In the X-chromosome linked form of the disease, the carrier state can sometimes be recognized by retinal pigment epithelial changes seen on fluorescein angiography, and by minor alterations in the electrical tests of retinal function. Many female carriers of the X-chromosome linked form of RP show some limited, but ophthalmoscopically detectable, disturbance of the pigment epithelium layer of the retina in the peripheral fundus.

Antenatal diagnosis of RP, as might be accomplished by amniocentesis, is not yet possible, since there is no chromosomal abnormality or chemical alteration that can be detected by this technique.

What, then, is new about this group of potentially blinding disorders? Basically, an improved approach to data collection and information organi-zation suited to computer analysis. This has been accomplished by the establishment of a Retinitis Pigmentosa Registry at the Jules Stein Eye Institute. This effort began in November, 1974, and in one year and a half, approximately 160 patients have been seen, extensively examined, their findings documented, and the data placed on questionnaire forms that have subsequently been transferred by a keypunch operator to IBM computer cards. Patient information contained on the punchcards is then computer analyzed according to pre-established programs designed to provide specific statistical information on a wide variety of variables and correlations. This has proven to be an extremely powerful research tool, insofar as it has given us a totally fresh look at the entity, retinitis pigmentosa, with statistical soundness. It has became apparent that a number of the features of retinitis pigmentosa that have been accepted for a hundred years or more were simply not true. In addition, we felt we saw correlations between the use of certain drugs and medications and the rate of progression of visual deterioration.

We became interested in the non-pigmented variety of the disorder, and very rapidly determined that rather than being a rare or atypical form of the disease, it almost seemed to be the universal state when the symptom of night blindness was of short duration (Pearlman, Flood & Seiff 1972). Overall, in our series, 22% of patients with clinically and functionally established retinitis pigmentosa showed no evidence of typical pigmentary migration within the fundus. When the nonpigmented state was correlated to duration of symptoms, the incidence of nonpigmented RP rose to 50% within the first 3 years after the onset of night blindness. Retinal function studies, such as the elctroretinographic response, visual field impairment, and dark adaptation function, were also less severely advanced in persons having shorter duration of symptoms. The appearance of typical bone-spicule pigmentation within the retina was quite variable in onset, but inevitably represented an advanced stage of the disease. Our findings statistically confirmed the observation of earlier workers in the field, including Leber and Nettleship, who postulated that all cases of retinitis pigmentosa would be without pigment if detected at an early enough stage in its natural history. Thus, the very feature which lent the name to the condition was of secondary importance, enabling the clinician to make the diagnosis on the basis of ophthalmoscopic appearance, but signifying relatively little from a functional point of view.

The implications of this observation for the pediatric patient are considerable. If, as we believe, retinitis pigmentosa in its earliest manifestations occurs without typical fundus pigmentation, an additional effort should be made to detect the presence of retinitis pigmentosa in childhood, especially where there is a positive family history for the disease. Early detection becomes an important factor, since there is now considerable evidence that exposure to light, of even moderate intensity, may 'overload' the visual pigment regeneration mechanism within the retinal pigment epithelial cells and the rod receptor cells (Kaitz, 1976). If the clinician knew early in a patient's life that retinitis pigmentosa was going to be a problem in the future, protection of the eyes from exposure to bright light, even daylight, could begin earlier and could, conceivably, prove to be a means of prolonging useful vision by, perhaps, a matter of years.

To test the theory of accelerated visual loss by exposure to bright ambient light, such as daylight, we have started a computer assisted project involving the use of a unilaterally worn contact lens of reduced light transmission and selected wave length. Three types of contact lenses are currently being tested: a cobalt blue one, a ruby red lens, and a neutral gray lens. All lenses reduce light transmission to approximately 13%. By allowing the contralateral eye to serve as a control, visual fields and dark adaptometry can be used to monitor the progression of the disease in each eye to see whether, over a period of several years, there will be an unequal acceleration of the disease between the two eyes. This type of experiment is feasible because of the basic symmetry of functional deficit between the two eyes. Goldmann fields are remarkably similar with respect to peripheral field limitations, and dark adaptation determinations of the rod absolute threshold are likewise virtually identical in one eye and the other. The computer analyzable contact lens study is clearly not one that can be applied to the pediatric patient, but it is used as an example of the type of experiment that can be done in a population of known retinitis pigmentosa patients, while other patients are given sunglasses to wear outside, from early childhood.

Another feature of retinitis pigmentosa that has been repeatedly emphasized to patients suffering from the disease, is the notion that while the disease basically attacks peripheral vision and spares central vision until late in the course of the disease, the RP sufferer may therefore look forward to being able to read and perform fine detailed visual functions late into life. Our information does not support such optimism. It would seem that between 40 and 45 percent of patients, regardless of age and duration of symptoms, have vision less than 20/50 in each eye. For persons so affected, the disease has to be a great deal more threatening, since the likelihood of total blindness is increased.

Our approach has also indicated that autosomal dominant transmission of the disease does not necessarily mean a milder form of the disease with less functional impairment and later onset (Duke-Elder & Dobree, 1967). With respect to this feature, it now becomes apparent that even within the autosomal dominant type of hereditary transmission, there is a good deal more pleomorphism in terms of functional deficit than has been previously realized.

The computer assisted program permits us to study groups of patients that have been on certain medications such as estrogens (including birth control pills) and thyroid hormone. By careful data collection and analysis, these and other aspects of retinitis pigmentosa can be reviewed systematically and in a statistically sound way. The Registry constitutes the main front of our current investigative effort to redefine retinitis pigmentosa and to search for meaningful ways of prolonging vision while basic science research is directed at answering questions at a molecular or enzymatic level.

REFERENCES

Duke-Elder, S. & Dobree, J.H.: System of Ophthalmology Vol. X ('Diseases of the retina') St. Louis, C.V. Mosby Company, p. 579. 1967.

Kaitz, M: Protection of the dystrophic retina from susceptibility to light stress. *Invest. Ophthalmol.* 15, *153-156*, (1976).

Pearlman, J.T., Flood, T.P. & Seiff, S.R.: Retinitis pigmentosa without pigment: Its clinical significance. *Am. J. Ophthalmol.* 81, *417-419* (1976).

Author's address:
Jules Stein Eye Institute
800 Westwood Plaza
Los Angeles, Cal. 90024
USA

ERG IN SECTORIAL PIGMENTARY RETINOPATHY

J. FRANÇOIS, A. DE ROUCK & A. GOLAN

(Ghent, Belgium)

We would present 7 cases of sectorial pigmentary retinopathy. In 5 patients, the ophthalmoscopically visible dystrophic lesions were localized to the inferior half of the retina. Three of them showed in addition a generalized cone dysfunction. In the last 2 patients, the dystrophic process seemed confined to the nasal sector of the retina.

In most of our patients the disease was discovered at a rather advanced age. The first subjective complaints were noted in the 3rd or 4th decade. In the group with cone dysfunction, however, the complaints were already present in early childhood. The main complaints were either poor vision or photophobia. Only one patient (case 6) complained of hemeralopia.

It must be stressed that in all our patients the lesions were strictly symetrical in both eyes. In the involved retinal area, small pigment deposits or osteoblastic clumps were seen, sometimes mixed with yellow dots. The optic discs were normal, except in one patient (case 6). The retinal vessels

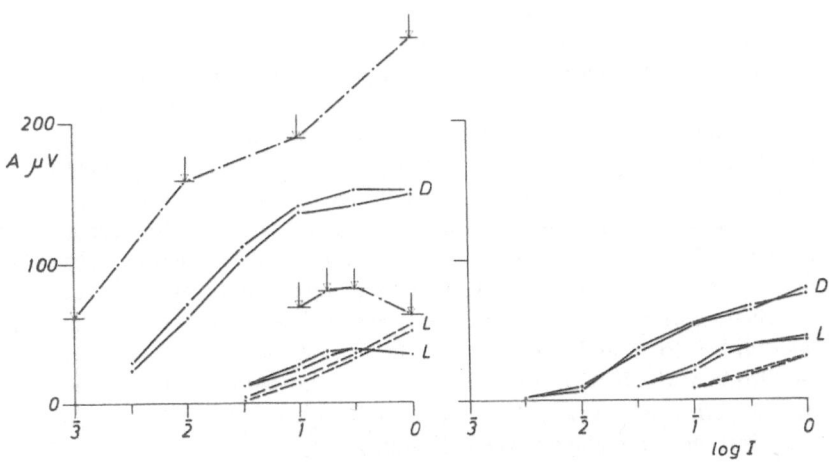

Fig. 1.   Case A. Amplitude curve. D: dark adapted state. L: light adapted state. *b*-wave. : –. *a*-wave: – · – · · m – 2 S (normal). On the right: amplitude curve 7 years later. later.

were normal, although slightly narrowed in 3 patients (cases 4, 5, 6). Macular lesions were seen in 2 patients (cases 3 and 7).

Fluorescein angiography revealed pigment epithelium defects with increased choroidal transmission. Its findings correlated very well with the ophthalmoscopic picture. Although it is known in the literature that the margins of the fluoro-angiographic lesions may extend beyond the ophthalmoscopically normal retina, this was not the case in our patients.

The extent of the dystrophic area showed individual differences in the group of patients with involvement of the inferior retina. In cases 1 and 3, the lower half of the retina was completely involved. In cases 4 and 5, the lesions were localized to the periphery. In case 2, only a small area in the extreme periphery showed the aspect of paucipigmentary retinopathy.

In most patients the visual field defects matched fairly well the dystrophic areas. They were, however, larger than could be expected. The ring scotomas in cases 1 and 3 extended beyond the horizontal meridian. Cases 2, 4 and 5 showed, in addition to the upper field defect, a concentric narrowing of the peripheral isopters.

The global light sense was normal in most of our cases. Nevertheless, the final threshold of the dark adaptation curves was slightly raised in 2 cases (2 and 6).

The color discrimination was either normal or showed a type I red-green defect. In the cases associated with a generalized cone dysfunction, the colour sense was severely impaired. All the EOG records were pathological. The maximal light/dark ratio did not exceed 145% (case 6). In one case (7), the EOG was even extinguished.

The ERG records were also pathological, and allowed the classification of our cases in 3 groups:
1. *Rod dysfunction.* The cone responses were normal (single flash response to white light in light adapted state, single flash responses to red light, flicker ERG). On the contrary, the rod responses were selectively impaired (single flash response to white light in dark adapted state, single flash responses to blue light in dark adapted state): cases 2 and 6.
2. *Rod-cone dysfunction.* Both cone and rod responses were pathological, but the rod responses were mainly involved (cases 1 and 7).
3. *Cone-rod dysfunction.* The cone responses were completely extinguished, and the rod responses severely reduced (cases 3, 4 and 5).

The temporal characteristics of the responses were usually normal. They were modified only in 2 cases. Case 1 showed a delayed implicit time of the rod responses, in white as well as in blue light, while the cone responses remained normal. Case 7 showed only residual potentials with delayed implicit times for cone as well as rod responses. It must be stated, that the amplitude of the ERG responses in case n° 1 showed a progressive reduction over a period of 7 years. The abnormal delayed implicit times of the scotopic responses remained nevertheless unchanged.

According to Wirth & Ponte (1964), 2 forms of sectorial pigmentary retinopathy can be distinguished. One is really sectorial and the ERG is altered proportionally to the affected retinal areas. The other is in fact a widespread dystrophy; the electrical results, as well as the other visual func-

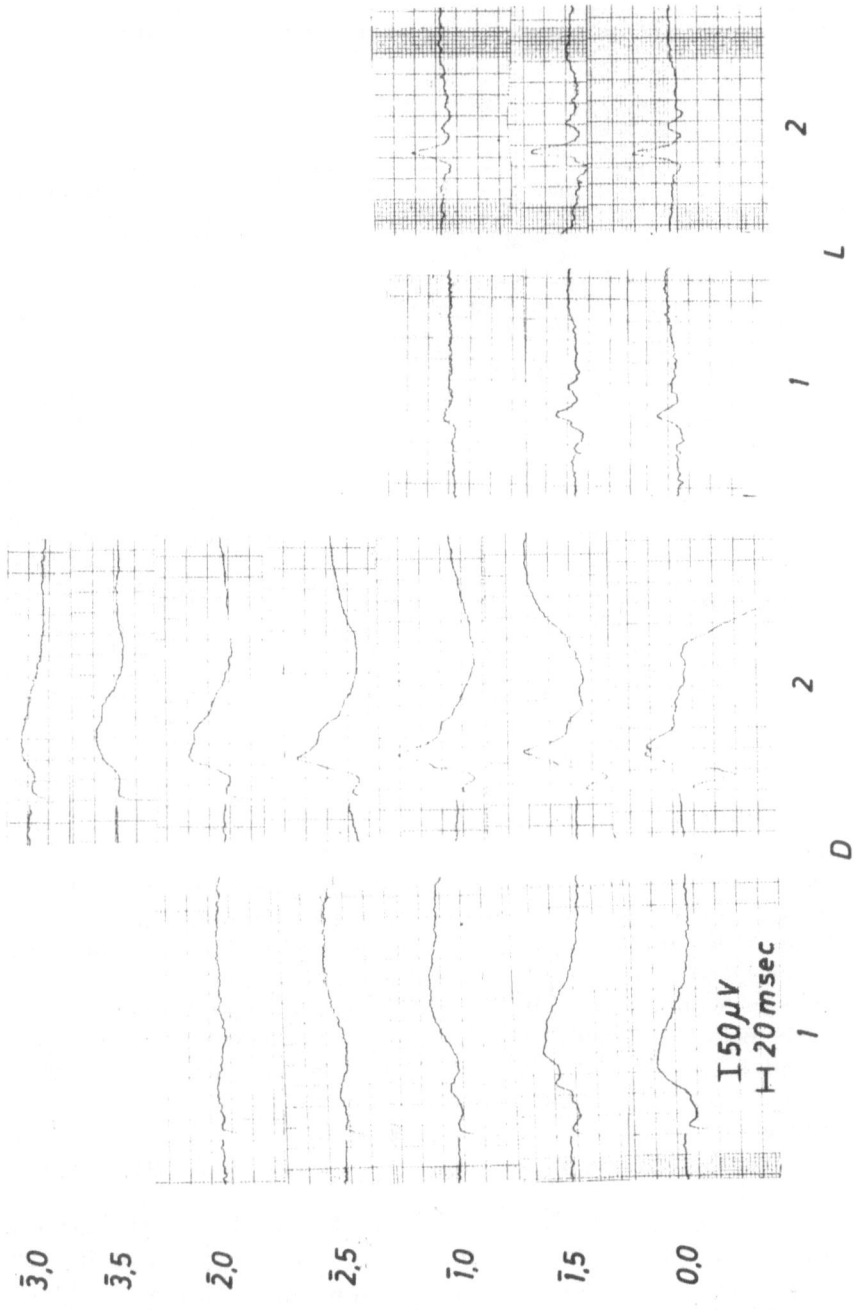

Fig. 2. ERG record in cases 1 and 2. A: dark adapted state. L: light adapted state. Xenon flashes: I in log. scale.

Table I. P = pathological, N = normal, r = photopic b-wave/scotopic b-wave relationship

Name	Age	Onset	Heredity	Location	Angiography	Refraction	V.A.	Visual Field	Dark adaption
E	55	?	–	inferior half	good correlation	–	1,0	annular scotoma of	$\bar{5},7$
							1,0	upper field	
				no change			1,0	no change	$\bar{5},6$
							1,0		
R	38	3y	–	extreme lower periphery	good correlation	– 1D −0,5D	1,0	constricted	$\bar{4},2$
D	8	Birth?	–	inferior half	–	–	0,3	central scotoma +	$\bar{5},4$
							0,3	annular scotoma of the superior half	
	16			no change	good correlation	–	0,3	no change	$\bar{5},4$
							0,3		
DB	26	Birth?	+ recessive	inferior half	not made	−5D −5,5D	0,8 0,8	irregular constriction mainly of superior half	$\bar{5},5$
DB	24	Birth?	+ recessive	inferior half	good correlation	–	0,3 0,8	irregular constriction mainly of superior half	$\bar{5},2$
W	43	a few years	+	nasal periphery		–	1,0 1,0	narrowing on temporal side	$\bar{4},5$
S	24	3y	–	nasal half	good correlation	+2 90° +3 90°	0,2 0,5	pericentral scotoma and loss of temporal field	$\bar{5},6$

tions do not correlate with the ophthalmoscopical extent of the lesions. Berson et al. (1968) have emphasized the importance of the implicit time in sectorial pigmentary retinopathy. The temporal characteristics of the response obtained in 'ganzfeld' stimulation remain normal, in contrast to the delayed implicit time of the widespread retinal dystrophy (Berson et al., 1968; Berson & Kanters, 1970). We were able to follow 4 of our patients for a period of several years. We did not find any modification either of the fundus lesions nor of the subjective visual functions. The bioelectrical results also remained unchanged, except in case 1.

Some facts suggest, nevertheless, that all our cases are in fact wide-spread dystrophies:

1. In cases 2 and 6, the raised threshold of the dark adaptation curve. Case 6 belongs to a family with dominant pigmentary retinopathy. The mother of the propositus has a typical pigmentary dystrophy with tubular visual fields, high monophasic dark adaptation curve and extinguished ERG.

2. In cases 1, 2, 3, 4 and 5 the defect of the visual field does not match strictly the fundus alterations. There is, in addition to the sectorial defects, a general constriction of the peripheral isopters.

3. The results of the electrical tests suggest that the dystrophy is more

color vision	ERG					temporal aspect	EOG	Follow-up	Evolution
	photopic	scotopic							
	μV	F3 μV	a-wave μV	b-wave μV	r				
No	40	–	55	150	0,26	P	130%	7y	no change in functional state,
	40	–	50	150	0,24	P	125%		but decrease of ERG and EOG
	45	–	30	80	0,56	P	118%		
	45	–	30	75	0,60	P	115%		
V_1 type I	120	40	160	220	0,54	N			? not known
	125	35	130	220	0,56	N			
V_1 type I	–	30	50	100	–	N		10y	no change
	–	45	65	125		N			
	–	25	45	95	–	N	120%		
	–	40	60	135	–	N	120%		
$V_1 b_2$	–	15	40	70		N	122%	8y	no change
	–	15	50	80		N	118%		
$b_2 a$	–	–	90	90		N	135%	3y	no change
	–	–	50	90		N	134%		
No	110	20	100	200	0,55	N	140%	–	not known
	90	30	110	180	0,50	N	145%		
B-Y	10	–	20	15	0,67	P	100%	–	not known
	10	–	20	20	0,50	P	100%		

widespread and also involves areas which are ophthalmoscopically normal: (a) the amplitude of the rod responses is reduced to less than half of the normal value (cases 1, 3, 4, 5 and 7); (b) case 1 shows a progressive reduction in amplitude of the ERG rod responses and of the EOG; (c) temporal characteristics are modified in cases 1 and 7.

The apparently healthy retinal quadrants are probably potentially dystrophic and may display functional impairment, which may later on progress and result in morphologically visible defects. On the other hand, the progress of the disease appears to be very slow in our patients, and consequently, the prognosis is rather good.

SUMMARY

1. Seven cases of sectorial pigmentary retinopathy are described.
2. There was no correlation between the electrophysiological and other functional symptoms.
3. According to the ERG findings, the cases could be classified in 3 groups: rod dystrophies, rod-cone and cone-rod dystrophies.

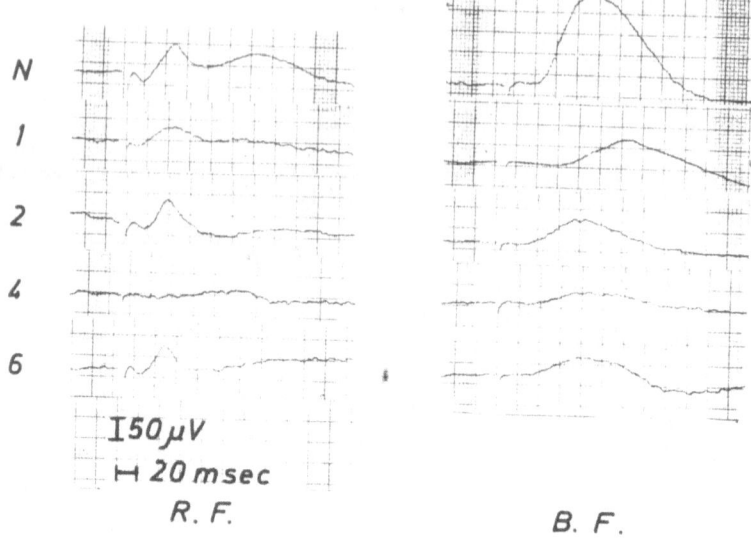

Fig. 3. ERG records in cases 1, 2, 4 and 6. N: normal subject. RF: red light. BF: blue light. Dark adapted state. The responses are not equivalent.

4. No progression of the visual impairment could be found, even after a period of 10 years.
5. The temporal characteristics of the ERG responses were abnormal in 2 cases.

REFERENCES

Berson, E.L., Gouras, P. & Gunkel, R.D.: Rod responses in retinitis pigmentosa dominantly inherited. *Arch. Ophthal. (Chicago)*, 80, *58-67*, (1968).

Berson, E.L., Gouras, P. & Gunkel, R.D.: Progressive cone-rod degeneration. *Arch. Ophthal. (Chicago)*, 80, *68-76*, (1968).

Berson, E.L. & Kanters, L.: Cone and rod responses in a family with recessively inherited retinitis pigmentosa. *Arch. Ophthal. (Chicago)*, 84, *288-297*, (1970).

Wirth, A. & Ponte, F.: Fisiopatologia e clinica dell' elettroretinogramma. Industria Grafica Nazionale, Palermo, Italia, 1964.

Author's address:
University Eye Hospital
135 De Pintelaan
Ghent
Belgium

SECONDARY RETINITIS PIGMENTOSA (SYPHILIS)

JOHN R. HECKENLIVELY

(Lexington, Kentucky)

This paper presents four cases of syphilitic chorioretinitis that meet the criteria generally used in the diagnosis of retinitis pigmentosa (RP): namely, suppressed electroretinogram (ERG), abnormal electrooculogram (EOG), constricted fields, nightblindness, and pigmentary degeneration. Findings that can help to differentiate syphilitic chorioretinitis from true retinitis pigmentosa are discussed.

Bone spicule formation or retinal pigment in a reticulated pattern may be associated with a large variety of inflammatory and noninflammatory diseases, including lattice degeneration, myotonic dystrophy, high myopia, and syphilis.

In addition to mimicking the pigmentary changes of retinitis pigmentosa, clinical findings in syphilitic chorioretinitis can also mimic RP; these can be vascular narrowing, nightblindness, and constricted visual fields. The nightblindness is a noteworthy finding, as this has been long regarded as a hallmark of retinitis pigmentosa. The effect is due to the diffuse atrophy of the retina, which usually spares the macula area and leaves a small central area on visual field (Duke-Elder, 1966).

Since the pathophysiologic basis of retinitis pigmentosa is unknown, it is impossible to differentiate clearly between persons with true hereditary forms of retinitis pigmentosa and persons diagnosed as RP with systemic diseases, e.g., Refsum's and mucopolyaccharridoses, in which clinical findings are identical to hereditary RP, but may be quite different on a biochemical and cellular location basis.

The electrophysiologic changes in syphilitic chorioretinitis are sparsely documented. Harden & Wright (1974) report a patient with syphilitic chorioretinitis with a ring scotoma and with bilateral loss of vision. Dr. Alec Harden kindly shared the electrophysiologic results of this patient: The EOG was OD 120%, OS 160% light rise, ERG was low normal in each eye, dark adaptometry reported normal threshold in each eye.

Krill (1972) in discussing pigmentary eye ground changes in infancy and early childhood, states that the ERG is normal or subnormal in the infant with hereditary syphilis and abnormal to a mild or modest extend in cases with luetic optic atrophy.

In the last two years, four cases of luetic chorioretinitis have been evaluated at the University of Kentucky Medical School Department of Ophthalmology. Two cases were congenital, and two cases were the acquired form. At the time of electrophysiologic evaluation, all cases were without evidence of active inflammatory disease. All four cases had retinal pigmentary changes similar to those in RP. The cases ranged from one in which the fundus changes were mild to three in which they were severe, yet in all cases the electrophysiologic findings were abnormal.

Case 1. A 15-year-old white girl was seen first in June 1970 with a history of nightblindness from the age of 2 (Fig. 1). She had visual acuities of OD 20/100, OS 20/70, mildly constricted visual fields, retinal pigmentary clumping, some arteriole narrowing, and a diminished photopic and scotopic ERG. There was no family history of night blindness or eye disease. A VDRL test was weakly reactive, and a fluorescent-treponemal-antibody absorption (FTA-ABS) test was positive. Her mother also had a positive FTA-ABS test, and the diagnosis was considered, therefore, to be congenital syphilis.

Case 2. A 45-year-old white woman was admitted first in 1967 with an attack of closed angle glaucoma. According to her history, both she and her mother were treated for 'bad blood' in 1940 when she was 9 years old. Visual acuity has remained in the 20/60 range OU. With surgical and medical treatment, intraocular pressure and cup/disc ratio have remained normal. Visual fields have remained unchanged, and they are severely constricted. Since cup/disc ratio has remained 0.2, the constricted visual fields can be attributed to luetic chorioretinitis.

Fundus examination reveals a salt and pepper appearance, a leaden hue, arteriole narrowing and sheathing, and mild optic and peripapillary atrophy. There is pigmentary clumping in the periphery.

Case 3. A 62-year-old white man was admitted to the eye clinic with a conjunctivitis, best corrected visual acuities of 20/70 and 20/60, and a history of being treated for syphilis 17 years previously.

Fundus examination (Fig. 2) revealed large areas of choroidal sclerosis, retinal pigment epithelial dropout, mild arteriole narrowing, and pigmentary clumping in the periphery. Fluorescein angiography demonstrated a deficit in filling of the choroidal vasculature in the macula area.

Case 4. A 67-year-old white woman was admitted to the eye clinic with a history of night blindness and poor vision in her right eye for at least 15 years. Her best corrected visual acuities were OD light perception, OS 20/50 + 2. She had been told elsewhere that she had retinitis pigmentosa. The FTA-ABS test was positive, and the patient recalled that her former husband had been treated for syphilis 20 years previously.

Fundus examination of the OD eye revealed yellow blanched choroidal vasculature seen clearly through large depigmented areas of retinal pigment epithelium. There was severe disruption of the macula and several small perimacular hemorrhages. While the clinical appearance would be called severe choroidal sclerosis, her fluorescein angiogram demonstrated a patent choroidal vascular system. The left eye gave an appearance of perimacular choroidal sclerosis, with pigmentary clumping and patchy thinning of the retinal pigment epithelium in the macular area.

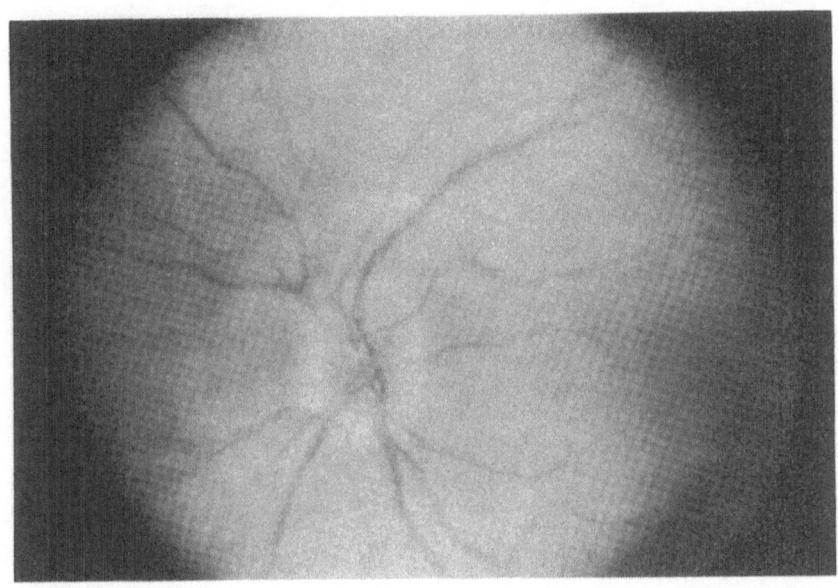

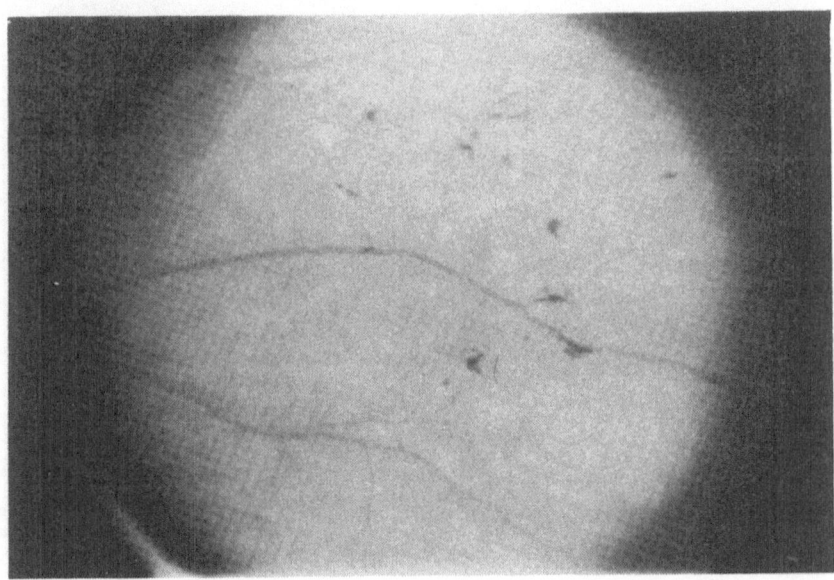

Fig. 1. (Heckenlively) – Case 1. Congenital syphilitic chorioretinitis with atrophic areas of the retina, peripapillary choroidal atrophy, mild arteriole narrowing, and scattered fine pigmented deposits ('bone spicules') in the periphery.

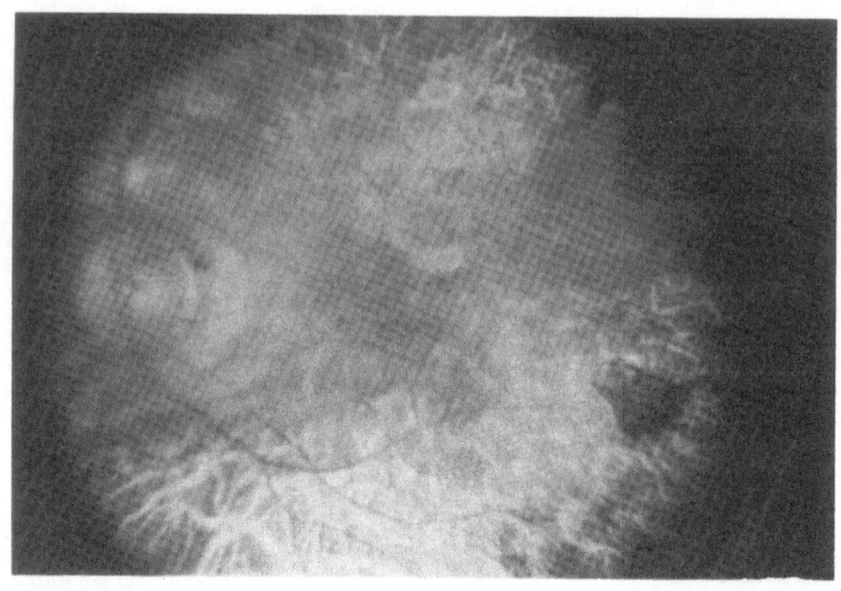

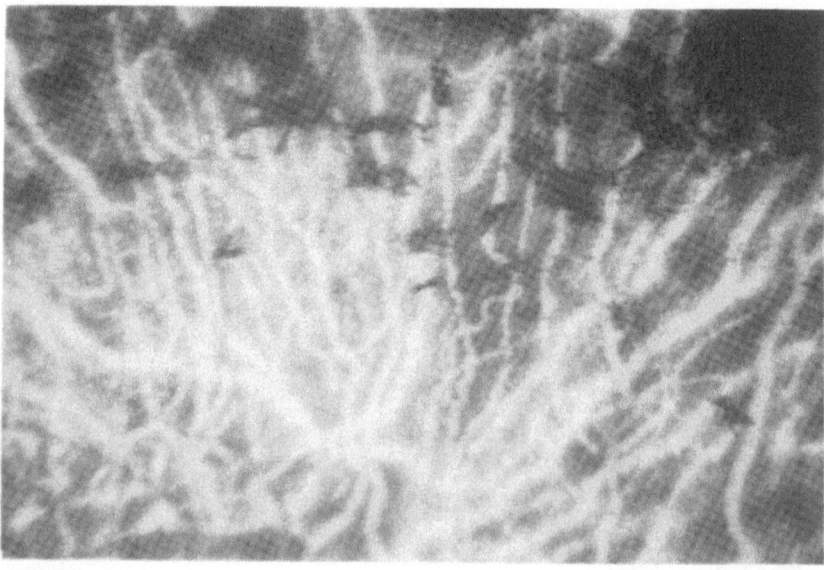

Fig. 2. (Heckenlively) – Case 3. Acquired syphilitic chorioretinitis treated 17 years previously, with large areas of choroidal sclerosis in the posterior pole, retinal pigment epithelial dropout, mild arteriole narrowing, and pigmentary clumping in the periphery.

METHODS AND MATERIALS

The ERG was recorded with Burian-Allen bipolar contact lens/electrode, using the Tetronix preamplifier and storage oscilloscope. A Grass P-2 strobe was used as the stimulus. Single flash photopic traces were done first with the l-16 setting; after the patient was dark adapted, the l-1 setting was used for scotopic tracing. A Sanborn two-channel recorded and the Tetronix preamplifier were used to perform the EOG.

DISCUSSION

Case 1 was diagnosed, initially, as having retinitis pigmentosa because of a 10-year history of night blindness, change in visual fields similar to those in RP, and a suppressed ERG. Visual fields tested between 1972 and 1974

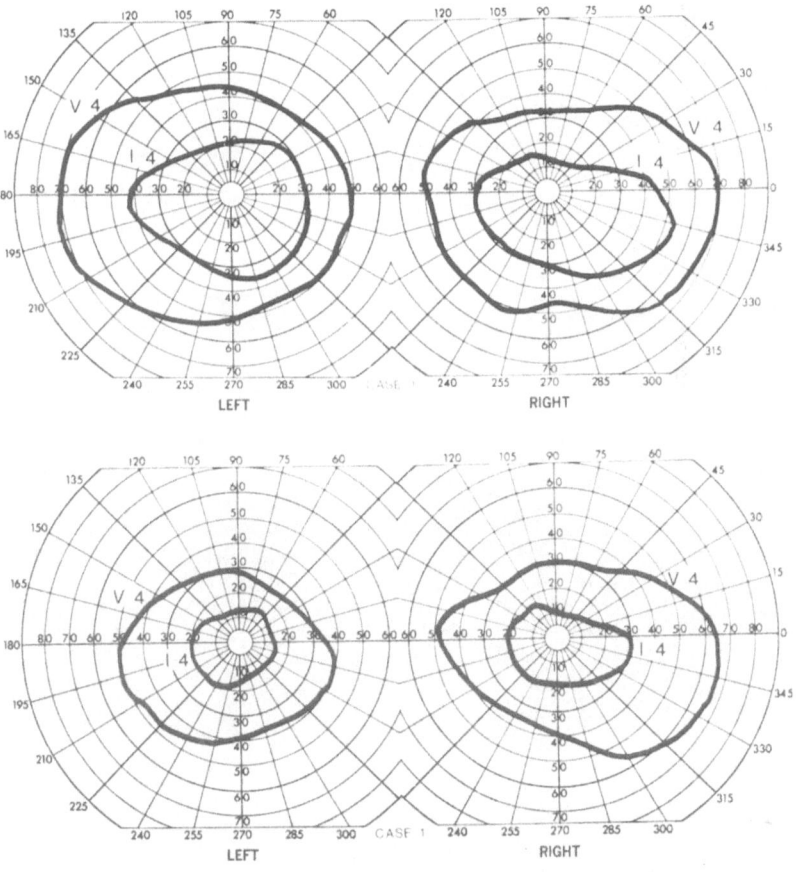

Fig. 3. (Heckenlively) – Case 1. Visual fields. *Top*, from November 1972. *Bottom*, February 1976; stable for two years since penicillin therapy.

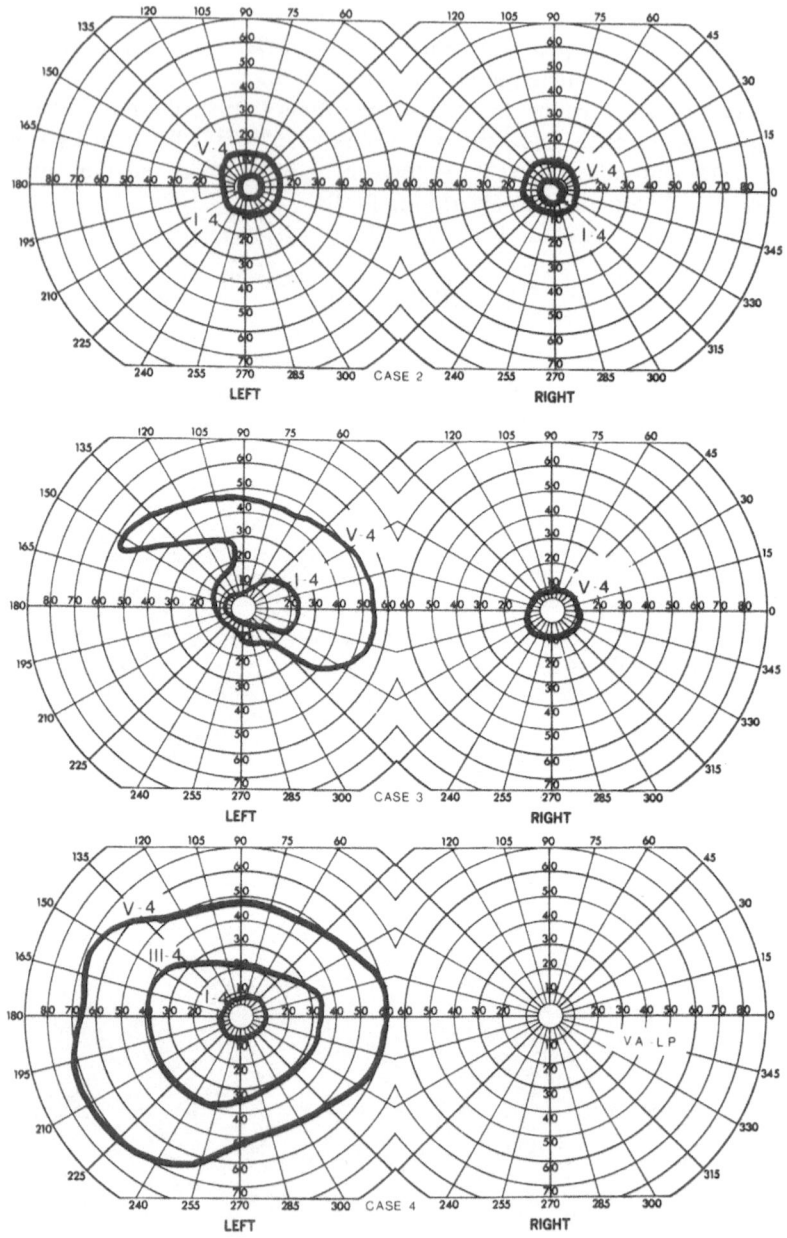

Fig. 4. (Heckenlively) – Visual fields. (a) Case 2. Severely constricted fields have remained unchanged since initial visit nine years ago. (b) Case 3. Severe constriction OD, with severe loss of inferior temporal field and pattern suggestive of partial ring scotoma OS. (c) Case 4. Constricted fields OS; LP vision prevented visual fields OS.

250

(Fig. 3) showed progressive constriction, but they stabilized in examinations subsequent to a course of penicillin in 1974.

The other three patient's visual fields show variability. Case 2, with congenital syphilis, has severely constricted fields, which have remained unchanged since the initial visit in 1967. Case 3, with acquired syphilis, is severely constricted OD, with severe loss of inferior temporal field and pattern suggestive of partial ring scotoma OS. Case 4, with acquired syphilis has only mildly constricted fields OS; L.P. vision prevented visual fields OS (Fig. 4).

Factors in case 1 that prompted looking for an alternative diagnosis were: no family history of RP, mild gliotic changes, sheathing of the retinal vasculature, and peripapillary ring-like atrophy. Contact lens examination showed a previtreoretinal haze. These factors do not negate the diagnosis of RP, but they do point to ruling out an inflammatory etiology. A VDRL test was weakly reactive, and the FTA-ABS test was positive. The

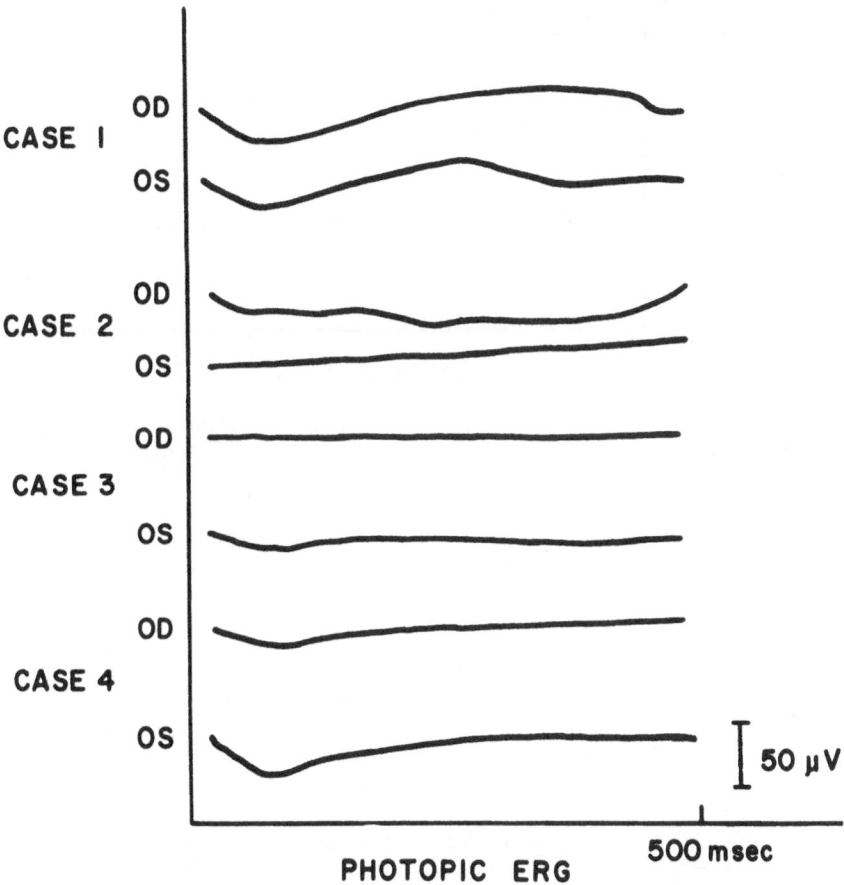

Fig. 5. (Heckenlively) – Photopic single flash ERG showing marked suppression of the b-wave in all four patients, with a-waves borderline abnormal in cases 1 and 4 and extinguished in cases 2 and 3.

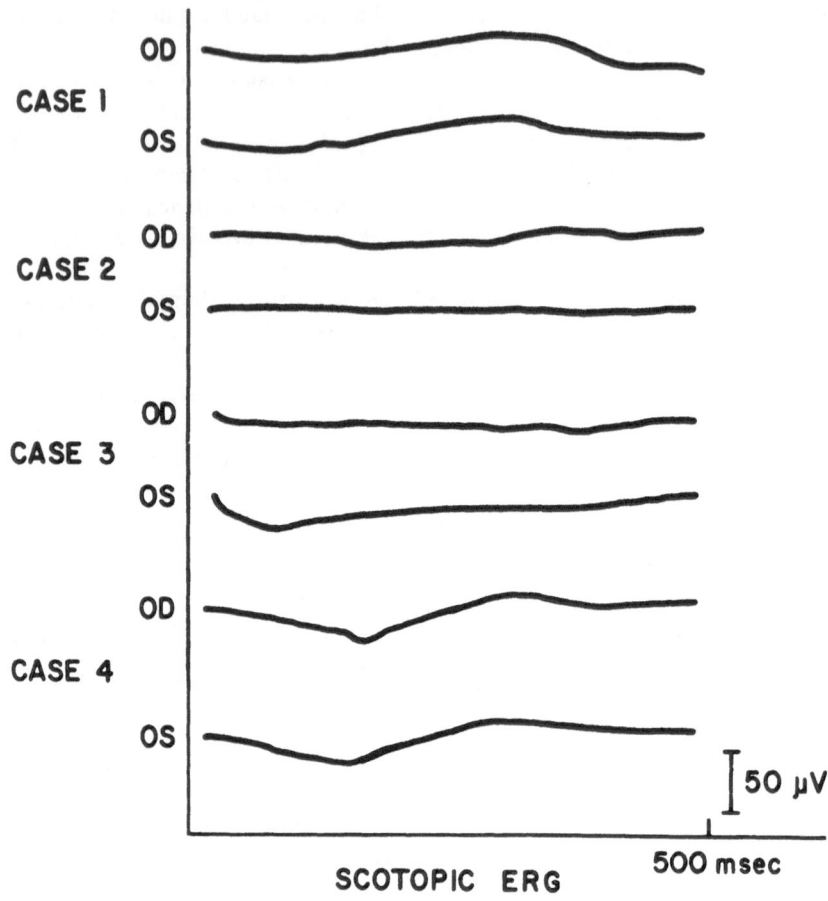

Fig. 6. (Heckenlively) – Scotopic single flash ERG showing extinction of both a and b wave components in all patients. Case 4 has prolonged stimulus a wave latency period, with late appearing, small b wave.

Table I. Summary of Four Cases of Secondary Retinitis Pigmentosa

Case No.	Age	Diagnosis	Family History	Comments
1	15	Congenital syphilis	Negative	Mother's FTA-ABS positive
2	45	,, ,,	,,	Patient and mother treated 1940's for glaucoma
3	62	Acquired syphilis	,,	
4	67	,, ,,	,,	

Table II. Comparison of Clinical Findings

Case No.	FTA-ABS	VDRL	Visual Fields	Best Corrected Visual Acuity	Interstitial Keratitis	EOG (L/D)		Color Vision	Intraocular Pressure
1	+	Weakly reactive	Constricted	20/50 OD 20/40 OS	No	OD 1.77	OS 1.75	WNL	WNL
2	+	Nonreactive	,,	20/60 OU	No	OD 1.14	OS 1.20	–	WNL (treated)
3	+	Weakly reactive	OD constricted OS atypical	20/70-OD 20/60+ OS	No	OD 1.50	OS 1.43	WNL	WNL
4	+	Nonreactive	Constricted	L. P. (SMD) 20/50+2 OS	No	OD N. I.	OS 1.42	WNL	WNL

253

Table III. Diagnostic clues for differentiating syphilitic chorioretinitis (secondary retinitis pigmentosa)

1.	Negative family history
2.	Atypical visual fields
3.	ERG not extinguished, though may be suppressed
4.	Decreased presenting visual acuity
5.	Evidence of retinal inflammatory disease

mother's FTA-ABS test was also positive, and the diagnosis was believed to be congenital syphilis.

In all cases, on single flash recordings (Fig. 5, 6) there was ERG activity, though minimal, in at least one eye. In all cases, including the first with minimal retina findings, the waveforms were greatly diminished both in the scotopic and the photopic states.

Dr. J. Lawton Smith (in a personal communication) states that in his experience the ERG is extremely depressed when the patient with syphilitic chorioretinitis is first seen; this may become extinguished in several years time. Dr. Smith emphasizes that the presence of some ERG activity helps to differentiate this disease from hereditary RP, although this can be a relative point of differentiation, since dominant RP also can have ERG activity in the early stages.

In all cases the EOG was abnormally low, though Case 1 might be considered borderline abnormal. The EOG in the right eye of patient 4 was not interpretable, due to extreme variability within the tracing from extraneous ocular movement. Unless a patient tells you of treatment for the disease, there may be no absolute indication for thinking of a diagnosis of syphilis, but there are some clues that can help to distinguish this secondary from true RP.

The ERG may be severely depressed, but usually it is not completely extinguished, although it may become so. The EOG is abnormal in both conditions, so that is not helpful. The presenting visual acuity, however, was down in all patients with syphilitic chorioretinitis. This may serve as a good clue, although by no means an absolute indication, since approximately 48% of RP patients with only moderately advanced disease will have visual acuities of less than 20/50 (Pearlman, Unpubl. data).

An important clue in all cases was a family history with no night blindness or hereditary eye disease. Evidence of inflammatory disease such as sheathing of the retinal vasculature, massive dropout of the retinal pigment epithelium, or changes in the choroidal vascular are suggestive of atypical RP.

Asymmetry of the visual fields is the final important clue, although the fields can be bilaterally constricted. Both syphilitic chorioretinitis and RP may have ring scotomas.

In summary, four patients were presented, with documented inactive syphilitic chorioretinitis, who had clinical and fundus changes similar to those that can be seen in retinitis pigmentosa. Two cases were congenital and two were acquired forms. Ages ranged from 15 to 67 years. All had negative family histories. All had positive reactions to FTA-ABS tests, while two were nonreactive VRDL tests. There was some variability, but visual fields were generally constricted. None of the patients had interstitial keratitis; all had abnormal EOG's; and in all cases, at least one eye had some ERG activity, although all ERG's were markedly suppressed.

ACKNOWLEDGEMENTS

The author wishes to thank Drs. Wilbur C.,Blount, Gerald D. Carp, and David J. Abbott of Lexington, Ky., for referring Cases 2, 3, and 4; Drs. J. Lawton Smith of Miami, Fla., and Alex Harden, Sussex Eye Hospital, Brighton, England, for sharing their valuable experience with this disease; and Verona Pettyjohn, Jules Stein Eye Institute, UCLA, for editorial assistance.

REFERENCES

Duke-Elder, S: Systems of Ophthalmology, Vol. IX. Diseases of the Uveal Tract. London, Kimpton, 1966, p. 301.

Duke-Elder, S.: Systems of Ophthalmology, Vol. X. Disease of the Retina. London, Kimpton, 1967, p. 598.

Harden, A.D. & Wright, D.J.M.: Clinical aspects of treponemal eye disease. A report of 21 cases. *Proc. R. Soc. Med.* 67, *817*, (1974).

Krill, A.E.: Hereditary Retinal and Choroidal Diseases, Vol 1. Evaluation. Hagerstown, Md., Harper & Row, 1972, p. 261.

Pearlman, J.T.: Letter to the editor. *Arch. Ophthal.*, accepted for publication, on data from a series of 200 cases of retinitis pigmentosa.

Author's address:
Dept of Ophthalmology
University of Kentucky
Medical Center
Lexington, Ky
USA

Reprint requests to:
Jules Stein Eye Institute
UCLA School of Medicine
Los Angeles, Cal. 90084
USA

RETINAL DEGENERATIONS, ELECTRORETINOGRAPHIC ASPECTS IN PATIENTS WITH MYOTONIC DYSTROPHY

B. STANESCU & J. MICHIELS

(Louvain, Belgium)

Steinert's myotonic dystrophy is an heredo-familial disorder that involves many organ systems.

Cataract is a well-known cardinal sign and has been the only ocular sign which has been associated regularly with the disease. Less known and only recently substantiated is the complex ophthalmological symptomatology including constant intra-ocular hypotonia (Brand 1950, Junge 1966, Babel & Tsacopoulos 1970) and retinal dystrophy (Burian & Burns, Junge, Stanescu & Wawernia, Babel & Tsacopoulos). Retinal alterations, macular and peripheral were seldom and sporadically reported to occur. Begaux & Decock (1952) and Franceschetti, François & Babel (1963) suggested for the first time that both diseases, muscular and retinal are produced by the same polyphenic gene. More recently Burian & Burns (1966) Junge (1967) and one of us (1970) revealed clear-cut impairment of the ERG, despite minor ophthalmoscopic changes.

The purpose of this study was to note changes in the ERG and specially to see if the implicit time is impaired in myotonic patients.

MATERIAL AND METHOD

Eleven patients, ranging in age from 30 to 54 years had well established myotonic dystrophy of the Steinert type. Thirty subjects, ranging in age from 2-68 years without abnormal ocular findings served as controls. None of our myotonic patients had been on quinine therapy.

The E.R.G. was recorded on a Van Gogh electroretinograph and for implicit time on a Tektronix cathode ray storage oscilloscope connected to the electroretinograph and Van Gogh photostimulator. The recording was done in Ganzfeld (full-field) with a single low intensity flash stimulation (intensity 1 of the photostimulator) and neutral filter that attenuated the stimulus light 200 times (−2,3 u.log) for the implicit time. The 'Ganzfeld' was realized by using a homemade translucent electrode. The tests for implicit time were recorded after 10 minutes of complete dark adaptation for scotopic conditions, and after one minute adaptation to a light of 750 Lux for photopic conditions, with the intensities 1 and 4 of the photostimulator. (It is known that the implicit time is not influenced by the intensity of the light, when no average, in photopic conditions). The implicit time was

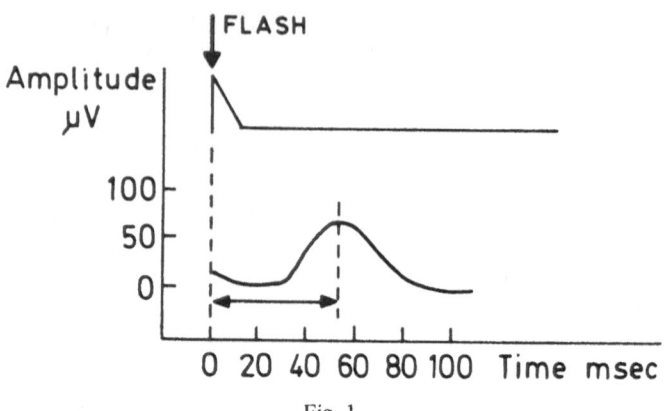

Fig. 1.

measured from the onset of the stimulus to the peak of the wave (Fig. 1). All patients had a complete ophthalmologic examination; visual acuity, slit lamp, Goldmann applanation tonometry, Goldmann perimetry, Friedmann central analyser scotometry and fundoscopy.

RESULTS

All of our 11 patients (22 eyes) with myotonic dystrophy had hypotonia, 8 of them had bilateral lens opacities and one was myopic. All had low intraocular pressure of 10 ± 2,1. In seven subjects, very minimal changes were observed in the macular areas. However in only one of eleven myotonic patients was there a serious impairement of visual acuity with a central relative scotoma, attributable to the macular involvement. No pigmentary clumping in the retinal periphery was seen. It is remarkable that the ERG of every myotonic patient was affected, with low voltage of the b-wave in photopic and scotopic conditions. Six of 11 patients had 'minimal' (less than 30 μV) (Krill 1972) photopic and scotopic ERG. The photopic implicit time was not measured since the amplitude of b-waves was too low in these patients. So an increased intensity (4 of our photostimulator) of the flash stimulation was used. Five of our patients had 'subnormal' photopic and scotopic ERG. We consider 'subnormal' less than 2 S.D., as Krill proposed in 1972. The photopic implicit time was normal but all myotonic patients had delayed scotopic implicit time (Fig. 2). The average value for amplitude and implicit time were significantly higher than the normal value (P < 001). (Table. 1, 2).

DISCUSSION

In contrast with minimal changes or rather normal fundoscopy in ten of eleven myotonic patients, all eleven showed a marked decrease of the b-wave amplitude of the ERG in photopic and scotopic conditions with delayed scotopic implicit time. It is relevant that no concordance exists between ophthalmoscopic appearance and ERG alteration. As none of our

258

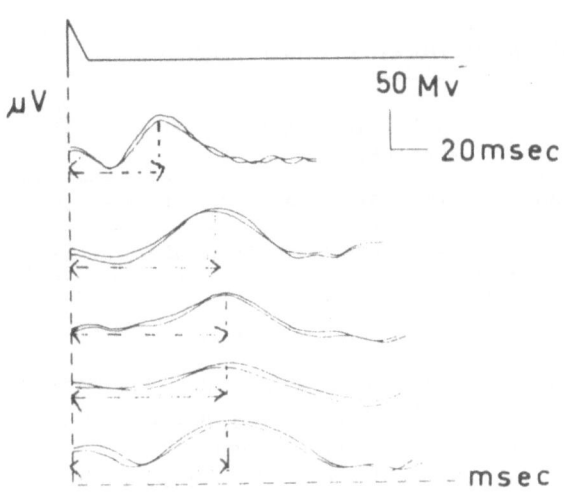

Fig. 2.

Table I.

No	SEX	AGE	PHOTOPIC b WAVE INTENSITY 2	SCOTOPIC b WAVE INTENSITY 2
			AMPLITUDE	
1	M	49	40	60
2	M	39	15	60
3	F	54	60	80
4	F	30	35	50
5	F	50	40	60
6	M	36	10	40
7	M	49	20	40
8	F	45	50	70
9	M	39	40	70
10	F	50	50	70
11	M	44	60	80
S.E.M.		44,1 ± 7,3	38,2 ± 17,1	61,8 ± 14
Normal values + S.D.			85 ± 14	148 ± 30

ERG IN PATIENTS WITH MYOTONIC DYSTROPHY

Table II.

IMPLICIT TIME[X] IN HEALTHY AND MYOTONIC SUBJECTS

	No of subjects	mean age	Photopic Intensity 1	Intensity 4	Scotopic Intensity 1	Intensity 4
HEALTHY SUBJECTS	30	34,2	41,3 ± 5,7	41,0 ± 6,0	60,0 ± 7,23	47,9 ± 8,9
MYOTONIC SUBJECTS	11	44,01	41,40 ± 5,7	41,25 ± 4,13	83,63 ± 6,34	53,81 ± 6

[X]Implicit time measured in milliseconds and S.E.M.

patients was on quinine therapy (Betten et al., 1975), we agree with the opinion of Mausolf and Burns that retinal abnormalities are part of the disease and not the result of an intoxication.

Berson et al (1969) and Brunette (1969) made distinction between voltage and temporal alterations of the E.R.G. Destruction of circumscribed retinal areas results in a reduced amplitude of the b-wave but not delayed implicit time, while alterations in amplitude and implicit time can be explained by generalized malfunction of all receptor systems, of cones or rods. The delayed scotopic implicit time in myotonic patients implicates primarily the rod system, that is a widespread functional alteration of rods, which explains the abnormal dark adaptation curves found by Burian & Burns (1966). We noted also the lenticular opacities and the decreased intra-ocular pressure in a majority of our patients. It is evident that in myotonic dystrophy there is a widespread involvement of the eye. Burian & Burns agreed that Steinert's myotonia is an abiotrophy, as Francheschetti, François & Babel (1963) had suggested. The question is, What is the basic defect in myotonic dystrophy?

Recently Roses & Appel (1973) have suggested that the fundamental defect in Steinert's myotonia is of membrane origin and considered it like a diffuse membrane disorder with manifestation in many tissues. Controlled scanning electron microscopic studies of erythrocytes, and abnormalities of endogenous membrane protein-kinase system (Roses et al., 1975) in myotonic patients support the idea of the widespread presence of metabolic alterations in membranes. Appel & Roses (1975) demonstrated on red bloods cells of myotonic patients the existence of abnormal Ca^+ that stimulated K^+ efflux. They considered that many membranes may be affected. Steinert's myotonia is due probably to an inborn error of metabolism, that is probably of membrane origin. This could explain the involvement of the eye; lens opacities, hypotonia and retinal dystrophy. In our laboratory, we are now trying to modify the permeability of the retinal cellular membrane in normal and myotonic subjects. We have only a few cases, so we are unable to have valuable conclusions yet.

CONCLUSIONS

— The ERG alterations confirm the existence of the retinal dystrophy in

Steinert's disease in contrast with minimal or no ophthalmoscopic modifications.
– The delayed scotopic implicit time suggests a predominant alteration of the rod system.

REFERENCES

Appel, S.H. Biochemical membrane changes in myotonic dystrophy. Lecture in the department of neurology. U.C.L. Louvain Belgium 1975.

Appel & Roses (1975) quoted in addendum by Roses et al., 1973.

Babel, J. & M. Tsacopoulos. Les lésions rétiniennes de la dystrophie myotonique. *Am. Oculist.* 203, *1049*, 1970.

Begaux, C. & Decock, G. Sur une souche de myotonie dystrophique dont au moins un des sujets atteints est porteur de dégénérescence tapeto-rétinienne atypique. *J. Genet. Hum.* 1, *95*, 1952.

Berson, E., Gouras, P. & Myrianthopoulos, M. Dominant retinitis pigmentosa with reduced penetrance. *Arch. Ophth.* 81, *226*, 1969.

Berson, E. & Kanters, L. Cone and rod responses in a family with recessively inherited retinitis pigmentosa. *Arch. Ophth.* 82, *228*, 1970.

Berson, E. Progressive cone-rod degeneration. *Am. J. Ophth.* 80, *68*, 1968.

Berson, E. Progressive cone degeneration dominantly inherited. *Arch. Ophth.* 80, *77*, 1968.

Betten, M.G., Bilchick, R.C. & Smith, M. Pigmentary retinopathy of myotonic dystrophy. *Amer. J. Ophthal.* 72, *720*, 1975.

Burian, H.M. & Burns, Ch. Electroretinography and dark adaptation in patients with myotonic dystrophy. *Amer. J. Ophthal.* 61, *1044*, 1966.

Burian, H.M. & Burns, Ch. Ocular changes in myotonic dystrophy. *Am. J. Ophthal.* 63, *22*, 1967.

Brand, J. Augendruck bei myotonicher dystrophie. *Ophthalmologica* 159, *157*, 1950.

Brunette, J.R. The human electroretinogram during dark adaptation. Implicit time and amplitude studies. *Arch. ophthalm.* 82, *495*, 1969.

Davidson, L. The eye in dystrophia myotonica. *B. J. Ophth.* 45, *182*, 1965.

Francheschetti, A., Francois, J. & Babel, J. Les hérédo-dégénérescences chorio-rétiniennes. Masson Paris 1963.

Francheschetti, A., Francois, J. & Babel, J. Chorioretinal heredo-degeneration. Ch.C. Thomas. Springfield, Illinois 1974.

Junge, J. Ocular changes in dystrophia myotonica. *Ophthalmologica* 155, *295*, 1968.

Krill, A. Hereditary retinal and choroidal diseases. Harper and Row publishers – Hagerstown. Maryland, 1972.

Manschot. Histological findings in a case of dystrophia myotonica. *Ophthalmologica* 155, *294-296*, 1968.

Mausolf, F. & Burns, Ch. Morphologic and functional retinal changes in myotonic dystrophy unrelated to quinine therapy. *Amer. J. Ophthal.* 74, *1141*, 1972.

Roses, A.D., Appel, S.H., Butterfield, D.A. & Chesnut, D.B. Membrane alterations in myotonic muscular dystrophy. New developments in electromyography and clinical neurophysiology (Desmedt, J.E. Tome 1). Karger – Basel 1973.

Roses & Appel (1975) quoted in addendunn in Roses & Appel et al (1973).

Stanescu, B. & Wawernia, E. Electroretinographic and electroencephalographic changes in dystrophia myotonica Steinert. *Ophthalmologica* 160, *157*, 1970.

Stanescu, B. & Michiels, J. Temporal aspects of electroretinography in patients with myotonic dystrophy. *Amer. J. Ophthal.* 80, *2*, 1975.

Authors' address:
Clinique Ophtalmologique
Hôpital St. Raphael
3000 Louvain
Belgium

CENTRAL AND PERIPHERAL RETINAL DEGENERATION IN A FAMILY: A STUDY OF THE ERG AND FIELDS

G. STEPHENS, A. CINOTTI, C. HWA, A. CAPUTO,
J. BASTEK & J.H. WHITE

(Newark, N.J.)

In a family with x-linked intermediate hereditary retinal degeneration, two variants of a degenerative process were found. In one family branch the degeneration was peripheral, and the second was the inverse type, central retinal degeneration.

FIGURE 1 IS THE PEDIGREE OF THIS FAMILY

An important fact to mention is that the first known carrier in this family, a great-grandmother (Generation I, # 1), had married twice. As a result of her first marriage, the affected members demonstrated primary peripheral retinal degeneration, and from her second marriage, one descendant demonstrated primary central retinal degeneration, while two others were known to have severe visual problems prior to their deaths.

METHOD

A history of the entire family was ascertained. Each of the members available received a standard complete ophthalmological examination, which included visual acuity, color vision, biomicroscopy, ophthalmoscopy, visual field with white and color test objects on the Goldman perimeter. In addition, dark adaptation tests and electroretinography were performed.

REPORT OF CASES

Case 1: The propositus of the family was A.B. (Generation III, # 16), who had a visual acuity of 5/200 OD and 2/200 OS. The fundi show black, bony, scattered, corpuscle-like pigment, excluding the macular area. The optic discs were slightly pale, and the caliber of the arteries was attenuated. The dark adaptation test showed only a 6.5 log unit elevation of the cone fraction of the curve. The EOG was of a low ratio: 1.0 OD and 1.12 OS. The ERG was extinguished. Similar data was found in F.B., the 45 year old brother of A.B. (Generation III, # 18).

Case 2: M.B., the 81 year old mother of A.B. (Generation II, # 4), a carrier, was seriously ill with lymphoma. Due to her general health status, her examination was incomplete. Five other members of the family were examined. The first two were from the family branch with peripheral retinal degeneration, and the other three were from the family with central degeneration.

Case 3: M.C. (Generation IV, # 34), the 28 year old daughter of the propositus, A.B., had a visual acuity of 20/20 OU. Both fundi were slightly

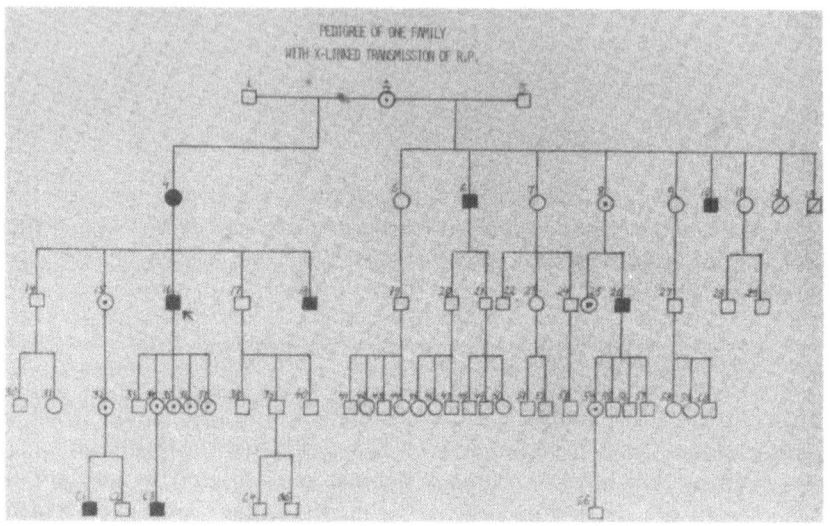

Fig. 1.

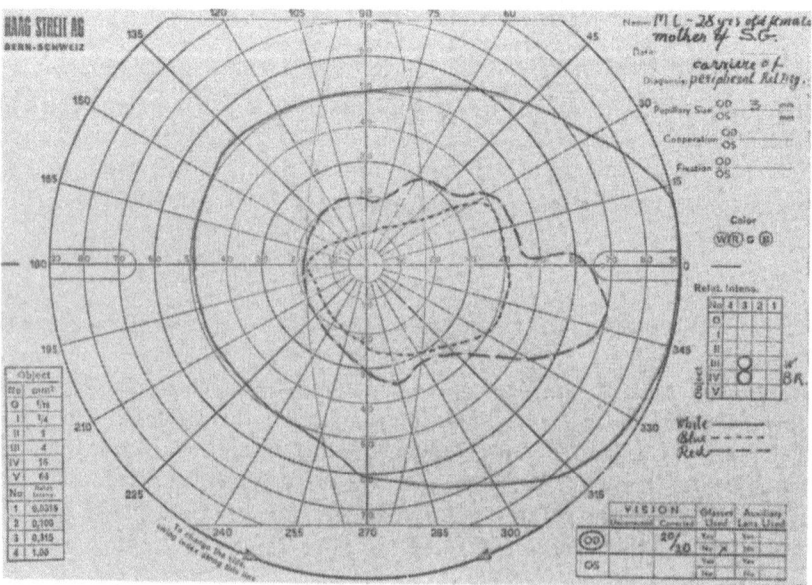

Fig. 2.

tigroid with some granularity at the equator and normal appearing vessels. Dark adaptation was within normal limits OU; the alpha point was present; the scotopic curve reached 2 log units, and the EOG ratio was 1.8. The dark-adapted ERG to white, red and blue light was within normal limits. *Figure 2* shows the remarkable aspect of the field of this patient, namely that the blue isopter was inward to the red, using test objects of exactly the same size and intensity for both colors.

Case 4: S.G. (Generation V, # 63), the five year old affected son of M.C. and grandson of A.B., had a visual acuity of 20/50 OU with correction. Both fundi showed some granularity at the equator. The macular areas appeared normal. The disc showed a small physiological cup, and biomicroscopy showed clear media OU. In dark adaptation OU, the alpha point was not very well marked, and the scotopic curve reached only 3 log units. The EOG ratio was low: 1.4 OD and 1.5 OS. The ERG was done with an acrylic hook and a gold point as the active electrode, since the skin electrode response was too small to be recorded. This small boy reacted strongly on the first trial use of the Burian-Allen contact lens, and his mother would not permit further trials. In the dark adapted state with the hook electrode, the ERG response to white light was: a-wave 16 μV, b-wave 52 μV. The culmination time of the b-wave was 45 msec. Response to red light in the dark adapted state was: a-wave 14 μV, b-photopic wave 19 μV, and b-scotopic wave 7μV. The culmination time of the b-photopic wave was 45 msec. Culmination time of the b-scotopic wave was 102 msec. Thus, the ERG response as recorded with the hook was diminished with some delay in the response. Figure 3 showed the visual field of this patient, S.G., to have more

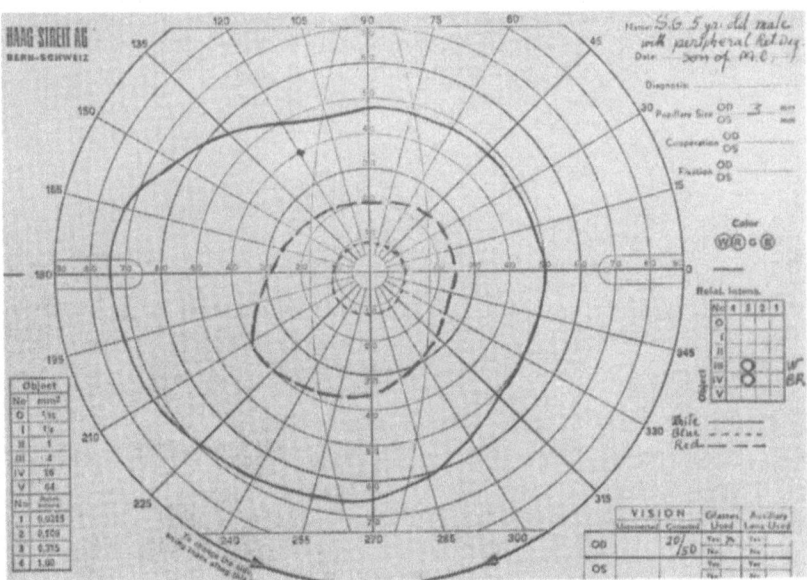

Fig. 3.

265

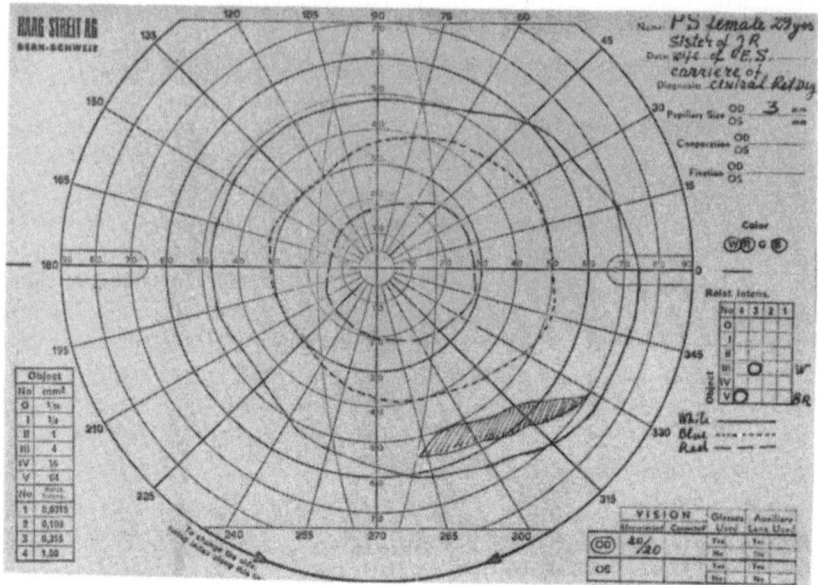

Fig. 4.

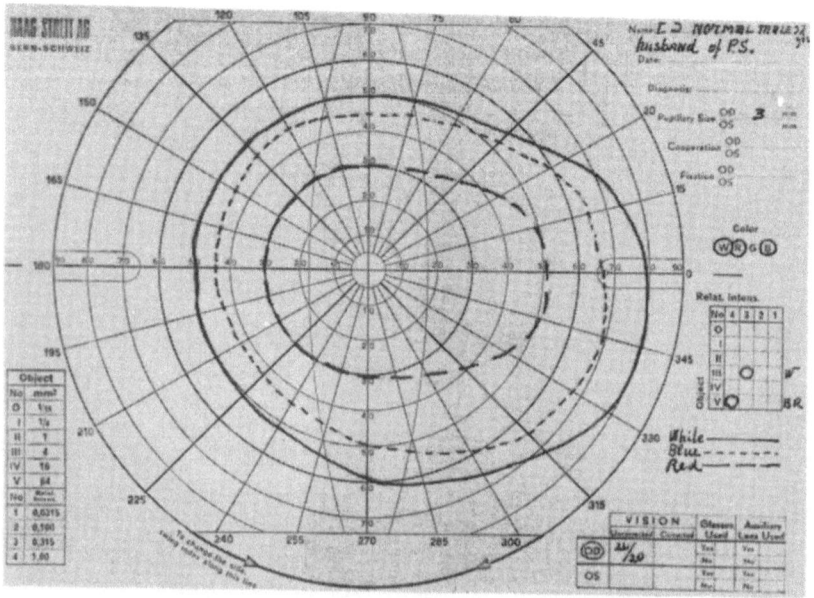

Fig. 5.

pronounced constriction of the blue isopter than the red isopter. When compared with the field of his mother, M.C., the blue isopter was more constricted than hers. This concludes the cases which we were able to examine in the family branch with peripheral degeneration.

From the second family branch with inverse (central) degeneration, we examined three members, one of whom had normal results.

Case 5: P.S. (Generation III, # 25), a 29 year old female carrier and sister of J.R., had a visual acuity of 20/20 OU. Her color vision was normal. The fundi showed some glistening reflections in the paramacular area and toward the equator. The disc appeared normal. On dark adaptation testing, the alpha point is present and the scotopic portion of the curve reached 2 log units. The EOG ratio was 1.96 OD and 2.0 OS. In the dark adapted state, the ERG responses to white, red and blue light were within normal limits. Figure 4 shows the field of P.S. Here, the red isopter was abnormally constricted (as is obvious when compared to the field of her husband in Fig. 5). There was also a small sectorial segmental defect inferotemporally.

Case 6: J.R. (Generation III, # 26), the 43 year old brother of P.S., was affected by the central type of degeneration and had a visual acuity of 20/200 OD and 6/200 OS. He did not recognize any Ishihara color plates. Biomicroscopy showed some vitreous floaters in each eye. Dark adaptation testing showed a lack of the cone plateau. The scotopic curve reached 2.5 log units. The fundi showed a well-circumscribed, roundish degenerative lesion of about 2 disc diameters at the macular area. This lesion looked slightly granular and had some scanty pigment inward. Additional dark pigmentation was seen at the border of this lesion. The rest of the fundus

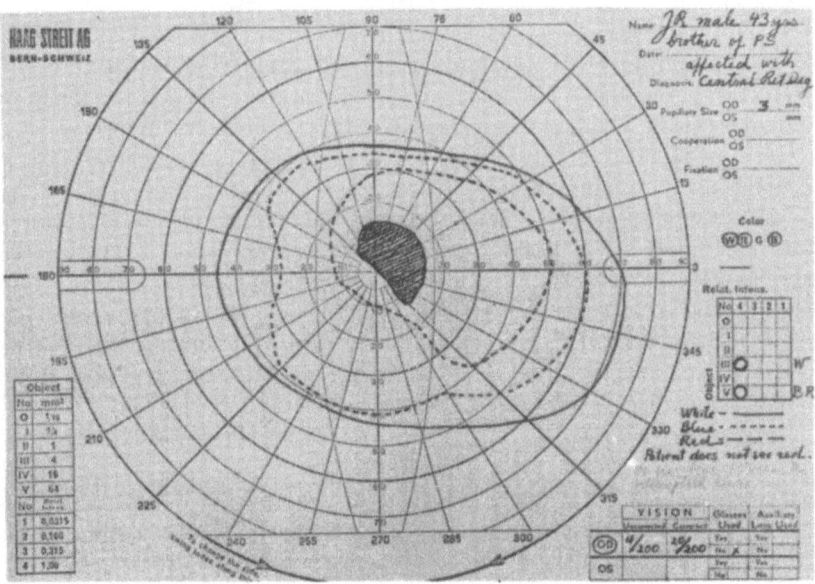

Fig. 6.

was tigroid. The EOG ratio was 1.25 OD and 1.4 OS. In the dark adapted state, the ERG with the Burian-Allen contact lens was: a-wave 52 μV, b-wave 138 μV. The culmination time of the b-wave was 48 msec. The response to red light was: a-wave 13 μV, b-photopic wave 6 μV (extremely small) and b-scotopic wave 40 μV. The culmination time of the b-photopic wave was 45 msec, and that of the b-scotopic wave was 98 msec. The response to blue light is: b-wave 122 μV, with a culmination time of 55 msec. The ERG photopic response is very small, but all other waves were within normal limits. There was a slight delay in the culmination time. Figure 6 shows the field of J.R. with a white test object of size 3 and intensity 4. The field was slightly constricted with a symmetrical eccentric scotoma located slightly superotemporally, touching the central fixation point. He did not see the red test object, of size 5, intensity 4. With a blue test object of the same size and intensity as the red, he was able to see an irregular ring-like area around the central area and scotomata. He did not have a ring scotoma. The field of the left eye was a mirror image of the field of the right eye.

Members of this family were also examined for certain trace elements. In affected members, we found decreased zinc and increased copper. The healthy carriers showed a reversed ratio. This idea to examine the trace elements was from J. Bastek (1975).

COMMENTS

The specific findings of the fundi, dark adaptation and the ERG in a sex-linked peripheral form of tapeto-retinal degeneration have been described by previous investigators (Berson et al., 1969). In our case of G.S. with the same form of the disease, we have obtained similar ERG findings, namely a diminished response with a slightly delayed culmination time. In the case of J.R. with the inverse (central) degenerative form of the disease, all responses except the photopic b-wave response to red stimulus were within normal limits. However, there was some slight delay in the culmination time of the other responses. The b-photopic red response was strongly diminished.

The EOG ratio in carriers was within normal limits, but in affected members of both family branches it was low.

In the visual field tests, the changes of the position of the color isopters (red and blue) could be indicative of peripheral or central tapeto-retinal degeneration. A matter of conjecture is the possible unfluence (or lack of it) of the gene of the first husband upon the gene of the carrier great-grand-mother in the formation of the family branch with peripheral tapeto-retinal degeneration, and the interaction of the second husband's gene to form the family branch with inverse tapeto-retinal degeneration.

REFERENCES

Bastek, J., Bogden, J., Cinotti, A., TenHove, W., Stephens, G., Marcopolous, M. & Charles, J., Trace elements in a family with sex-linked retinitis pigmentosa. Report given at ARVO Meeting, Atlantic Section, Symposium on Retinitis Pigmentosa at Durham, N.C., November 1975.

Berson, E., Gouras, P., Gunkel, K. and Mirianthopoulus, N., Rod and cone responses in sex-linked retinitis pigmentosa. *Archives of Ophthalmology* 81, *215*, Feb. 1969.

A CASE OF UNILATERAL RETINITIS PIGMENTOSA SINE PIGMENTO

G. STEPHENS, A. CINOTTI, C. HWA, A. CAPUTO,
J.H. WHITE & L. VINCENTI

(Newark, N.J.)

This is a follow-up report of a case of unilateral retinitis pigmentosa first published in 1962 by Jacobson & Stephens (1962).

Francois (1952, 1961) reviewing the subject of unilateral retinitis pigmentosa, felt that in order to make this diagnosis: 1. The affected eye must show all the classical symptoms and signs of R.P.; 2. The other eye should have no trace of the disease; 3. The patient should be observed for a sufficiently long period to preclude the late development of the disease in the fellow eye; and 4. A secondary R.P. should be ruled out.

This patient, first seen at age 27, showed unilateral retinitis pigmentosa since pigmento OS. When first seen, she gave a history that six years previously, during the fourth month of her pregnancy, she noticed some difficulty with vision in her left eye. She was told at that time that she did not have toxemia of pregnancy. There was no evidence or history of hereditary disease or consanguinity in her family. Her general health status was good, and her VDRL was negative. The only medication she had been taking was Fiorinal for migraine headaches.

Her visual acuity was 20/30 with −5.5 correction OD, and 20/30 with −7.0 correction OS. On fundus examination of the right eye, the disc was normal except for a few yellowish spots at its margin. There were some myopic changes. The macular reflex was slightly blurred, but the vessels in this eye were normal.

The left disc was slightly paler than the right. There were a few myopic changes near this disc, and two small black pigment spots near the nasal border. The macular reflex was not very clear. The arteries were slightly narrowed, but no abnormal pigment was in evidence here. Biomicroscopy OU − slight vitreous floaters.

As you see in Fig. 1, the Visual Field of the right eye was normal; but, the field of the left eye was reduced to 5 degrees with a small arcuate segment preserved inferiorly. The adaptation test showed a normal cone curve and a normal rod curve in the right eye. The left eye showed only the cone portion of the curve. In Fig. 2, the ERG of the right showed a normal response. The ERG of the left eye was non-recordable.

In February 1976, fourteen years after the first publication of her case and seventeen years since the first examination, we saw this patient again. She is now 44 years old. Her general health has been good. She no longer

269

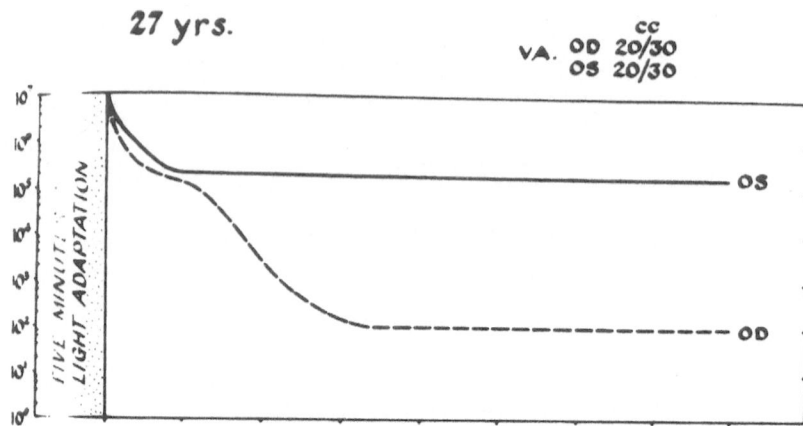

27 yrs.

VA. OD 20/30 cc
OS 20/30

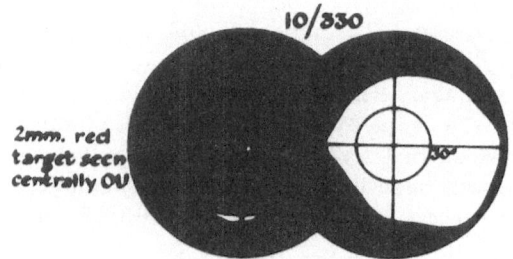

10/330

2mm. red target seen centrally OU

Fig. 1.

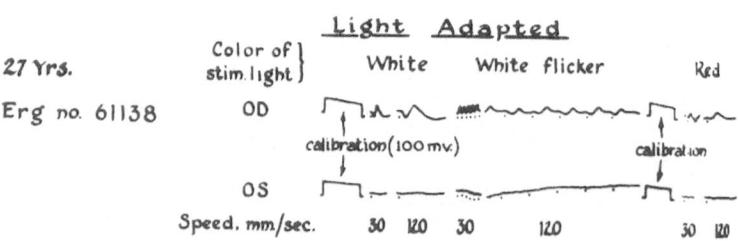

Light Adapted

27 Yrs.

Erg no. 61138

Color of stim. light

| | White | White flicker | Red |

OD — calibration(100 mv.) — calibration

OS

Speed, mm/sec. 30 120 30 120 30 120

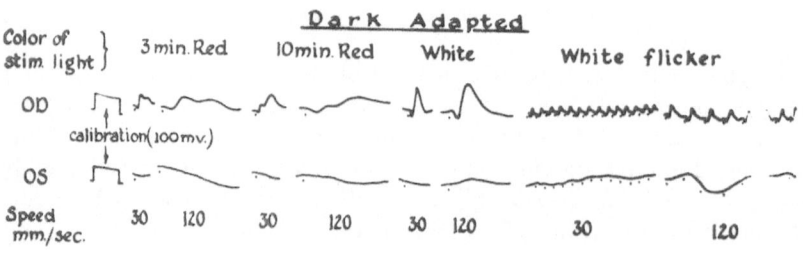

Dark Adapted

Color of stim. light } 3 min. Red   10 min. Red   White   White flicker

OD — calibration(100 mv.)

OS

Speed mm/sec. 30 120 30 120 30 120 30 120

Fig. 2.

270

complains of the migraine headaches and therefore is no longer taking the Fiorinal. However, subjectively the patient seemed more nervous and impatient.

On examination, her vision with correction was still 20/30 OD. However, the vision of the left eye was reduced to light perception with uncertain projection.

The fundus of her right eye was unchanged. The fundus of the left eye was difficult to visualize in detail because of a now-advanced nuclear cataract. Once again, we were not able to detect pigmentation looking through the clear peripheral edge of her lens at the periphery of her fundus. The cataract precluded good fundus photography. The visual field and adaptometry of the right were again normal. These tests were impossible to do on the left eye because of the cataract. Fig. 3 shows the results of the ERG examination which was done with the skin electrode method. In a dark adapted state, the response to white light was: a-wave = 15 μV; b-wave = 82 μV; a-wave culmination time = 19 msec; b-wave culmination time = 42 msec. The response was within normal limits.

The response with the Burian-Allen contact lens was: a-wave = 66 μV; b-wave = 205 μV. This response is about three times greated than that with

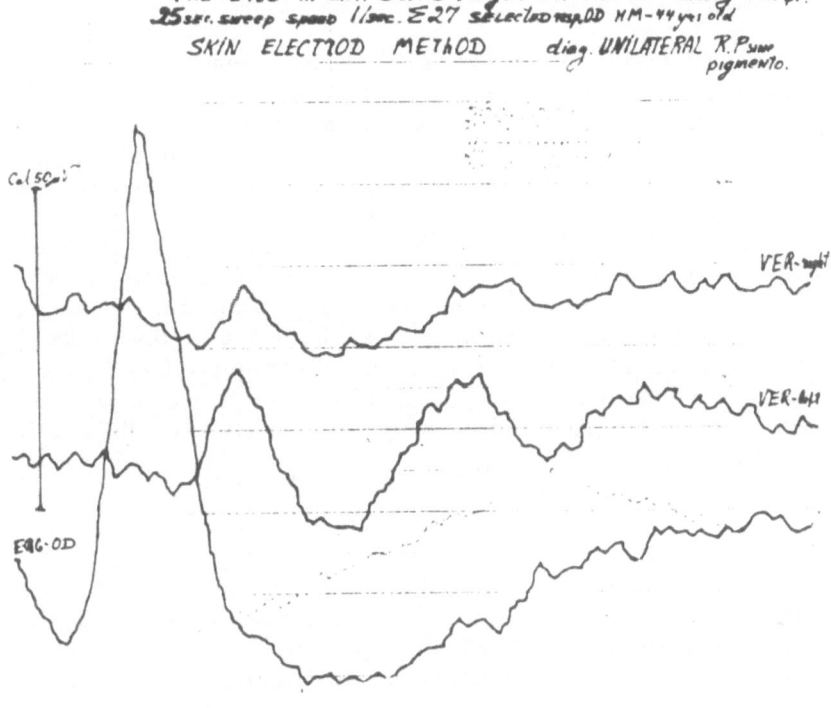

Fig. 3.

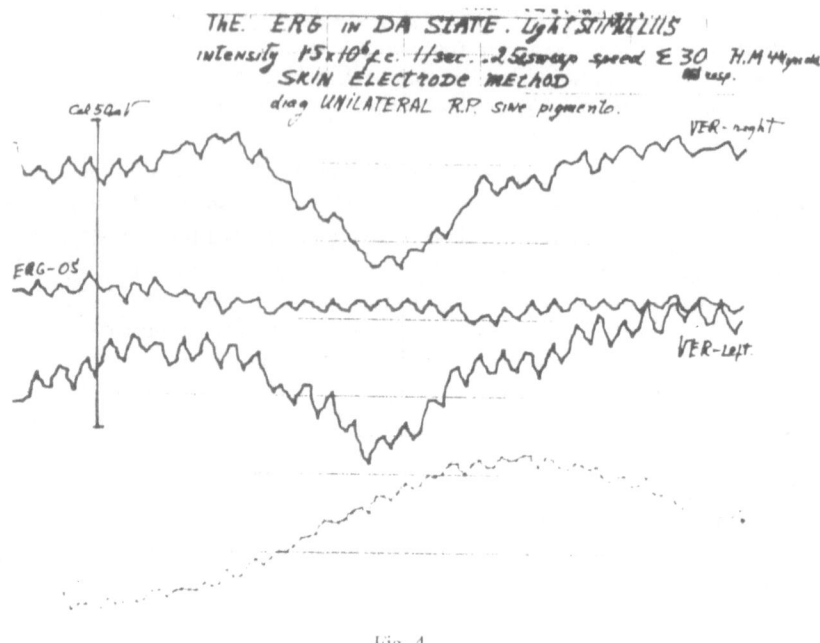

Fig. 4.

the skin electrodes. The configuration of this response is similar to that withthe skin electrodes. The visual evoked response recorded simultaneously with the ERG was well-formed and with good voltage.

The ERG response of the left eye was again non-recordable. However, the patient perceived light with this eye. The VER response obtained was abnormal in configuration. (Fig. 4 below).

The patient declined the use of the contact lens in the OS. The ERG and VER results of the right eye were obtained by summation after preliminary analysis of each response and elimination of those resulting from inadequate visual stimulation due to blinking, eye movement or distortion of the EEG base line. It was not possible to apply the selective proceeding for the left eye because of the lack of any recordable response. Here we have no information as to whether the stimulation was adequate, and the ERG and VER were summated without editing.

SUMMARY

All classical symptoms and signs of retinitis pigmentosa, namely: 1) night blindness, well-documented by the adaptometry result; 2) a strongly constricted field with a small vestige of annular segment; and 3) a non-recordable ERG were found in the left eye at the first examination of this then 27 year old female. Seventeen years later, her right eye remains normal, while the left eye has progressed with loss of vision and cataract formation, as well as retinal degeneration, but still no noticeable pigmentation.

REFERENCES

Francois, J. and Verriest, G. Retinopathy pigmentair unilaterale. *Ophthalmologica* 124, 65, 1952.

Francois, J. Hereditary in ophthalmology. St. Louis, C.V. Mosby Co., 1961, p. 455.

Jacobson, J.H. & Stephens, G. Unilateral retinitis pigmentosa sine pigmento. *Archives of Ophthalmology* 67, *456*, 1962.

Authors' address:
Dept of Ophthalmology
New Jersey Medical School
100 Bergen Street, Room 1401
Newark, N.J. 07103
USA

ABNORMAL ERG FINDINGS IN A CASE WITH FUNDUS FLAVIMACULATUS WITH TYPICAL STARGARDT'S MACULAR DEGENERATION

HIDEKI NAKANO M.D.

(Tokyo)

INTRODUCTION

Since the first description of seven patients from two families with juvenile hereditary macular degeneration by Stargardt in 1909, many cases with this disease, have been reported by subsequent workers. And the disease described in Stargardt's original publication has been termed Stargardt's prototype for a specific disease or Stargardt's juvenile macular degeneration. However, several conditions were included in the Stargardt's disease category in the past literature, and this confusion is well illustrated by Stargardt himself in a subsequent publication (Stargardt, 1913).

Recently Krill & Deutman (1972) evaluated the conditions under the diagnosis of Stargardt's disease precisely and classified them into several different diseases. They advocate that the condition initially described by Stargardt (1909) is identical to fundus flavimaculatus described by Franceschetti in 1962, especially with atrophic macular degeneration (Krill & Deutman, 1972).

Only a few cases of fundus flavimaculatus have been reported in Japan (Yuri, Akabane & Tajima, 1969; Ogino, Hasebe, Uchino & Yoshida, 1970; Watanabe, Tamai & Matsuura, 1971), and their functional studies were unsatisfactory. Neither of them had apparent macular degeneration.

This paper presents a case of fundus flavimaculatus with typical Stargardt's macular degeneration. The ERG revealed severe photopic dysfunction, while scotopic function was mildly affected.

METHODS

The evaluation consisted of personal and family history, visual acuity, slit-lamp examination, fundus photography, fluorescein angiography, visual fields with a Goldmann perimeter, dark adaptation with a Goldmann-Weekers adaptometer, color vision tests (the Ishihara, Ohkuma and TMD pseudoisochromatic plates, the Farnsworth Panel D-15 and 100-hue test), and ERG.

Electroretinographic testing consisted of the single-flash photopic responses elicited by scotopically and photopically balanced, red and blue colored stimuli, modified methods of Berson et al. (1968) and of Ohba (1974), were presented at various levels of light adaptation, as well as dark-adapted responses at increasing intensities of a white stimulus, as described

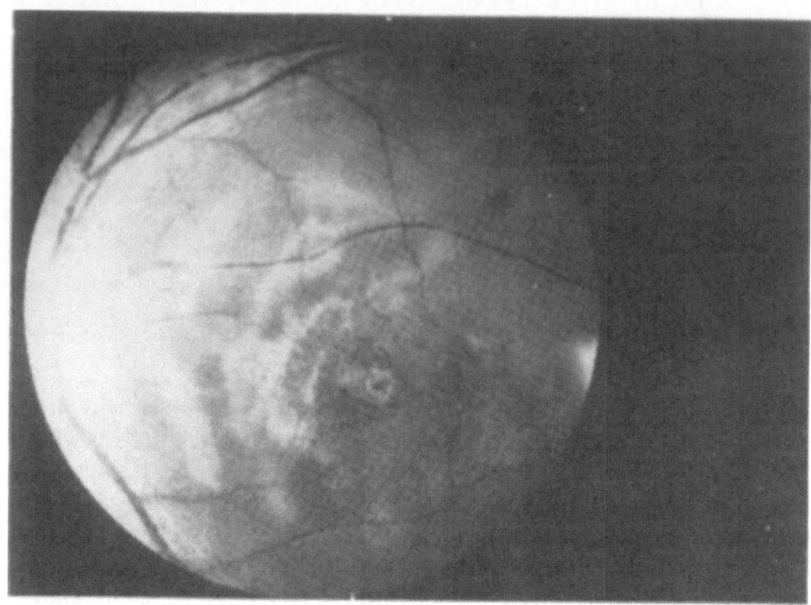

Fig. 1. The fundus of the left eye. Note the typical macular degeneration. Both fundi were similar.

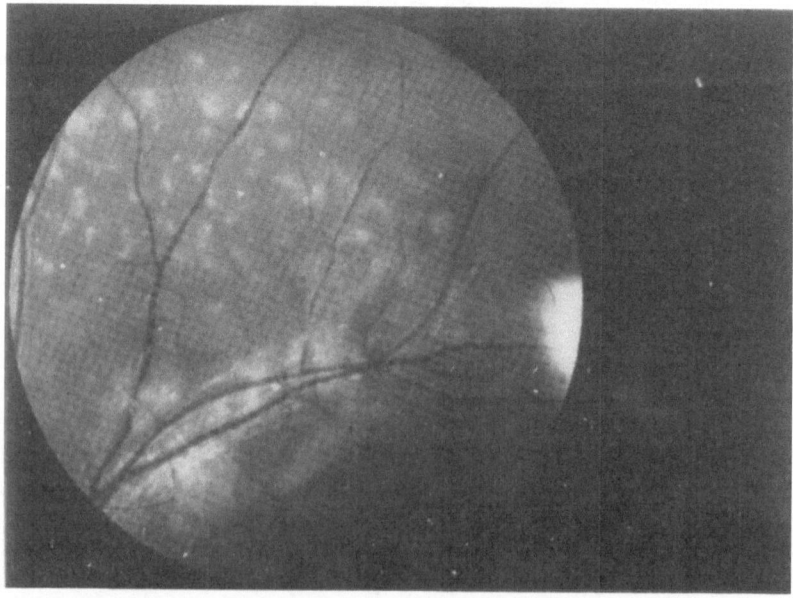

Fig. 2. Upper temporal area of the left fundus. Many scattered flavimaculatus flecks, some of them confluent into various patterns.

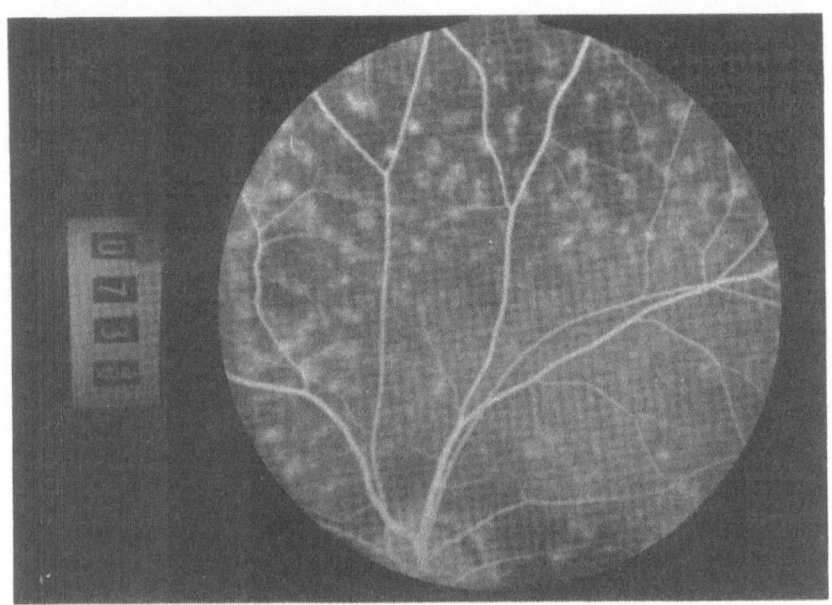

Fig. 3. Same eye as fig. 2, during late venous phase of fluorescein angiography. Apparent increase of number of flecks. Faint or no fluorescence in conspicuous, more isolated lesions of fig. 2.

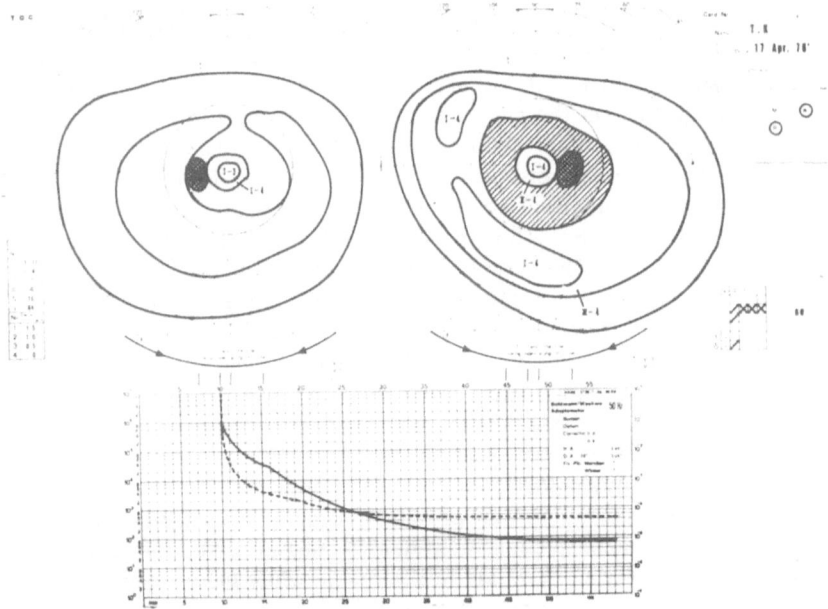

Fig. 4. Top: Peripheral visual fields of both eyes. Bottom: Dark adaptation curves. Solid line indicates right eye's and dashed line left.

277

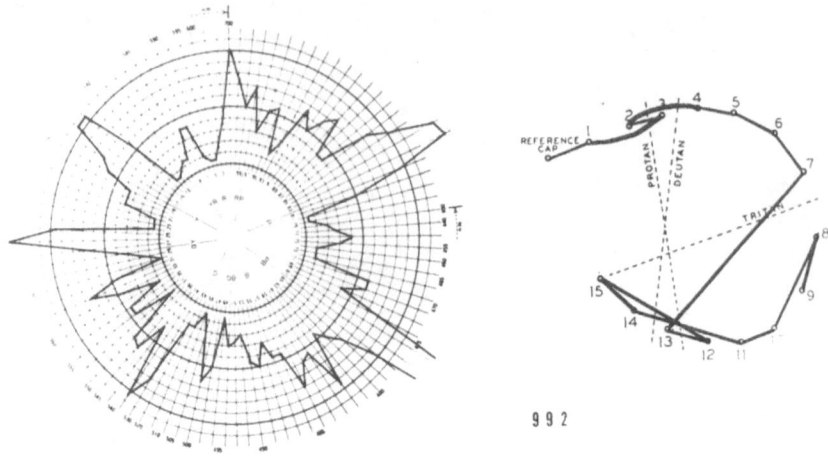

Fig. 5. Results of Farnsworth Panel D-15 and 100-hue test. Number in the center of the bottom is the total error scores of 100-hue test.

in detail previously (Nakano, 1976). In addition, the recovery of the ERG during dark adaptation (Merin & Auerbach, 1970) was examined in this study.

RESULTS

A boy, aged 15 years, complaining of poor vision, was referred to our clinic for investigation of his loss of visual acuity, which had gradually deteriorated from the age of about 8. There was some consanguinity in his family, i.e. his grandmother on the maternal and his father were in the relationship of cousins. But his mother stated that all other members of the pedigree except for him had good visual acuity and normal color vision.

His best corrected visual acuity was: RE; 0.1 with sph. −2.75D. cyl. −1.25D. ax. 30° and LE; 0.15 with sph. −3.25D. cyl. −1.75D. ax. 180°. No nystagmus was noted. The anterior segments, the media and the optic discs were normal. The macular area was covered by an atrophic patch, about 3 PD wide, showing a yellowish gray metallic color and stippled by fine and coarse dusty pigment (fig. 1). Deep yellowish flecks varying in shape, size, some of pisciform of round shape, were scattered over the paramacular and midperipheral regions (fig. 2). There was a tendency for confluence of the flecks and the borders were occasionally fuzzy with the lesions having a dirty appearance of the color. Both fundi were similar.

Fluorescein studies showed an increased number of flecks in areas which were occupied by inconspicuous confluent lesions in ophthalmoscopy, but more isolated pisciform and round flecks seen in white light showed little or no fluorescence (fig. 3). Peripheral visual fields were normal, but partial ring and paracentral scotomas were obtained. The isopters with the smaller target were constricted (fig. 4).

278

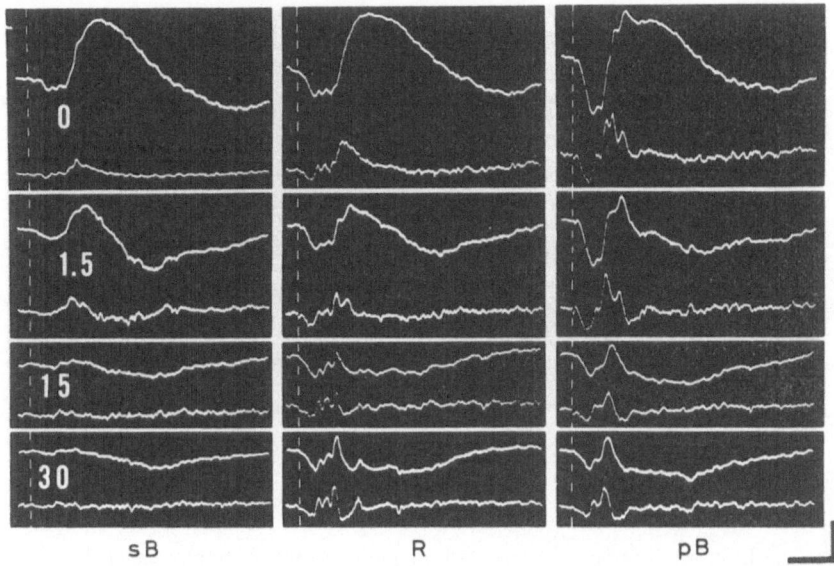

Fig. 6. a) Normal electroretinogram elicited by red and blue coloured stimuli of various background intensities. The sB-blue and R-red flash, and pB-blue and R-red flash equated scotopically and photopically each other. Vertical hatched line indicates stimulus onset. Numbers on the left end of column: Intensity of the adapting white light (cd/m^2). Calibration: 40 msec, 200 μv in each.

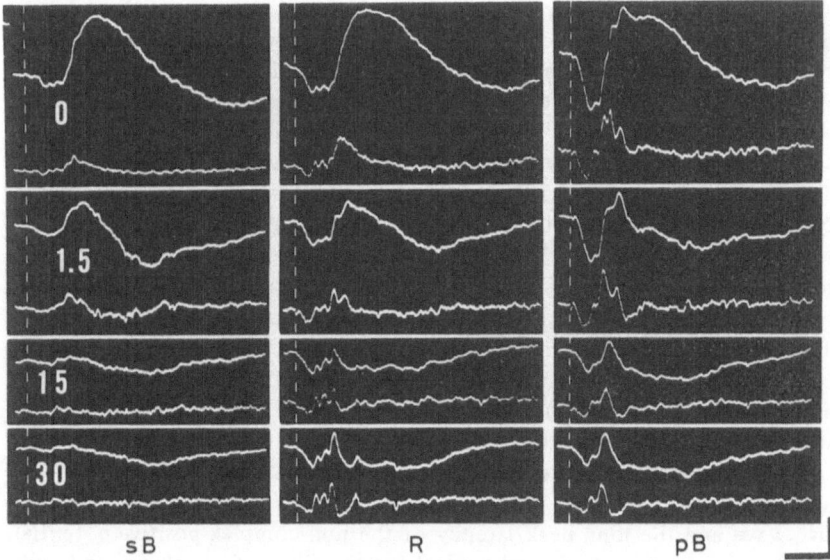

Fig. 6.b) Electroretinogram of the patient under same test condition on a). The upper and lower records in each pair represent responses obtained by different time constant (upper; 0.1 sec., lower; 0.003 sec.) at the same time. Left eye was recorded.

279

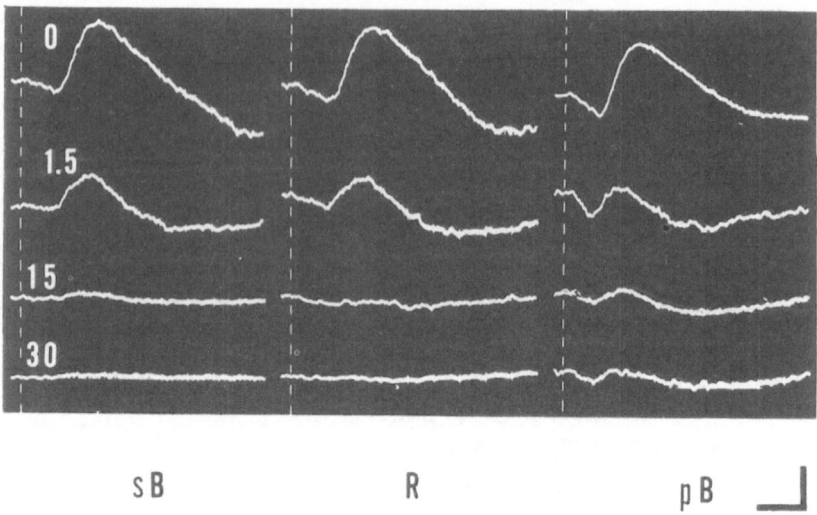

SB   R   pB

Fig. 7. Electroretinogram of a case with progressive cone dystrophy under same condition on fig. 6.

The dark-adaptation study revealed a slightly elevated and shortened cone plateau, but an almost normal final threshold was observed, on the right eye. On the left eye, there were absence of cone plateau and a mildly elevated final threshold (fig. 4)

Color-vision tests showed a tendency to green defects on the Ishihara charts and other pseudisochromatic plates but those abnormalities were not specific to any of the congenital types of color-blindness. The Farnsworth Panel D-15 test showed the 'scotopic' line. With the 100-hue test, total error scores were high, but error patterns were not specific (fig. 5).

The ERG revealed very subnormal function of the photopic mechanism. The single-flash photopic ERG responses elicited by a pair of photopically balanced colored stimuli by Berson and others (1968) were practically absent at any level of light adaptation, whereas slightly diminished scotopic responses were apparently recorded with both scotopically and photopically balanced colored flashes at various intensity of the adapting light (fig. 6). These results are quite similar to those of the progressive cone dystrophy (fig. 7) and or of a congenital total color blindness. The scotopic ERG with a white stimulus at increasing intensities in a fully dark adapted condition was subnormal in a- and b-wave amplitudes, and revealed significantly less marked oscillatory potentials (fig. 8). The recovery of the ERG during dark adaptation was quite different from normal (fig. 9) The long extended negative wave and the long peak latency of the non-complex positive potential, which are purely scotopic and typical for the ERG of an achromate (Auerbach & Merin, 1974), were recorded in this case. Besides, unlike an achromate, the scotopic positive potentials hardly recovered during dark adaptation (fig. 10).

DISCUSSION

The present case showed ophthalmoscopically typical macular changes for Stargardt's disease, as well as flavimaculatus flecks scattered over the paramacular and midperipheral regions. After fluorescein injection many more fleck lesions were seen than in ophthalmascopy, but they did not exactly corespond (Klien & Krill, 1967; Irvine & Wergeland, 1972) to the individual yellowish flecks. These findings are apparently similar to those of previously reported fundus flavimaculatus (Franceschetti, 1963), especially

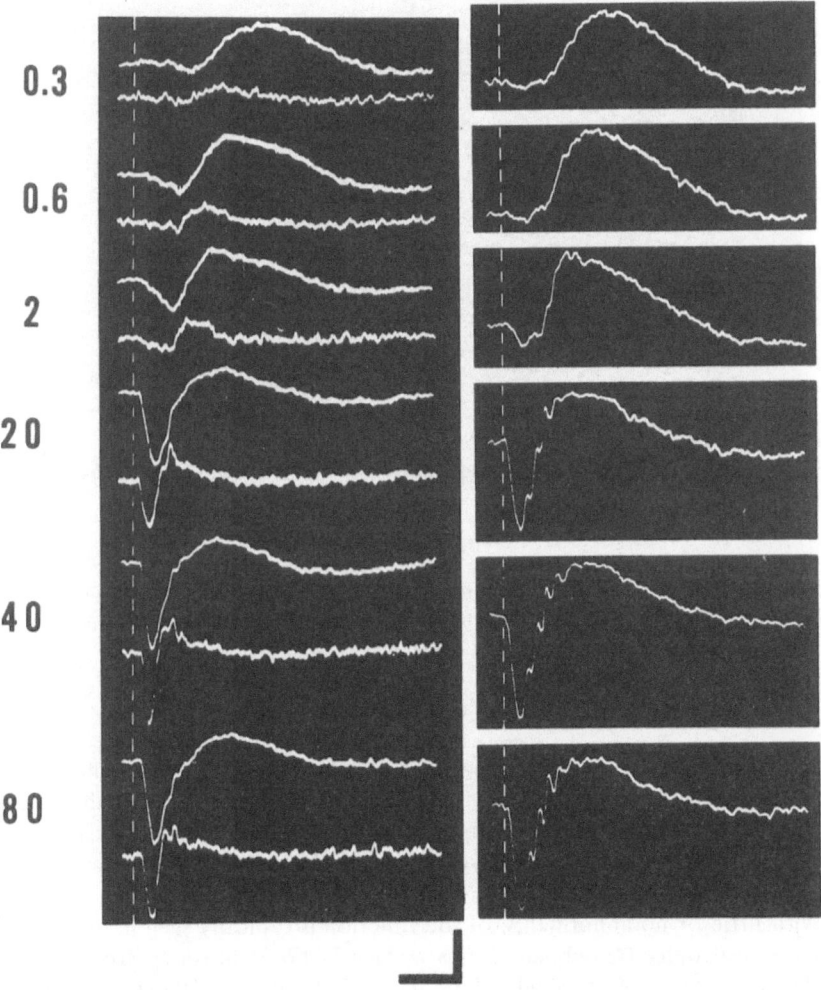

Fig. 8. The scotopic ERG with a white light at increasing intensities in a fully dark adapted condition. Left column: the present case; right: a normal control. Numbers on the left: stimulus intensity (joule).

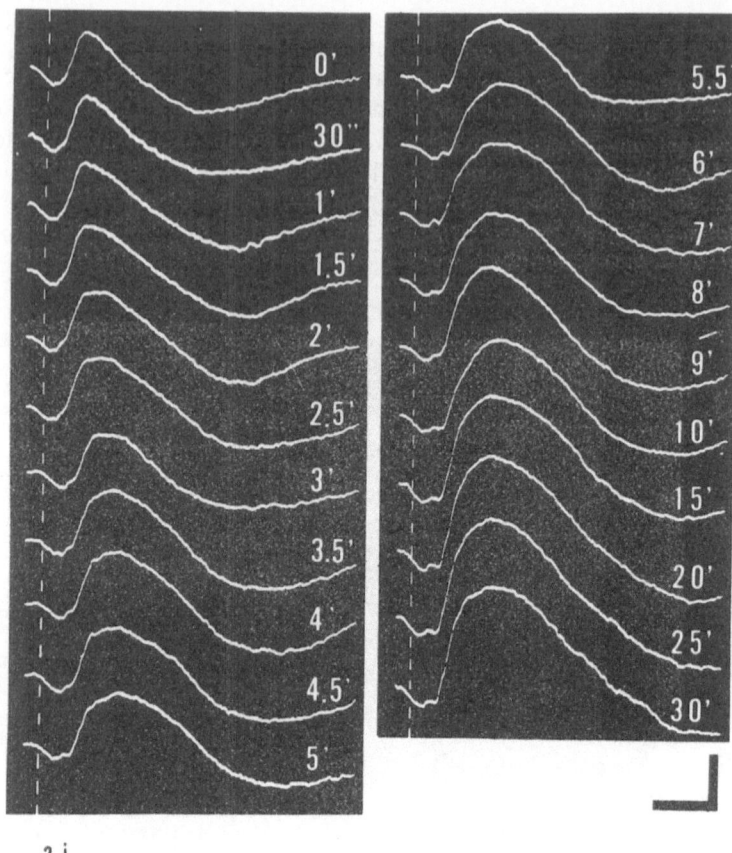

2 j

Fig. 9. Normal recovery of ERG during beginning of dark adaptation after the room light switched off. Time in dark (minutes and seconds) at which each record was made is given at right of each column. Stimulus intensity: 2j.

those with atrophic macular degeneration reported by Klien & Krill (1967).

Retinal function tests including peripheral visual field, dark-adaptation and color-vision, revealed severe photopic and milder scotopic dysfunction (Krill & Deutman, 1972; Merin & Auerbach, 1970; Merin & Landau, 1970). It is well known that severe and selective involvement of photopic system with little or no abnormality of rod function is typically seen in progressive cone dystrophy (Goodman, Ripps & Siegel, 1963; Sloan & Brown, 1962; Berson, Gouras & Gunkel, 1968; Krill & Deutman, 1972), but fundus changes have been reported to be lesser than functional disturbance (Ohba, 1974; Goodman, Ripps & Siegel, 1963; Sloan & Brown, 1962; Babel & Stangos, 1973). Recent investigations of Krill et al. (1972) using fluorescein angiography, however, have demonstrated clear fundus changes, the most frequent appearance being a bull's eye lesion occuring at the macular region. Krill et al. also noted in the same report that nine of forty-five patients had flavimaculatus flecks and seven of nine had macular lesion.

Krill & Deutman stated in another paper (1972) that a few patients with fundus flavimaculatus (Group II-B) might have identical findings to cone dystrophy.

Severe photopic ERG abnormalities in the presence of only a mild abnormal scotopic ERG occuring in the progressive cone dystrophy (Ohba, 1974; Nakano, 1976; Merin & Auerbach, 1970; Berson, Gouras & Gunkel, 1968; Krill & Deutman, 1972; Babel & Stangos, 1973; Krill, Deutman & Fishman, 1973; Yokoyama, Ui & Yoshida, 1974) were recorded in this case.

The present case is proved to be a typical representative of fundus flavimaculatus Group II-B by Krill & Deutman.

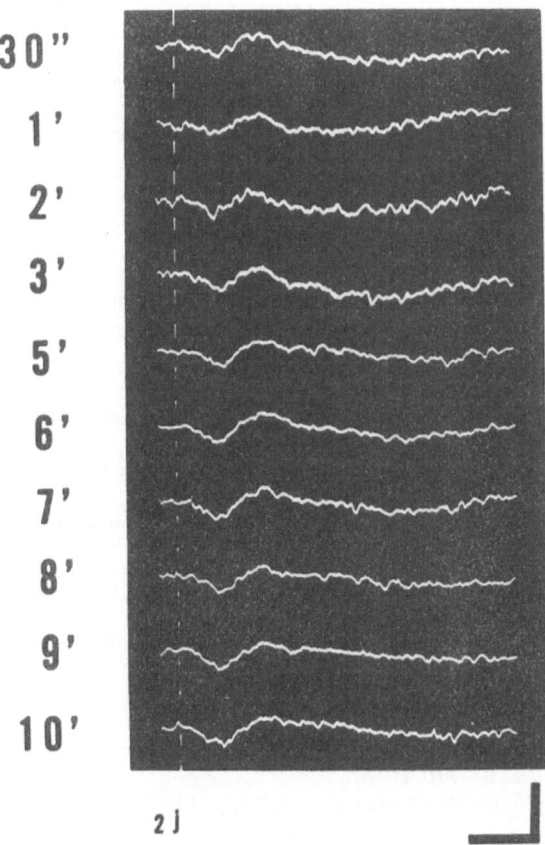

Fig. 10. In contrast to the normal ERG (fig. 9), the response of the present case is dominated by a slow positive wave essentially composed of a scotopic component.

SUMMARY

A case was described having a typical Stargardt's hereditary macular degeneration. Deep yellowish flecks, some of pisciform or round, were also seen, scattered over the paramacular and midperipheral regions. Psychophysical and ERG studies showed severe photopic dysfunction like that seen in progressive cone dystrophy or in congenital achromatopsia, while scotopic function was mildly depressed. This case resembles the cases of fundus flavimaculatus Group II-B described by Krill & Deutman, both clinically and electroretinographically. Such associated changes in this condition were, to the best of my knowledge, not described until now in our country.

ACKNOWLEDGEMENT

The author wishes to thank Professor J. Otsuka of the Tokyo Medical and Dental University for his encouragement during the course of this work.

REFERENCES

Auerbach, E. & Merin, S. Achromatopsia with amblyopia, I. A clinical and electro-retinographical study of 39 cases. *Doc. Ophthal.*, 37, 79, (1974).

Babel, J. & Stangos, N. Progressive degeneration of the photopic system. *Am. J. Ophthal.*, 75, 35, 511, 1973.

Berson, E.L., Gouras, P. & Gunkel, R.D. Progressive cone degeneration, dominantly inherited. *Arch. Ophthal.*, 80, 77, 1968.

Berson, E.L., Gouras, P. & Gunkel, R.D. Rod responses in retinitis pigmentosa, dominantly inherited. *Arch. Opthal.*, 80, 58, 1968.

Franceschetti, A., Ueber tapeto-retinale Degenerationen im Kindesalter, in Entwicklung und Fortschritt in der Augenheilkunde, Stuttgart, Enke Verlag, 1963, 97-120.

Goodman, G., Ripps, H. & Siegel, I.M. Cone dysfunction syndromes. *Arch. Ophthal.*, 70, 214, (1963).

Irvine, A.R. & Wergeland, Jr., F.L. Stargardt's hereditary progressive macular degeneration. *Brit. J. Ophthal.*, 56, 817, (1972).

Klien, B.A. & Krill, A.E. Fundus flavimaculatus; Clinical, functional and histopathologic observations. *Am. J. Ophthal.*, 64, 1, 3, (1967).

Krill, A.E. & Deutman, A.F. The various categories of juvenile macular degeneration. *Tr. Amer. Ophthal. Soc.*, 70, 220, 1972.

Krill, A.E. & Deutman, A.F. Dominant macular degenerations; The cone dystrophies. *Am. J. Ophthal.*, 73, 3, 352, 1972.

Krill, A.E., Deutman, A.F. & Fishman, M. The cone degenerations. *Doc. Ophthal.*, 35, 1, 1, 1973.

Merin, S. & Landau, J. Abnormal findings in relatives of patients with juvenile hereditary macular degeneration (Stragardt's disease). *Ophthalmologica*, 161, 1, (1970).

Merin, S. & Auerbach, E. The central and peripheral retina in macular degenerations. *Arch. Ophthal.*, 84, 710, (1970).

Nakano, H. Aquired color dysfunction and color ERG. *Acta Soc. Opthalm. Jap.*, 80, 3, 177, (1976).

Ogino, T., Hasebe, N., Uchino, M. & Yoshida, M. A case of fundus flavimaculatus. Gankarinshoiho, 64, 4, 43, 1970.

Ohba, N. Progessive cone dystrophy; four cases of unusual form. *Jap. J. Ophthal. 18*, 50, (1974).

Sloan, L.L. & Brown, D.J. Progressive retinal degeneration with selective involvement of the cone mechanism. *Am. J. Ophthal.* 54, *629*, 1962.

Stargardt, K. Ueber familiäre, progressive Degeneration in der Makulagegend des Auges. V. Graefe. *Arch. Ophthal.*, 71, *534*, 1909.

Stargardt, K. Ueber familiäre, progressive Degeneration in der Makulagegend des auges. *Z. Augenheilk.*, 30, *95*, 1913.

Suzuki, Y. & Chiba, Y. A case of fundus flavimaculatus combined with albipunctate dystrophy. *Jap. J. Clin. Ophthal.* 27, 9, 5, 1973.

Watanabe, T., Tamai, A. & Matsuura, H. Three cases of fundus flavimaculatus. *Nihong-ankakiyo*, 22, 2, *88*, 1971.

Yokoyama, M., Ui, K. & Yoshida, T. The spectral response in the retina with progressive cone dystrophy. *Jap. J. Clin. Ophthal.*, 28, 6, *805*, 1974.

Yuri, H., Akabane, N. & Tajima, Y. A case of fundus flavimaculatus. *Jap. J. Clin. Ophthal.*, 23, 5, *5*, 1969.

Author's address:
7-2-305, 2-chome Nakane
Meguro-ku
Tokyo
Japan

THE SCOTOPIC AND PHOTOPIC BAR-PATTERN ERG – CONTRIBUTIONS OF THE CENTRAL AND PERIPHERAL RETINA*

THEODORE LAWWILL, CANDACE WALKER & S. CROCKETT

(Louisville)

ABSTRACT

The alternating phase bar-pattern ERG is used to investigate the contribution of specific retinal areas,and specific retinal components to the ERG. Photopic and scotopic bar-pattern ERG's are recorded under proper lighting conditions. The photopic ERG response is found to be proportional to the number of cones in the retinal area stimulated out to 18° from fixation and not to the total number of receptors.

Most previous studies using the bar-pattern ERG response from discrete areas of the retina have centered on the photopic response (Johnson, et al., 1966). In addition, Armington (1968) showed that under appropriate conditions a scotopic response could be elicited. We wished to determine if the activity of a given receptor population could be associated with a response produced under a given set of stimulus area and luminance conditions. We have compared the scotopic and photopic b-wave responses to the number of cones and rods in different areas of the retina to determine the relative contributions of these elements. The alternating phase bar-pattern stimulus was used because it eliminates the problem of scattered light and allows the stimulation of a specific area of retina without stimulating the rest of the retina.

MATERIALS AND METHODS

The pupils of the subjects were fully dilated and the eyes were adapted to the stimulus luminance level prior to each recording session. The bar-pattern stimulus alternated every half second, and 200 responses were collected for computer averaging each trial. The area stimulated was varied by changing the field diameter or by changing the diameter of a center stop to selectively exclude either the central or peripheral retinal area. The width of each bar was 1.4°. The field outside diameter varied from 10° to 60°. The luminance of the lighted bars was varied in one log unit steps from 0.01 to 100 foot lamberts. The contrast between dark and light bars was 1.4 log units.

* Supported in part by NIH NEI Grant No. EY 00412.

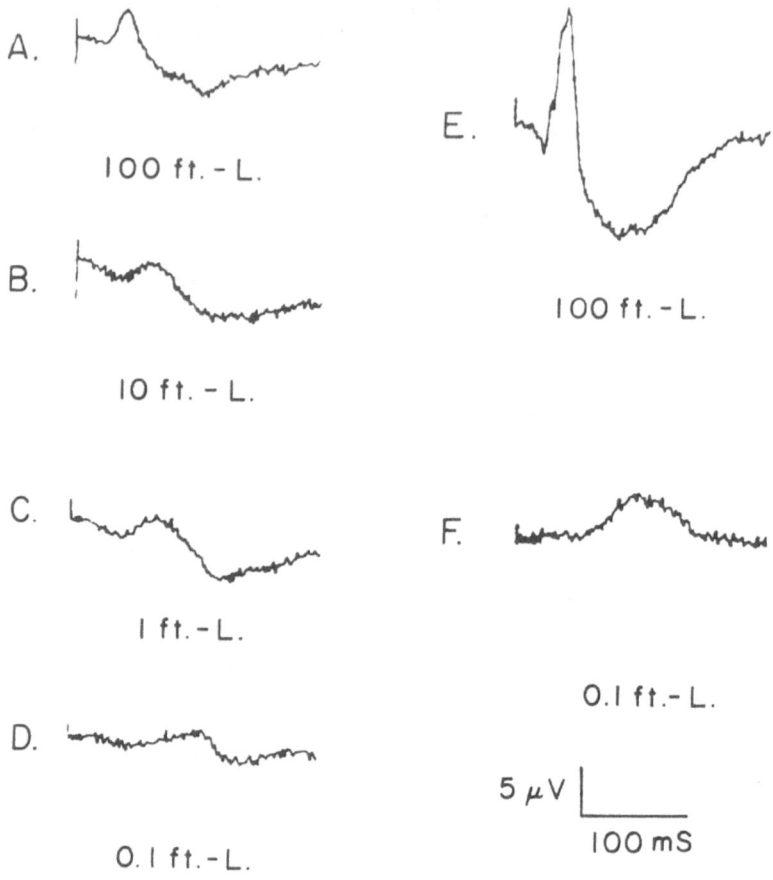

A.

100 ft.-L.

B.

10 ft.-L.

C.

1 ft.-L.

D.

0.1 ft.-L.

E.

100 ft.-L.

F.

0.1 ft.-L.

5 μV

100 mS

Fig. 1. Bar-pattern ERG's using 1.4° bar width and 60° outside diameter field. In traces A-D the center 40° are blacked out leaving a concentric band of retina stimulated. In traces E and F, the full 60° field is stimulated. The traces are the average of 200 responses. The stimulus occurred 10 msec following the beginning of each trace.

RESULTS

The ERG responses, recorded with a luminance level of 100 foot lamberts for the lighted bars, have photopic characteristics. The b-wave peak latencies are comparable to those seen with the light adapted red flash ERG.

As the luminance level decreases to ten foot lamberts, the peak latency and duration of the response increases, as shown in Figure 1, and increase further as the luminance is decreased to one foot lambert. At one foot lambert, the peak latency is still shorter than usually seen in the dark-adapted flash ERG. These levels appear to be intermediate where the response is neither entirely photopic nor scotopic, and there is a gradual transition as the photopic response fades into the scotopic response. When the luminance is decreased to 0.1 foot lamberts, the peak latency increases still further as shown in trace D. This peak latency is comparable to that seen in the dark adapted flash ERG. Further decreases in luminance generally extinguish the bar-pattern ERG, but on occasions where a small response is still present, no further increase in peak latency is seen.

Traces A thru D of Figure 1 show the ERG's from one subject obtained using a bar pattern stimulus covering the concentric retinal area between 20° and 30° from fixation. The luminance was 100 foot lamberts for trace A, ten foot lamberts for trace B, one foot lambert for C and 0.1 foot lambert for D. Traces E and F are from a second subject. Here the stimulus was a full-field bar-pattern of 60° diameter centered on the macula. The luminance of the bright bars was 100 foot lamberts for trace E and 0.1 foot lamberts for trace F.

The peak latencies for the scotopic b-waves are equal in the two subjects. Blocking the central 20° of the stimulus has a relatively greater effect on the amplitude of the photopic response compared to the scotopic.

Figure 2 shows a graph of average photopic ERG amplitude as a function of total receptors in the area stimulated. The number of receptors stimulated was calculated from the data of Osterberg, et al. (1935), and both the

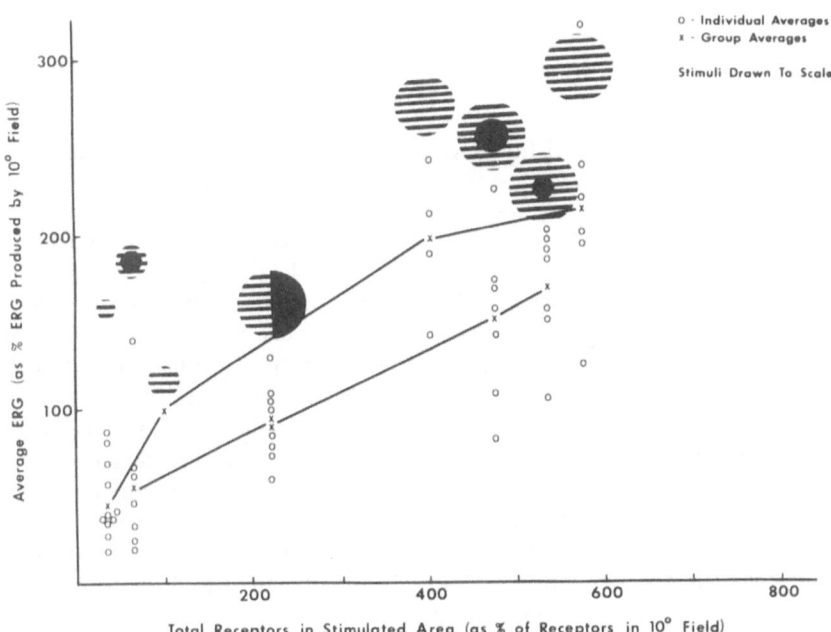

Fig. 2. The amplitude of ERG responses are plotted as percent of the response for that subject for a 10° solid bar pattern field. The number of receptors are plotted as a percent of the receptors in the 10° central field. The x's represent the group mean and the o's represent the normalized data for each subject. The stimulus pattern for each group of data is drawn to scale.

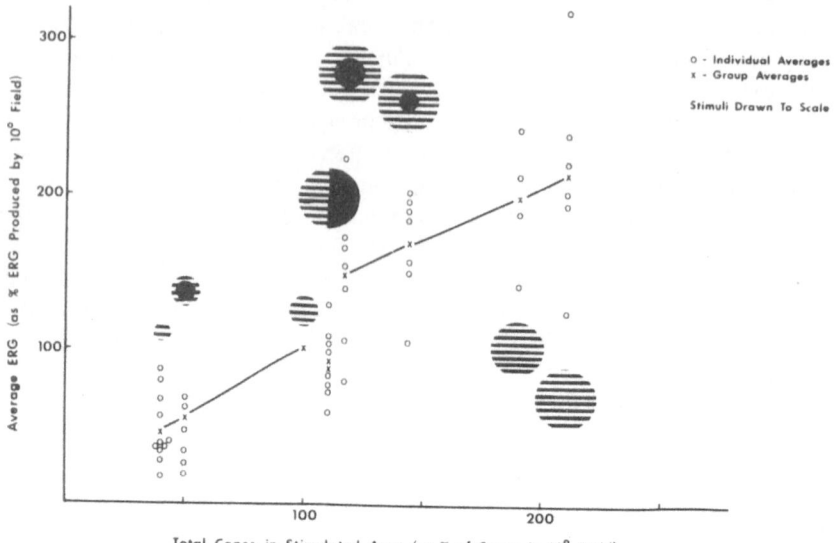

Fig. 3. The data in Figure 2 has been redrawn with the number of cones in the area stimulated instead of the number of retinal receptors in the area stimulated. The data is normalized on the 10° solid bar pattern field. The x's represent group means and the o's represent individual subjects' responses. The pattern of the stimulus field is drawn to scale.

numbers of receptors and the ERG magnitude are normalized by expressing them as a percent of the value found for the solid 10° field centered on the macula. The open circles represent the averages for each individual subject, and the x's represent the average responses of all subjects combined. Due to the normalization, there are no open circles at the point representing 100% on both ordinate and abscissa. The different stimulus configurations used in collecting these data are diagrammed to scale above the data. There appear to be two distinct curves. One is nearly linear and includes the data collected with all or part of the central stimulus blacked out. The other curve rises more rapidly and then flattens out. This second curve includes data collected using different size stimuli which all include the central area.

In Figure 3, the same data are presented where the average photopic ERG amplitude is plotted as a function of total cones instead of total receptors in the stimulated area. The data follow a single curve, which is nearly linear. The only point significantly off the line is for a split field, and fixation may have been a slight problem here.

DISCUSSION

A linear relationship between the number of cones stimulated and the magnitude of the resulting ERG has been shown by Armington to hold over the central 5° of retina. We have found that response magnitude also increases

290

with increasing number of receptors stimulated in the periphery. The fit is better with number of cones than with total receptors stimulated.

There appear to be two separate curves for increasing retinal area depending on whether or not the central part of the retina is included in the stimulated area. The curve followed by data obtained with the central retinal area included always lies above that followed by data collected with this central area blocked out. There is also a greater slope of this curve over the part where the amount of central retina stimulated is increasing. This indicates that in the central retina there is a greater increase in response magnitude per receptor stimulated than there is in the periphery, and this may be related to the higher proportion of cones to rods in this area. This set of curves is made into a single line when the same responses are plotted against the number of cones stimulated. This is consistent with there being no rod contribution to the bar ERG at this luminance.

A pure scotopic ERG has been produced at 0.1 foot lambert using the bar pattern system. Evidence has been presented against rod system contribution to the photopic bar-pattern ERG, but evidence is given for selective rod system contribution to the scotopic bar-pattern ERG.

Key words

Bar-pattern ERG
ERG

BIBLIOGRAPHY

Armington, John C.: Simultaneous electroretinograms and evoked potentials. *Am. J. Optometry and Arch. Am. Academy of Optometry 47, 450-459*, 1970.
Johnson, E. Parker, Riggs, Lorrin A. & Schick, Army M.L.: Photopic retinal potentials evoked by phase alternation of a barred pattern. *Vision Research* 6 (suppl. 2), *75-91*, 1966.
Osterberg, G.: Topography of the layer of rods and cones in the human retina. Acta Ophthalmologica Supplementum VI, 1935.

Authors' address:
Dept of Ophthalmology
University of Louisville
School of Medicine
Louisville, Ky 40202
USA

THE FOVEAL LOCAL ERG RESPONSE TO TRANSIENT AND STEADY STATE FLICKERING STIMULI

WILLIAM S. BARON

(Menlo Park)

The photoreceptors are the first neural elements in the visual system, and an appreciation of their response characteristics can greatly assist our understanding of higher order neural processes. The extent to which photoreceptor activity can be monitored in primates by means of a nearly normal preparation will directly effect our ability to attain this goal. It was in pursuit of such a preparation that this study was undertaken.

The foveal local ERG (LERG) is dominated by the late receptor potential (LRP) (Brown & Watanabe, 1962), and its plateau in response to a rectangular pulse stimulus longer than 250 msec reflects or is the LRP plateau (Baron & Boynton, 1974). This quality of the foveal LERG allows the monitoring of the LRP with discrete stimuli, but not necessarily with steady state flickering stimuli. If the LRP could be monitored with flickering stimuli via the foveal LERG studies of cone function addressable only with this type of stimulus could be undertaken without having to use physiologically traumatic techniques, e.g., clamping the central retinal artery, to isolate the LRP. Using sinusoidally flickering stimuli Baron & Boynton (1975) demonstrated (by the waveform of the response and voltage versus modulation functions) that the foveal local ERG (LERG) was linear for amplitudes of less than 60 μV. They eliminated the b-wave by injecting sodium aspartate into the vitreous, and found the temporal sensitivity of the system to be similar before and after the injection. This suggests that the foveal LERG consisted only of the LRP. However, the sodium aspartate may have effected the functioning of the receptors.

The present work was undertaken as a preliminary study to further identify the source of the foveal LERG as obtained with sinusoidally flickering stimuli.

METHODS

As previously described (Baron & Boynton, 1975), the foveal LERG was recorded by placing a micro-electrode within the foveal pit of a cynomolgus macaque, and positioning it within the retina at the level where the LRP obtains its greatest amplitude. Stimuli consisted of 10° fields of 580 nm light centered on the fovea, and were obtained by means of a three channel Maxwellian view stimulator (Baron, 1973).

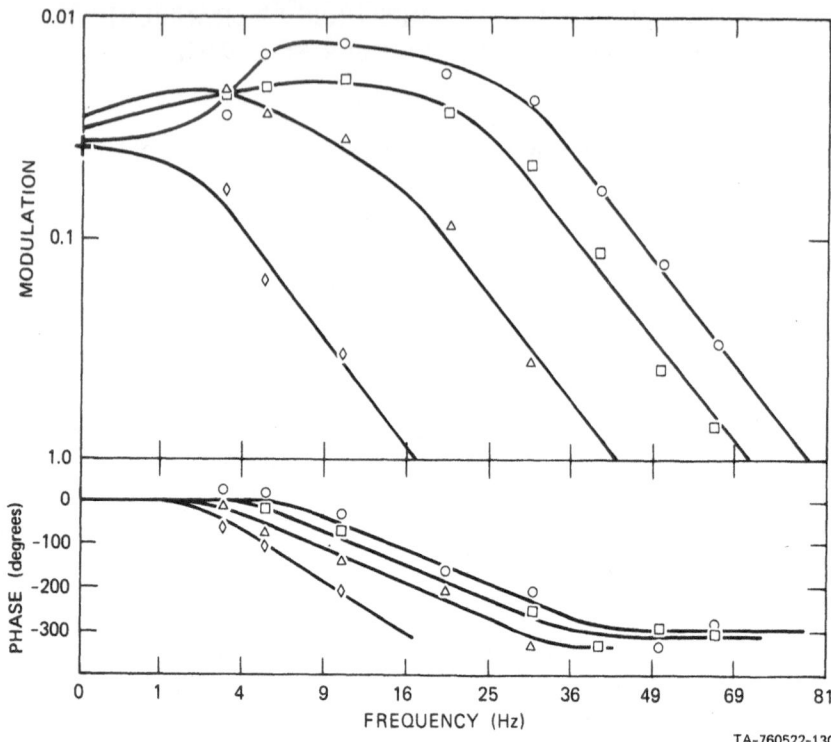

Fig. 1. Upper graph, modulation sensitivity on a log scale, and, lower graph, phase both plotted against frequency on a square root scale. The fitted curves indicate the functions used to compute the impulse response. The data at other than zero frequency is from Baron and Boynton, 1975, for adaptation levels of 100 td, ◇; 1000 td, △; 10,000 td, □, and 89,000 td, ○. The + indicates the mean sensitivity of 14 responses to rectangular pulse stimuli.

RESULTS

The temporal modulation transfer function (MTF) amplitude and phase data for the foveal LERG from Baron & Boynton (1975) are replotted in Figure 1. Here we have also plotted a zero-frequency point derived from the plateau height of responses obtained with 10 percent increment rectangular pulse stimuli of 400 msec duration superimposed upon backgrounds of 100 td, 1000 td, 10,000 td, and 89,000 td. As with the previously taken flicker data, the 'modulation' for this point was determined by interpolation between the amplitude of these responses and zero. Since this value did not vary significantly as a function of adaptation level, the four determinations (each derived from 3 experimental sessions) have been averaged to obtain this initial point. In Figure 1 frequency is plotted on a square root scale and modulation on a log scale. On these coordinates, the high frequency data are well fit by straight lines according to a model derived from psychophysical studies (Kelly, 1969, 1971; Baron & Boynton, 1975).

294

The inverse Fourier transforms of these data were computed using the Cooley-Tukey fast-Fourier transform algorithm. Functions fitted by eye were used as input for a 3 point smoothing algorithm, and the smooth curves drawn through the data represent the resulting functions that were used for the transform. The impulse responses, resulting from the transform, were then integrated over a 400 msec period to yield theoretical rectangular pulse responses for each adaptation level. Such calculations are legitimate only for systems that behave linearly. The foveal LERG's linearity to steady state flicker has previously been demonstrated for the small perturbations in the prevailing adapting level used in the flicker experiments. The calculated pulse responses are compared in Figure 2 to incremental responses obtained experimentally at each adaptation level. The derived pulse responses, indicated by the dotted lines, have been scaled vertically to cor-

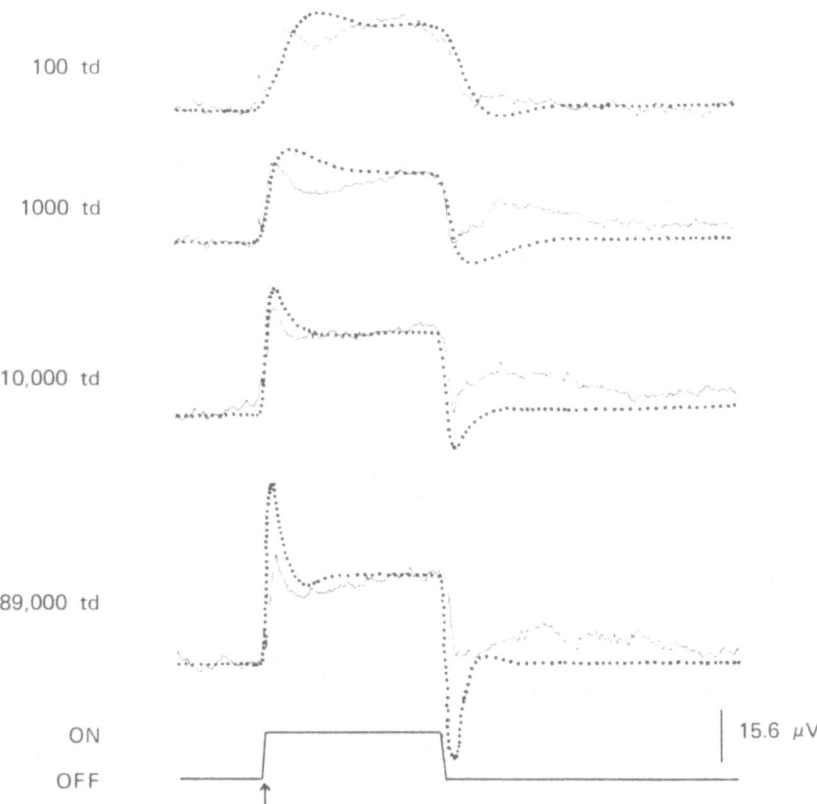

Fig. 2. Solid lines, recorded responses to 10 percent increment rectangular pulse stimuli 400 msec duration superimposed on 100 td, 1000 td, 10,000 td, and 89,000 td backgrounds. Dotted lines, the 400 msec rectangular pulse integrated impulse responses derived from the data of Fig. 1. The vertical calibration is 15.6 μV; 128 responses were averaged for each record.

respond to the plateau heights, since the plateau height corresponds to the 0 Hz threshold.

DISCUSSION

A comparison of the derived response and the experimentally obtained response at stimulus on set for the 100 td and 1000 td conditions suggests that there is a b-wave present in the experimentally obtained response but not in the derived response. This suggests that the b-wave may not be triggered by the sinusoidally flickering stimuli. The differences between the experimentally obtained and derived responses at 10,000 td and 89,000 td occur at latencies too short to be attributed to the b-wave (especially for the 89,000 td condition). Recent evidence from gecko photoreceptors indicates that the initial transient in the LRP is due to horizontal cell feedback (Kleinschmidt & Dowling, 1975); thus the differences at 89,000 td may be due to changes in horizontal cell feedback between the flicker data and the responses obtained with by rectangular pulse stimuli. The initial overshoot and eventual return to a plateau of the derived responses are characteristic of the LRP.

For a linear system the off response will be the complement of the on response, if the pulse is of sufficiently long duration. Accordingly, off sets of the derived responses are complements of their on sets, and thus have a negative component of amplitude equal to the initial peak. The experimentally obtained responses have no negative component even though the initial peak for the 10,000 td and 89,000 conditions is higher than the plateau. The 100 td and 1000 td responses also have non-symmetrical on sets and off sets. This non-symmetry and the lack of agreement between the derived and experimentally obtained responses demonstrates the foveal LERG's lack of linearity for rectangular pulse stimuli despite its linear behavior when tested with sinusoidally flickering stimuli.

While more data needs to be obtained before a firm conclusion can be reached, this preliminary analysis suggests that the b-wave contributes to the foveal LERG to a lesser or similar extent when using sinusoidally flickering stimuli than when using rectangular pulse stimuli.

ACKNOWLEDGEMENTS

This work was supported by NIH Grant RO1 EY01579-01. The author would like to thank Donald Kelly for helpful discussions.

REFERENCES

Baron, W.S. Maxwellian View Stimulator for Electrophysiological and Psychophysical Work, *Applied Optics*, 12, *2560-2562* (1973).

Baron, W.S. & Boynton, R.M. The Primate Foveal Local Electroretinogram: An Indicator of Photoreceptor Activity. *Vision Res.* 14, *495-501* (1974).

Baron, W.S. & Boynton, R.M. Responses of Primate Cones to Sinusoidally Flickering Homochromatic Stimuli. *J. Physiol. (Lond.)* 246, *311-331* (1975).

Brown, K.T. & Watanabe, K. Isolation and Identification of a Receptor Potential From the Pure Cone Fovea of the Monkey Retina. *Nature, (Lond.)* 193, *958-960* (1962).

Kelly, D.H. Diffusion Model of Linear Flicker Responses. *J. Opt. Soc. Am.*, 59, *1665-1670* (1969).

Kelly, D.H. Theory of Flicker and Transient Responses, I. Uniform Fields. *J. Opt. Soc. Am.* 61, *537-546* (1971).

Kleinschmidt, J. & Dowling, J. Intracellular Recordings From Gecko Photoreceptors During Light and Dark Adaptation. *J. Gen. Physiol.* 66, *617-648* (1975).

Author's address:
Stanford Research Institute
333 Ravenswood Ave
Menlo Park, Cal. 94025
USA

MACULAR ERG'S ELICITED BY
CHECKERBOARD PATTERN STIMULI

SAMUEL SOKOL & BENJAMIN H. BLOOM

(Boston)

Bar-pattern electroretinography was first investigated in detail by Johnson, Riggs & Schick. (1966) More recently, Lawwill (1973, 1974) has used this technique clinically in a large series of patients with various forms of macular dysfunction. This paper reports some of our recent work with checkerboard-pattern electroretinography of the macular region.

The stimulus used in our studies in a back-illuminated checkerboard pattern of Polaroid filters made by the Vectograph technique. (Sokol, 1977) The checks alternate sinusoidally at a rate of 12 per second and the average luminous flux of the entire screen is constant. The stimulus luminance was 75 foot-Lamberts and at a viewing distance of 75 centimeters subtended a visual angle of 12 degrees. The maximum contrast ratio of the checks was 75%.

Because we are particularly interested in the electrical signals generated by patterned stimuli which subtend small fields, e.g. 6 degrees, and are comprised of small checks, e.g. 15 minutes of visual angle, the contact lens electrode must induce very little optical distortion. Previous work in patterned electroretinography with corneal electrodes has employed the scleral lens, or Riggs type of electrode (Riggs, 1941) and the speculum contact lens, or Burian-Allen type of electrode. (Burian & Allen, 1954) The Riggs electrode provides a clear optical path but must be custom molded to fit each subject. The Burian-Allen lens is very easily applied but in our experience has not provided the optical clarity necessary for use with fine patterns. Fig. 1 shows a combination hard-soft contact lens electrode of our own design which induces very little optical distortion and is comfortable and convenient enough for clinical studies (Bloom & Sokol, 1977). After electrode placement, an acceptance refraction is performed and lenses are placed in a trial frame to provide optimal visual acuity. With this electrode we are also able to obtain flash-elicited ERG's which are indistinguishable from those obtained with a Burian-Allen lens.

Because long recording sessions and signal averaging are needed to record patterned ERG's, a substantial amount of artifact is generated by changes in fixation and by eye blinks. This is adequately removed from the data by an artifact rejection buffer, which is a software algorithm which has been programmed into the input stages of the averaging computer. The output of the electrode pre-amplifier is fed through an active narrow band-pass filter with

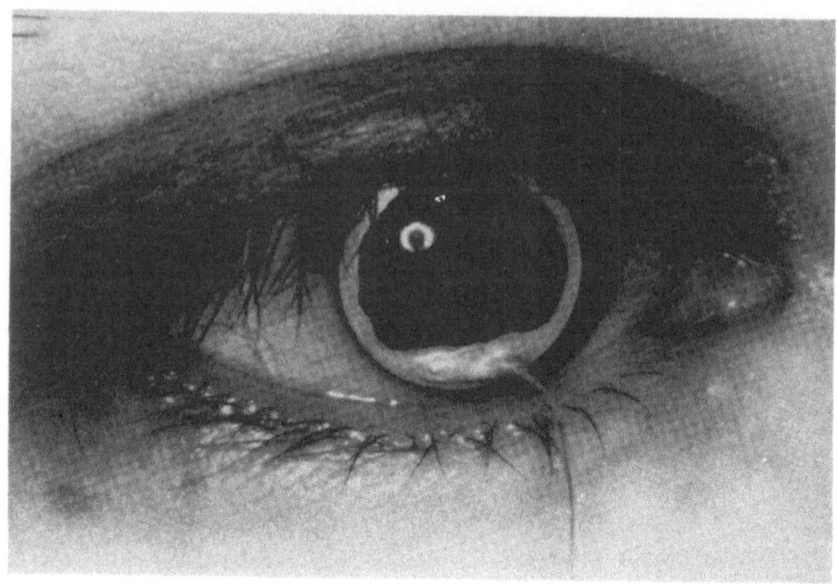

Fig. 1. The hard lens electrode placed onto a 14 mm. hydrophilic contact lens with the gold wire positioned inferiorly to avoid contact with the upper lid. No anesthesia or methylcellulose is used.

a 'Q' of 10 and then fed into the computer. The pass band is centered at the stimulus frequency of 12 Hz. This filter provides effective rejection of unwanted signal energy from such unrelated sources as slow eye movements and cortical alpha rhythm. The filtered signal is nearly sinusoidal and may be analyzed by measurement of the peak-to-trough amplitude. The output of the pre-amplifier is also fed directly into the computer. All of the data is stored on disk and off-line power spectrum analysis can then be performed. As the field size is reduced, the signal-to-noise ratio becomes smaller and a larger number of accumulations is needed. The use of power spectrum analysis enables one to obtain information from ERG's elicited by small stimuli when amplitude measurement of the stimulus related signal is unreliable due to small signals and/or high noise levels. With power spectral analysis of the unfiltered records one can also examine other frequencies, e.g. harmonics of the 12 Hz component, slow eye movements and alpha rhythm. Another advantage of treating the data by filtering and power spectral analysis is that one can look at the filtered records during the recording session and make immediate decisions regarding amplitude and phase and subsequently make changes in the stimulus conditions. On the other hand, events occurring at other frequencies can be examined when the recording session is completed.

Fig. 2 shows patterned ERG's taken from two normal subjects. The subjects wore the electrodes on both eyes and binocularly fixated on the center of a 6 degree square containing 30 minute checks. Visual acuity in each subject with the electrodes in place was 20/16 OU. The unfiltered signals were analyzed by calculating their power spectral density and comparing the amount of ERG power at 12 Hz in the left eye with that in the right eye. For these normals, this ERG power ratio between eyes is close to one.

As an evaluation of the optical properties of the contact lens electrode a spherical refraction was performed using the patterned ERG. (Millodot & Riggs, 1970) The subject had a refractive error of minus 3.75 diopters in his right eye and an accommodative amplitude of 8 diopters. The subject's right eye was cyclopleged with tropicamide and viewed the stimulus at a distance of 75 centimeters. The stimulus field subtended 12 degrees of visual angle and 15 minute checks were used. A sequence of ophthalmic lenses was placed in the trial frame beginning at + 3 diopters and proceeded in 1 diopter increments to −11 diopters; the left eye was occluded. The data points in Fig. 3 represent the relative power in the ERG taken from the 12 Hz peak in the response frequency spectrum at each of these refractive conditions. The curve peaks at −2 diopters which is the refractive error for this subject at this viewing distance. The calculated peak value is −2.42 diopters.

The effect of stimulus area on the ERG is shown in Figs. 4 and 5 in

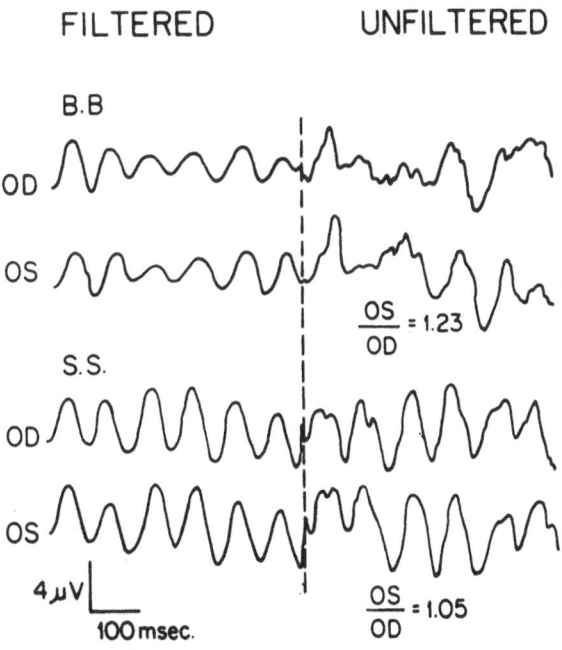

Fig. 2. ERG's obtained from two normal subjects using an alternating checkerboard stimulus. Field size: 6 degrees; check size: 30 minutes; number of accumulations: 64. Records were obtained simultaneously from both eyes using the left ear as a reference. The ratios compare the relative power in the unfiltered signals from each eye at 12 Hz with the larger signal placed in the numerator.

which the subjects fixated on a series of stimuli subtending several field sizes while binocular ERG's were recorded. The data points represent the relative power in the ERG at 12 Hz with all curves drawn to scale and normalized to a maximum value of 100. As expected, and in agreement with Armington's findings, (1968) the amplitude of the ERG is directly related to the stimulus area and there is good agreement between eyes.

Using this technique we have studied several patients who have well documented unilateral macular scars. Fig. 6 shows records obtained from

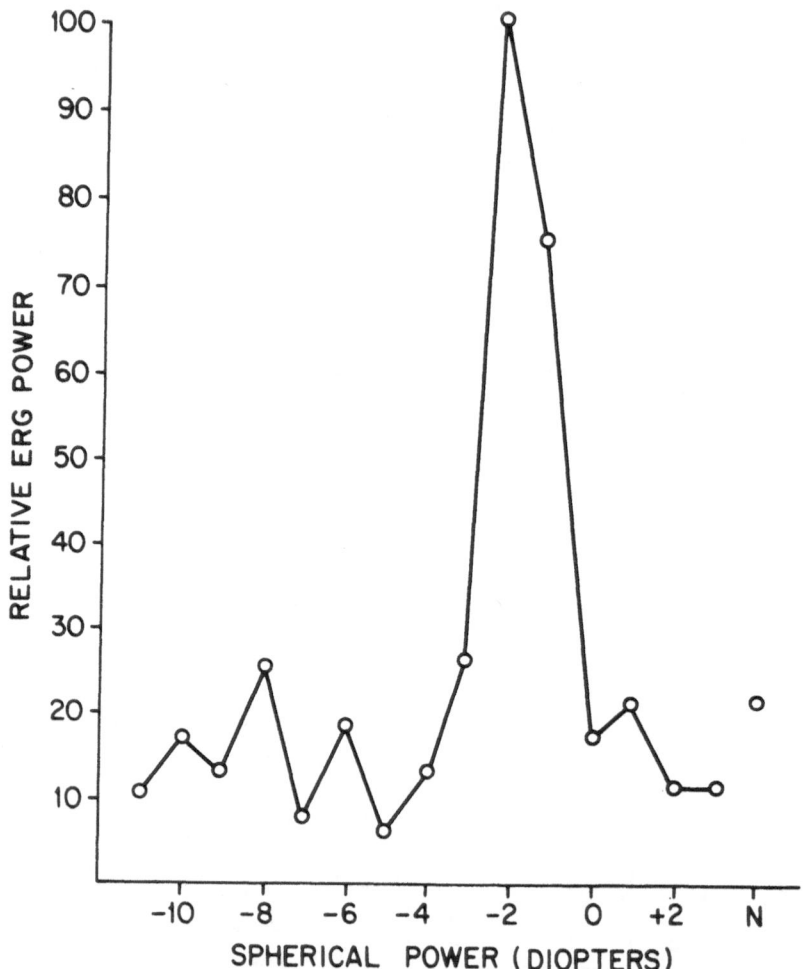

Fig. 3. Relative ERG power at 12 Hz as a function of dioptric strength recorded from a subject with a refractive error of −2.42 D at a 75 cm. viewing distance. Field size: 12 degrees; check size: 15 minutes; number of accumulations: 64. Records were obtained from the right eye after administration of tropicamide. The left eye was occluded and the reference electrode was on the cheek near the outer canthus. The power at 12 Hz with the stimulus light off is shown at N.

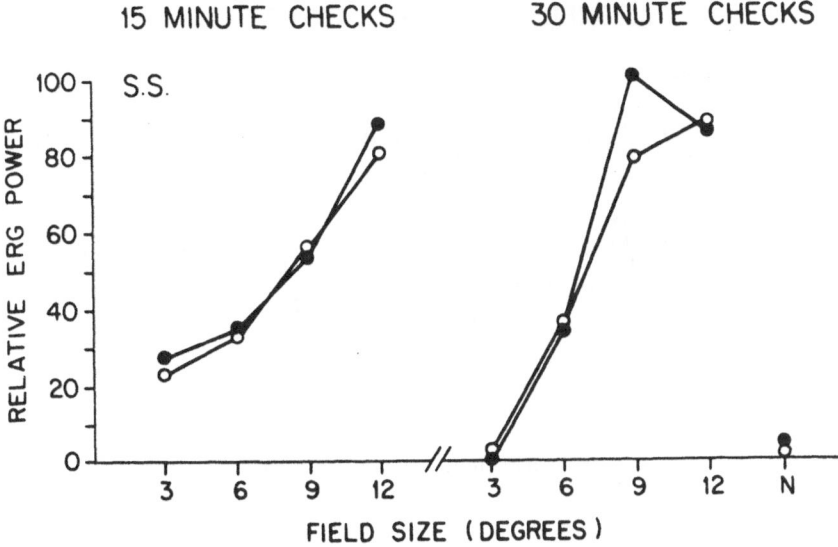

Fig. 4. Relative ERG power at 12 Hz as a function of stimulus area recorded from a normal subject. Number of accumulations: 64. Records were obtained simultaneously from both eyes using the left ear as a reference. Closed circles – right eye; open circles – left eye. The power at 12 Hz with the stimulus light off is shown at N.

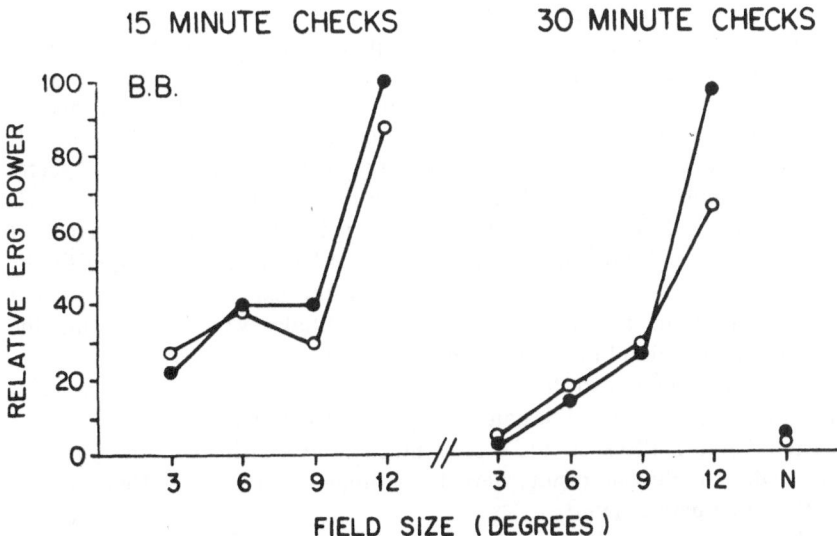

Fig. 5. Relative ERG power at 12 Hz as a function of stimulus area recorded from a second normal subject. Stimulus conditions identical to those in Fig. 4.

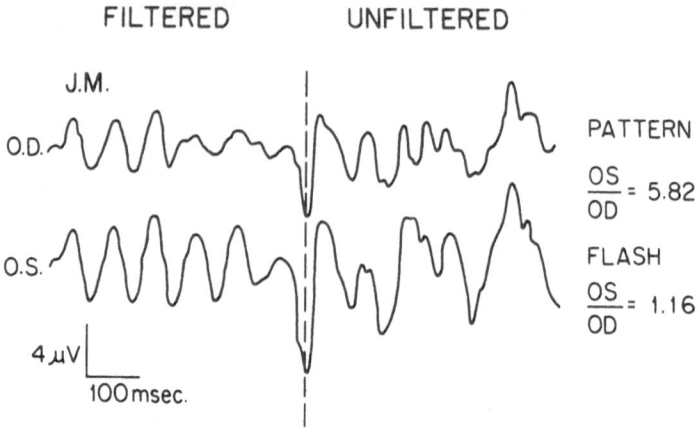

FILTERED   UNFILTERED

J.M.

O.D.   PATTERN

$\dfrac{OS}{OD}$ = 5.82

O.S.   FLASH

$\dfrac{OS}{OD}$ = 1.16

4 μV

100 msec.

Fig. 6. ERG's obtained from patient J.M. Field size: 6 degrees; check size: 30 minutes; number of accumulations: 128. Records were obtained simultaneously from both eyes with the patient fixating on the center of the stimulus with his better eye; the left ear was the reference. The pattern ratio compares the relative power of the unfiltered signals from each eye at 12 Hz. The flash ratio compares the amplitude of the flash-elicited photopic b-waves (not shown) from each eye.

J.M., a 47 year old white male with inactive congenital toxoplasmosis OU. There is surgical aphakia present OU and an ophthalmoscopic examination showed a circular scar about 1 disk diameter in size, located approximately centrally in the macula of the right eye as well as several old chorioretinal scars in each retinal periphery. Visual acuity with glasses was counting fingers at 6 feet OD and 20/30 −2 OS. Visual acuity with the ERG electrodes in place OU was counting fingers at 4 feet OD and 20/35 OS. The patient fixated on the center of a 6 degree spatially alternating stimulus with 30 minute checks for a total of 128 accumulations. The unfiltered signals are difficult to interpret by inspection but after this signal has passed through the narrow band-pass filter it is clear that the signal from the left eye is noticeably larger than that from the right eye. When power spectra are calculated from the unfiltered signals it is seen that the ratio of the ERG power in the left eye compared to the right eye is 5.82 which in our laboratory is a significantly abnormal ratio. Flash-elicited photopic ERG's were also obtained from this patient using white light after two minutes of light adaptation. The photopic b-wave amplitudes were each within the normal range and did not differ significantly from one another.

These data demonstrate that the flash-elicited ERG may be insensitive to the presence of a focal lesion in the macular region. The checkerboard pattern-elicited ERG in this case is much more sensitive to the patient's visual deficit. Similar results have been obtained in several other patients with similar pathology.

In summary, we have shown that patterned ERG's may be recorded using a new contact lens electrode and a checkerboard stimulus of small field size and small check size. The patterned ERG was recorded from normals as well as from several patients with focal macular pathology and in these cases provided a sensitive index of macular function.

ACKNOWLEDGEMENT

This work was supported by National Institutes of Health Research Grant EY-00926 and a Career Development Award EY-70275-01A1 to S.S. B.H.B. was supported by National Institutes of Health Training Grant 5 TO1 EY00054.

REFERENCES

Armington, J.C.: The electroretinogram, the visual evoked potential, and the area-luminance relation. *Vision Res.* 8, *263-276*, (1968).

Bloom, B.H. and Sokol, S.: A corneal electrode for patterned stimulus electroretinography. *Am. J. Ophthal.* (In Press).

Burian, H.M. and Allen, L.: A speculum contact lens electrode for electroretinography. *EEG Clin. Neurophysiol.* 6, *509-511*, (1954).

Johnson, E.P., Riggs, L.A., and Schick, A.M.L.: Photopic retinal potentials evoked by phase alternation of a barred pattern. In: Clinical Electroretinography, Burian, H.M. & Jacobson, J.H. (Eds.) Oxford, 1966, Pergamon Press, pp. *75-91*.

Lawwill, T.: Pattern stimuli for clinical ERG. In: Proc. 11th ISCERG Symposium, May 1973, Dodt, E. & Pearlman, J.T. (eds.) The Hague, 1974, Dr. W. Junk b.v. Publishers, pp. *353-362*.

Lawwill, T.: The bar-pattern electroretinogram for clinical evaluation of the central retina. *Am. J. Ophthal.* 78, *121-126*, (1974).

Millodot, M. and Riggs, L.A.: Refraction determined electrophysiologically. *Arch. Ophthal.* 84, *272-278*, (1970).

Riggs, L.A.: Continuous and reproducible records of the electrical activity of the human retina. *Proc. Soc. Exper. Biol. and Med.* 48, *204-207*, (1941).

Sokol, S.: Visual evoked potentials to checkerboard pattern stimuli in strabismic amblyopia. In: Visual Evoked Potentials in Man: New Developments of the Human Brain. Desmedt, J.E., editor. Oxford University Press, *410-417* (1977).

Authors' address:
Dept of Ophthalmology
Tufts — New England Medical Center
Boston, Mass. 02111
USA

Reprint requests to Dr. S. Sokol at the above address.

EFFECTS OF ATROPINE ON ERG AND OPTIC NERVE
RESPONSE IN THE CAT

G. NIEMEYER & L. CERVETTO

(Zürich, Switzerland)

Histochemical (Koelle et al., 1952; Francis, 1953; Nichols & Koelle, 1967, 1968; Dickson et al., 1971; Lam, 1972; Vogel & Nirenberg, 1976) and physiological (Noell & Lsansky,   ; Müller-Limmroth, 1959; Valtsev, 1966; Strashill, 1968; Ames & Pollen, 1969; Murakami, Ohtsu & Ohtsuka, 1972; Zak & Lelekova, 1975; Masland, Ames & Livingstone, 1975) evidences suggest the presence of cholinergic transmitting mechanisms in the retinae of a variety of vertebrates. The distribution of Acetylcholine-receptors in the outer and inner plexiform layers varies among these species. In mammals, in contrast to birds, a higher cholinergic activity seems to be confined to the inner as compared to the outer plexiform layer (Francis, 1953; Vogel & Nirenberg, 1976).

In order to study the effects of synaptically active chemicals on mammalian retina we used the arterially perfused eye of the cat (Gouras & Hoff, 1970; Niemeyer, 1975, 1976). This preparation offers several advantages over *in vivo* experiments: (1) the biochemical input to the isolated eye can be controlled completely, and (2) electrical signals from all layers of the retina and from the optic nerve are easily accessible (Niemeyer & Gouras, 1973; Niemeyer, 1975).

EXPERIMENTAL PROCEDURES

Eyes from thiamyal-anaesthetized and heparin-anticoagulated adult cats were enucleated and connected to a perfusion system in a plastic chamber. The perfusate consisted of oxygenated, serum-enriched tissue culture medium which was buffered to a pH 7.4 and maintained at 37.5°. The retina was stimulated with pulses of monochromatic light of 20 to 1000 msec in duration delivered in Maxwellian view via a modified Zeiss-ophthalmoscope. Experiments were carried out on dark adapted preparations. Fig. 1 illustrates the arrangement of the recording electrodes schematically, an ERG and an optic nerve signal. The optic nerve response in Fig. 1 represents both ON and OFF effects which reflect complex interactions of single axons. ON-responses, consisting of monophasic, negative, temporally dispersed action potentials, were recorded in all preparations with good reproducibility. OFF effects, observed at stimulus durations longer than 100 msec, consisted of more complex and variable, polyphasic

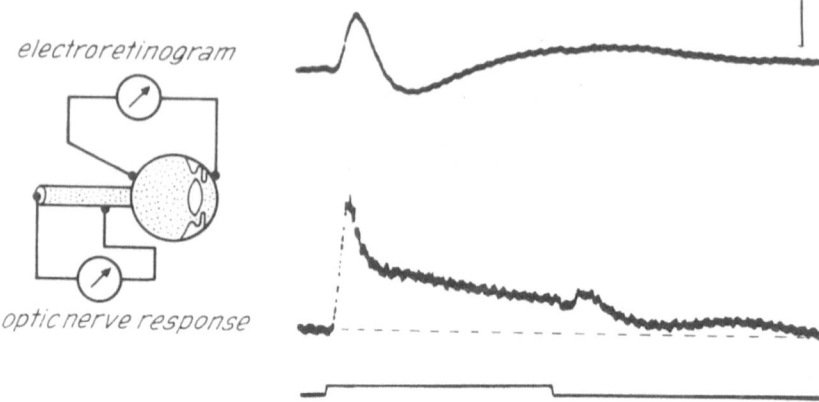

Fig. 1. Electrode arrangement, ERG and optic nerve response in the perfused cat eye. The stimulus was a pulse of monochromatic (λ max 620 nm) light of 400 msec in duration. Negativity is displayed upwards in this and in subsequent optic nerve response traces, and the stimulus is indicated by an upward deflection in the bottom trace. Calibrations: 200 μV (ERG) and 100 μV (optic nerve) DC recordings.

deflections. The polarity, configuration and amplitude of the OFF effect in the controls was found to depend on intensity, duration and wavelength of the stimulus an could also be influenced by changing the geometry of the recording electrodes (Niemeyer, 1976). For further details of the methods the reader is referred to the publication by Niemeyer, 1975.

RESULTS

I. Effects of atropine on the ERG

Injections of atropine into the perfusion reproducibly induced dose-dependent and reversible changes in the b-wave of the ERG. Low doses (0.1-0.5 mM) initially induced increases in the amplitudes of the b-wave, frequently followed by slight depressions (Fig. 2, see also plots in Fig. 4, top). During the period when the b-wave amplitude was increased, there was also an increase in its implicit time. Higher concentrations (1-5 mM) decreased the amplitudes of the b-waves. These effects were reversible.

II. Effects of atropine on the optic nerve responses

Atropine, in concentrations ranging from approximately 0.1 to 5.0 mM depressed the ON effect of the optic nerve response. This depressant action was dose-dependent and completely reversible as shown in Figs. 3 to 5. Fig. 3 shows a sequence of responses from the optic nerve, recorded before, during and after an injection of atropine for two minutes. A gradual de-

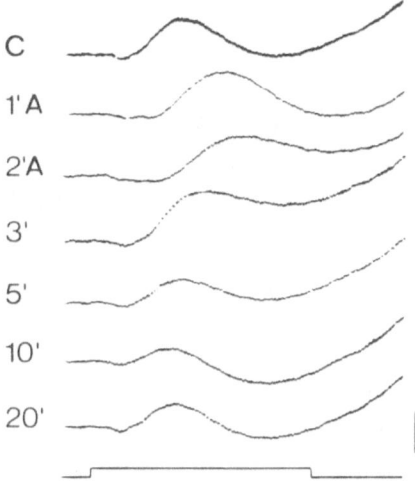

Fig. 2. Effects of atropine (concentration in the perfusate o.2 mM) on the ERG. In this as in subsequent figures: C = control, A = atropine sulfate; numbers on the left indicate time in minutes after onset of drug-injection. Stimulus duration: 200 msec, calibration 200 μV.

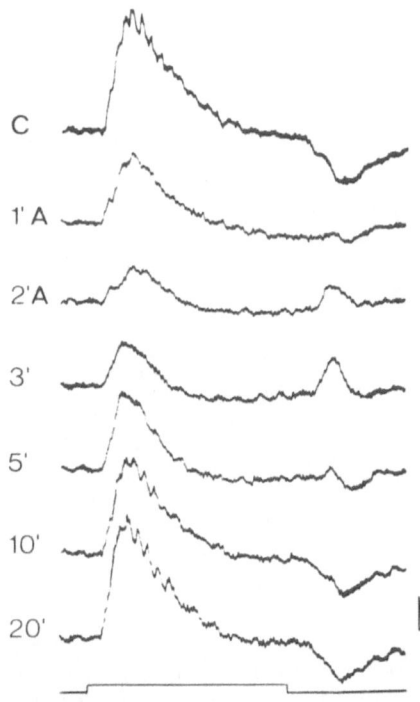

Fig. 3. Effects of atropine (0.2 mM) on the optic nerve responses. The stimulus duration was 200 msec; calibration 50 μV. Wavelength 620 nm.

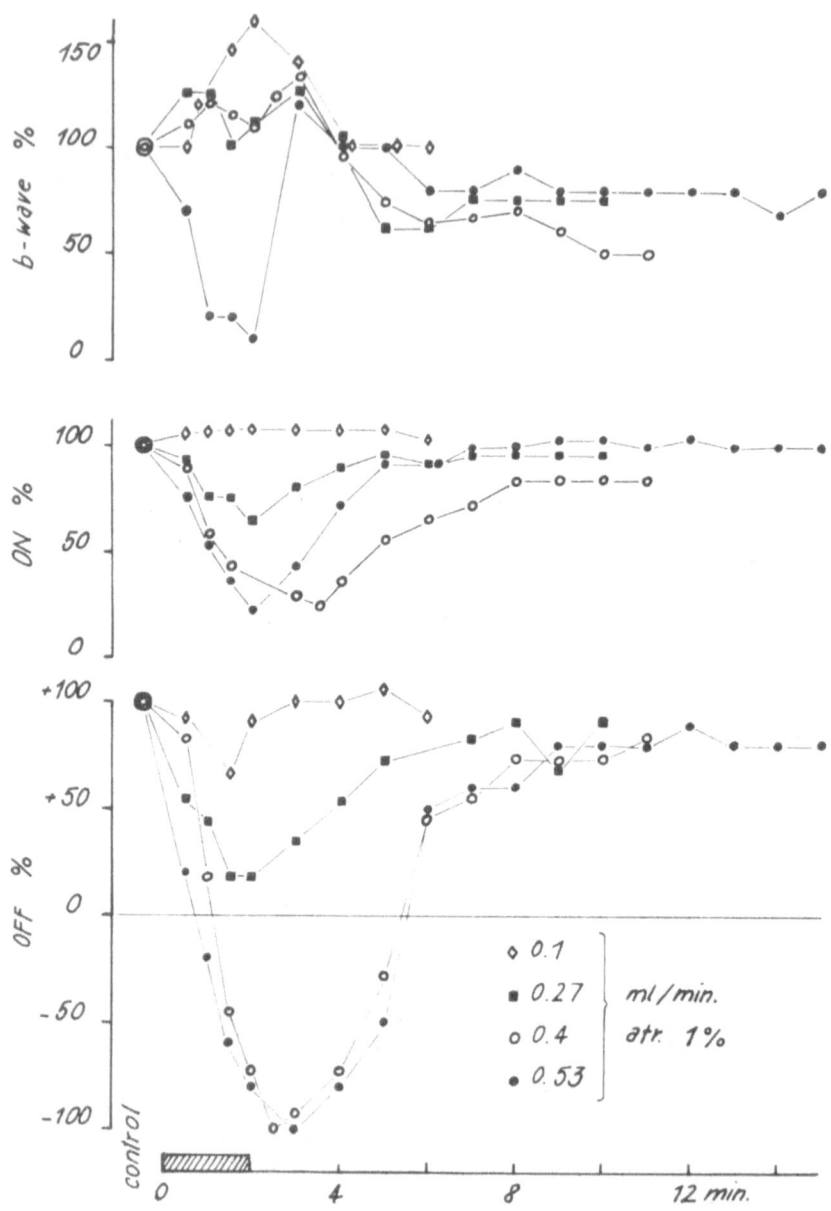

Fig. 4. Plots of the effects of atropine sulfate (1% solution) on the function of the retina. Top: amplitude of the b-wave; middle: amplitude of the ON effect of the optic nerve response; bottom: amplitude of the OFF effect of the optic nerve response. The dashed field on the abscissa indicates injection of atropine for two minutes at 4 different rates as indicated in the inset (right lower corner).

310

crease in amplitude and loss of the oscillatory components of the ON effect can be seen. Recovery was observed 18 minutes after the termination of this injection of atropine into the perfusate.

The OFF effect in uppermost trace in Fig. 3 (control), consisting of a positive deflection, was affected by atropine in a more complex way. Negative components appeared to be enhanced, whereas positive components were concurrently suppressed. These changes were also reversible.

The diagrams in Fig. 4 summarize the effects of brief (two minutes) injections of atropine at 4 different concentrations. The plot of the OFF effect (Fig. 5, bottom graph) does not quantitatively reflect all of its components, but emphasizes the change in polarity which occurs.

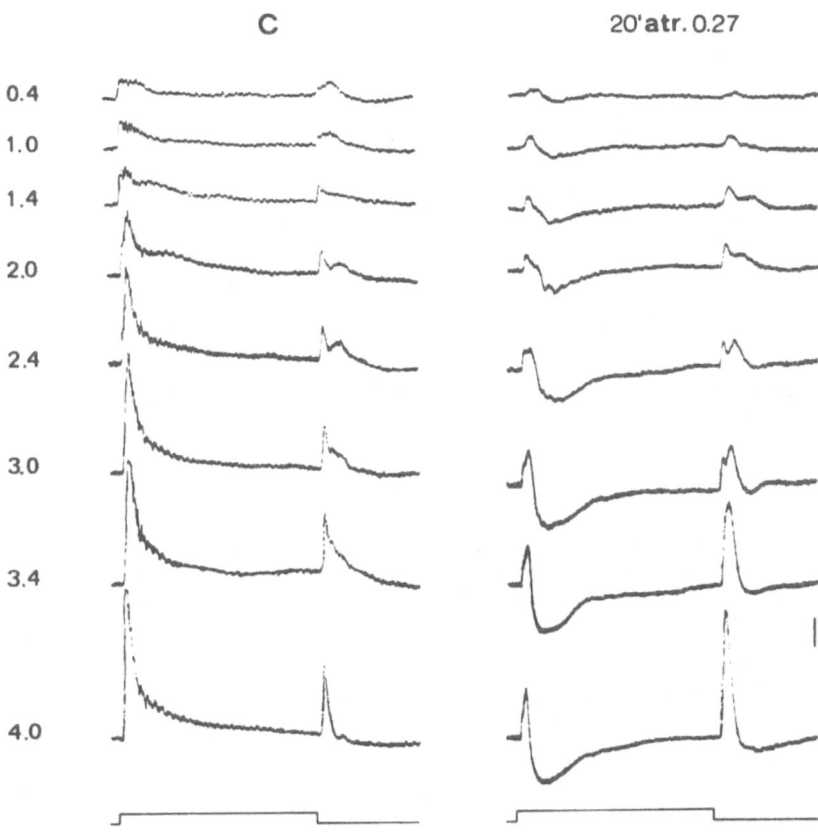

Fig. 5. Effects of a prolonged application of atropine on the optic nerve responses. Left column: control (C) intensity-response series to a red (λ max 620 nm) pulse of 600 msec in duration. The numbers on the left indicate the relative intensity in Log units. Right column: Intensity-response series under the influence of a continuous injection of atropine for 20 minutes. Note drastic changes in both ON- and OFF effects at higher intensities under identical stimulus conditions. Calibration 100 μ V.

Atropine-induced effects on the optic nerve could be maintained by injecting the drug continually (20-30 min.) at low rates. Controls and atropine-effects on the optic nerve as reflected in intensity-response series, are shown in Fig. 5. The controls showed negative ON and OFF effects at all intensities of light from threshold to relatively high suprathreshold levels (3.6 log units). All components of these responses appeared to be affected by atropine as seen in the right column. The ON effects became smaller and biphasic, particularly at high intensities. The OFF-effects were considerably increased after 20 minutes of continuous atropine injection.

The summed responses recorded from the optic nerve in the perfused eye are the resultant of both excitation and inhibition in the firing patterns of all the participating axons. These would presumably include all types of ganglion cells in the cat retina as described previously by numerous investigators. Our understanding of the changes in the optic nerve responses, as induced by a cholinergic blocking agent, is based upon this interpretation. The drug-induced changes thus consist essentially of processes which alter the balance between excitatory and inhibitory events in the retinal output as reflected in the optic nerve. Phase shifts between these excitatory and inhibitory events seem to be particularly prominent in the OFF effects.

Preliminary data on the effects of atopine on the responses of both single ganglion cells and optic nerve axons support this interpretation (Niemeyer & Albani, unpublished material).

The results on atropine therefore reveal effects in both the outer plexiform layer (the b-wave alteration) and the transmission to the ganglion cells (changes in the optic nerve responses). Curiously, the OFF components of the optic nerve response appeared to be affected differently than the ON components, suggesting some preferential influence of atropine on one of these two retinal channels.

ACKNOWLEDGEMENTS

The authors wish to thank Prof. R. Witmer for his support and Dr. P. Gouras for his stimulus to investigate the possibility of neuropharmacologically dissecting the retina. Dipl.-Ing. C. Albani contributed to the analysis of the data as well as to technical improvements of the experimental system. Mrs. R. Fessler provided reliable technical assistance

L.C. was supported by Schweiz. Fonds zur Verhütung der Blindheit as a visiting scientist in Zürich. Supported by Swiss National Science Foundation, grant 3.0630.73 to G.N.

REFERENCES

Ames, A. III & Pollen, D.A.: Neurotransmission in central nervous tissue: a study of isolated rabbit retina. *J. Neurophysiol.* 32, *424-442* (1969).

Dickson, D.H. et al., Ultrastructural localization of cholinesterase activity in the outer plexiform layer of the newt retina. *Brain Res.* 35, *299-303*, 1971.

Francis, C.M.: Cholinesterase in the retina. *J. Physiol.* 120, *435-439*, 1953.

Gouras, P. & Hoff, M.: Retinal function in an isolated, perfused mammalian eye. *Invest. Ophthal.* 9, *388-399*(1970).

Koelle, G.B. et al., *Am. J. Ophthalmology* 35: 2, *1580-1584*, 1952.

Lam, D.M.K.: Biosynthesis of Acetylcholine in Turtle Photoreceptors. *Proc. Nat. Acad. Sci. USA.*, Vol 69, No. 7, *1987-1991*, July 1972.

Masland, R.H., Ames, A. III & Livingstone, C.: Synthesis, Release, and Electrophysiological effects of Acetylcholine in mammalian Retina. Neuroscience Abstracts: 5th Ann. Meeting N.Y. 1975, 173: page 110.

Müller-Limmroth, W.: Elektrophysiologie des Gesichtssinns. Springer-Verlag Berlin (1959).

Murakami, M., Ohtsu, K. & Ohtsuka, T.: Effects of Chemicals on Receptors and Horizontal Cells in the Retina. *J. Physiol.* 227, 899-913 (1972).

Nichols, C.W. & Koelle, G.B.: Acetylcholinesterase – method for demonstration in amacrine cells of rabbit retina. *Science* 155, *477-478*, 1967.

Nichols, C.W. & Koelle, G.B.: Comparison of the localization of Acetylcholinestase and non-specific cholinesterase activities in mammalian and avian retinas. *J. Compar. Neurol.* 133, *1-16*, 1968.

Niemeyer, G. & Gouras, P.: The perfused mammalian eye as a preparation for electrophysiological studies. Xth Symposium, I.S.C.E.R.G., Los Angeles, 1972. Docum. Ophthal. Proc. Series, Vol. 2, pp. 261-268 (1973).

Niemeyer, G.: The function of the retina in the perfused eye. *Docum. Ophthal.* 39; 1, *53-116* (1975).

Niemeyer, G.: Effects of aspartate and glutamate on the function of the cat retina. *Experientia*, in press (1976).

Niemeyer, G.: Retinal physiology in the perfused eye of the cat. Symposium Neural Principles in Vision. F. Zettler & R. Weiler, ed., pp. 158-172 (1976), Springer, Berlin.

Noell, W.K. & Lasansky, A.: Effects of electrophoretically applied drugs and electrical currents on the ganglion cell of the retina. *Federation Proceedings* 18: *115* (abstract No. 453) (1959).

Since this Symposium two papers of particular relevance to the topic have been published:

Masland, R.H. & Livingstone, C.J.: Effects of stimulation with light on synthesis and release of Acetylcholine by an isolated mammalian retina. *J. Neurophysiol.* 39, *1210-1219* (1976).

Masland, R.H. & Ames III, A.: Responses to Acetylcholine of ganglion cells in an isolated mammalian retina. *J. Neurophysiol.* 39, *1220-1235* (1976).

Strashill, M.: Actions of Drugs on Single Neurons in Cat's Retina. *Vision Res.* 8, *35-47* (1968).

Vogel, T. & Nirenberg, M., *Proc. Natl. Acad. Sci. USA* 73, *1806-1810* (1976).

Valtsev, V.B.: Role of cholinergic structures in outer plexiform layer in the electrical activity of frog retina. *Federation Proc. Translation Suppl.* 25, T765-766 (1966).

Zak, P.P. & Lelekova, T.V.: Effect of acetylcholine on the membrane potential of goldfish retinal horizontal cells and frog electroretinogram. *Neurophysiologia* 717, *60-65*, 1975 (in Russian, Engl., summary).

Authors' address:
Neurophysiology Laboratory
Augenklinik, Kantonsspital
CH-8091, Zürich
Switzerland

RELATIONSHIP BETWEEN ERG AND O_2 CONSUMPTION
IN THE ISOLATED PERFUSED BOVINE EYE

Y. TAZAWA, Y. TAKAHASHI, T. OTSUKA & K. MATSUDA.

(Morioka, Japan)

I. INTRODUCTION

It is well known that oxygen plays an important role in the retinal meta-bolism. There have been many reports concerning this, (Granit, 1947; Noell, 1952; Brown, 1957; Tazawa & Seaman, 1972); only a few reported upon the quantitative relationship between the oxygen supply, oxygen consumption in the eye and the ERG wave form (Bauereisen, 1958; Brno, 1966).

A technique of maintaining the metabolism of a perfused isolated bovine eye had been accomplished in authors' laboratory (the Living Extracorporeal Bovine Eye (Tazawa & Seaman, 1972)). Studies on the relationship between retinal metabolism and the ERG have been performed by using this experimental preparation (Imaizumi et al., 1974; Mera, 1972; Otsuka, 1973). The minimum oxygen supply necessary for maintaining the ERG and oxygen consumption of the isolated eye, and the relationship between ERG wave form and oxygen consumption were investigated in the present paper.

II. MATERIALS AND METHODS

1. Perfusion of isolated eyes and ERG recording (Fig. 1).

The methods of perfusing an isolated bovine eye and recording the ERG are the same as that discribed previously by Tazawa & Seaman (1972).

The ciliary artery of an enucleated bovine eye was canulated with a 20-gauge polyethylene tube, immediately after the animal was sacrificed. During the transportation to the laboratory the perfusion of the whole eye was carried out through the tube with heparinized fresh bovine blood, saturated with 100 per cent oxygen, using a drop infusion apparatus at a perfusing pressure of 800 mmH_2O and a flow rate of 2.0 ml/min.

The eye was placed in a shielded dark box, having been dark-adapted during all the experimental course and the temperature was maintained at 32° C.

In the laboratory, the perfusate was changed to Krebs solution which was saturated with 100 per cent oxygen by bubbling in the container.

A pair of Zn-Zn sulfate electrodes, one on the cornea and the other on the sclera near the optic nerve, were connected to a differential amplifier (Nihon Kohden Kogyo Co., AVB 2). A flash light stimulus, intensity 1,730 candelas was given to the perfusing eye using a xenon strobo-

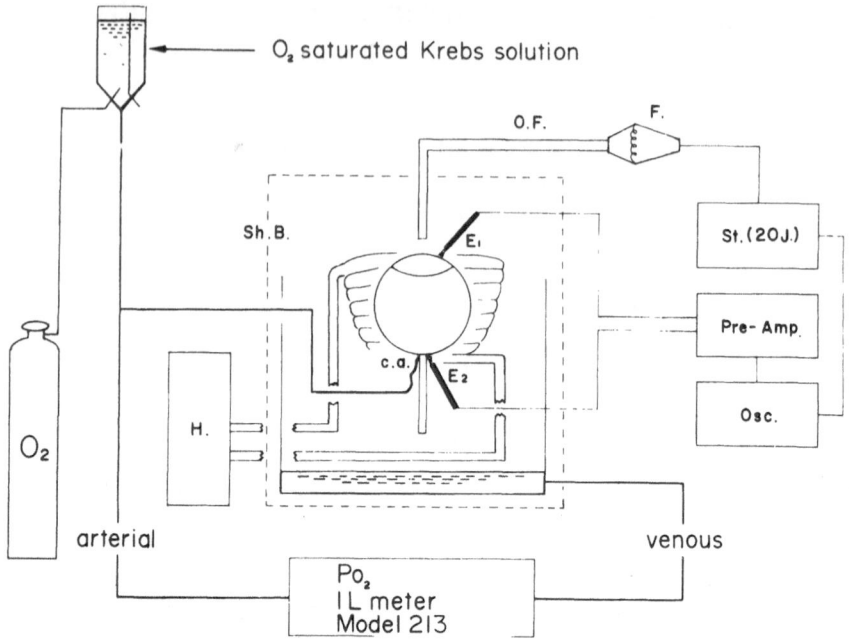

Fig. 1. Diagram of ERG recording of the living extracorporeal bovine eye and Po_2 determination of the perfusate.

scope (Nihon Kohden Kogyo Co., MSP-2R). The ERGs were displayed on a cathode ray oscilloscope (Nihon Kohden Kogyo Co., VC-7). The time constant was set at 0.3 seconds.

2. Measurement of the oxygen supply

The oxygen volume necessary for maintaining control ERG was determined by reducing the perfusion pressure to 650, 500, and 350 mmH$_2$0, and observing changes of ERG wave form. The flow rate at each perfusion pressure was measured by counting drops per minute in the drop infusion apparatus. The oxygen volume supplied to the eye was calculated by applying Po$_2$ value of the arterial perfusate and the flow rate to Henry's law (0$_2$ Vol. = 0.0243 x Po$_2$/760 x Solution Vol.). For Po$_2$ measurement, Asthrup's method by using an I.L. Meter, Model 213 (I.L.Co.) was employed.

3. Measurement of the oxygen consumption

The eye was placed in liquid paraffine (Matuishi Soyaku Co.) in a beaker. The venous outflow was collected under the liquid paraffine for measuring the venous Po$_2$. Prior to the experiment, it had been proved that the liquid paraffine prevented oxygen from diffusing from the solution to the air. The arterial and venous Po$_2$ values were thus measured on the eyes demonstrating various ERG wave forms; intact, b-wave extinguished or both

316

a- and b-wave extinguished. Oxygen consumption was calculated by applying the value of arterio-venous P_{O_2} difference and the flow rate to Henry's
law.

III. RESULTS

1. ERG during Krebs perfusion (Fig. 2, Fig. 3)

On switching the perfusion from blood to Krebs solution, the amplitudes of
the a- and b-waves increased gradually and reached 185 and 170 per cent of
those observed during the blood perfusion respectively. These values were
maintained for 120 minutes. The average flow rate increased to 7.8 ml/min
in Krebs perfusion. Hereafter, this perfusing condition and this ERG wave

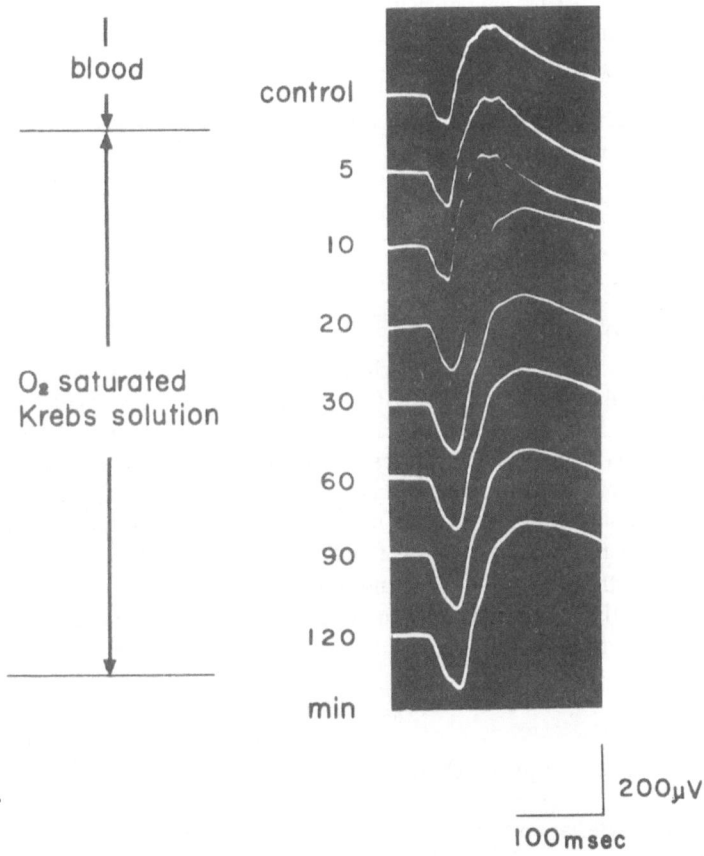

Fig. 2. ERGs recorded in the living extracorporeal bovine eye perfused with oxygen
saturated Krebs solution. Numbers at the left of each trace indicate the perfusing time
in minutes. Stimulus intensity: 20 joule. Stimulus interval: 30 sec.

317

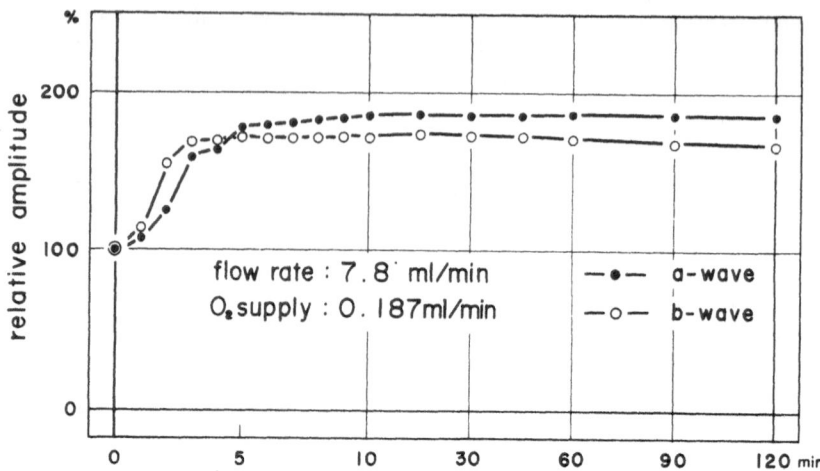

Fig. 3. Variations in amplitude of a- and b-waves recorded from eyes perfused with oxygen saturated Krebs solution. Ordinate: per cent amplitude of ERG. Abscissa: perfusing time in minutes.

form are regarded as control. The average Po_2 of the arterial perfusate was 750 mmHg. From the Po_2 of 750 mmHg and the flow rate of 7.8 ml/min, the average oxygen supply at this control stage was calculated to be 0.187 ml/min/eye.

2. Minimum necessary oxygen supply (Fig. 4 ~ 9)

On reducing the pressure of perfusion with Krebs solution to 350 mmH_2O the amplitudes of a- and b-waves showed a rapid decrease within 5 minutes and reached about 65% and 60% of the control value respectively. Perfusion at pressure of 500 mmH_2O also reduced the amplitudes of a- and b-waves to 75% of the control at 5 minutes. Elevating the perfusion pressure to 650 mmH_2O resulted in no significant change in ERG. It was obvious from the above that the necessary perfusion pressure for maintaining the ERG wave form of the isolated eye was from 500 to 650 mmH_2O. As the average flow rates at the pressure of 500 and 650 mmH_2O were 5.6 and 6.7 ml/min respectively, the minimum oxygen supply necessary for maintaining ERG was estimated to be in the range of 0.134 to 0.161 ml/min/eye.

3. Oxygen consumption

a) Oxygen consumption where the control ERG was produced (Table 1)

The average arterial and venous Po_2 values of the eye in the stage where the control ERG was produced were 744 mmHg and 573 mmHg respectively. As the arterio-venous Po_2 difference was 171 mmHg, and the average flow rate was 7.3 ml/min, the average oxygen consumption in this stage was found to be 0.039 ml/min/eye.

318

b) Oxygen consumption where the b-wave vanished (Table 2)

The a-wave was isolated by keeping the eye in hypoxia for a certain period. The average venous Po_2 value in this stage was 556 mmHg. From the average arterio-venous Po_2 difference of 151 mmHg, and the average flow rate of 5.7ml/min, the average oxygen consumption in this stage was 0.028 ml/min/eye.

c) Oxygen consumption where both a- and b-waves vanished (Table 3)

Persistent hypoxia for much longer period than the previous case resulted in vanishing of both a- and b-waves. The average venous Po_2 value measured in

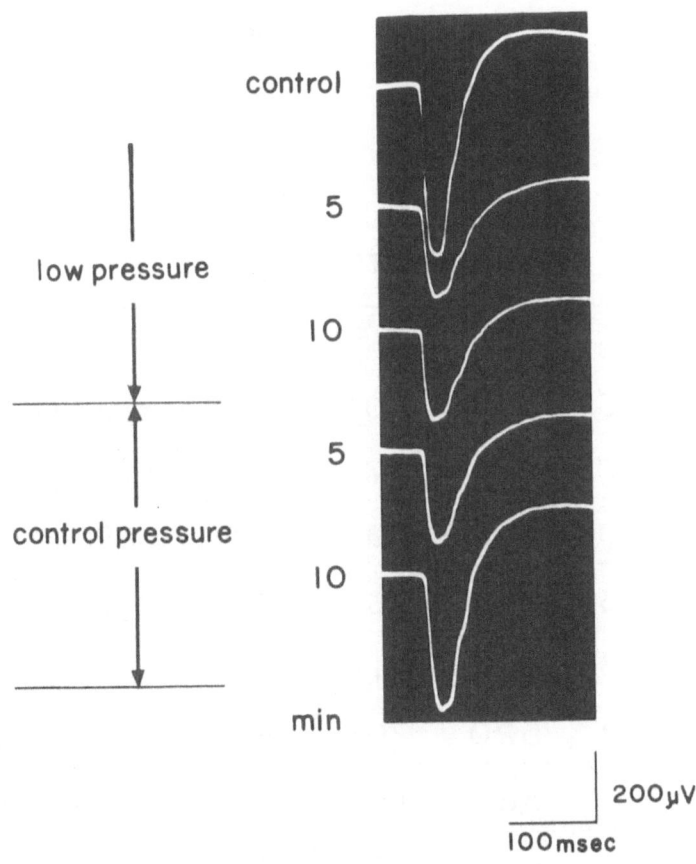

perfusion pressure : 350 mmH$_2$O

control

5

low pressure

10

5

control pressure

10

min

200μV

100msec

Fig. 4. ERGs recorded in the living extracorporeal bovine eye perfused by the low pressure of 350 mmH$_2$O.

319

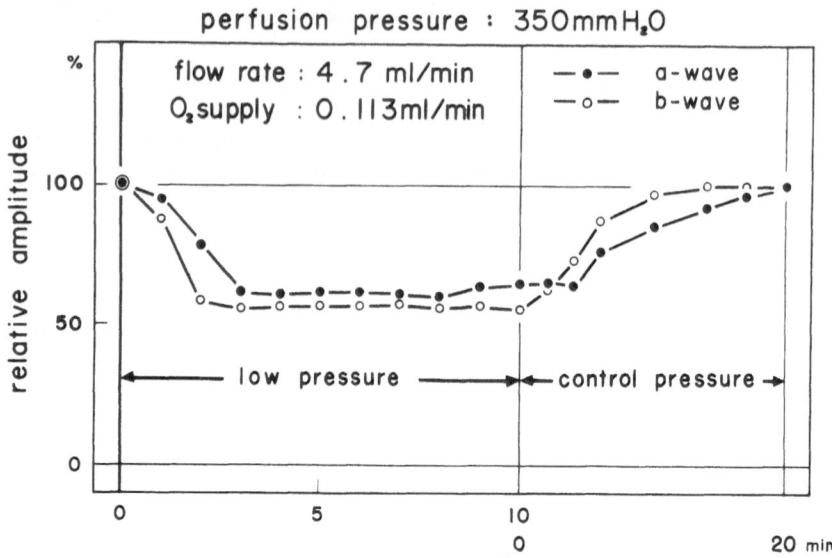

Fig. 5. Variations in amplitude of a- and b-waves recorded from eyes perfused by the low pressure of 350 mmH$_2$O.

control stage

eye No.	PA O$_2$ (mmHg)	PvO$_2$ (mmHg)	A-V diff. (mmHg)	flow rate (ml/min)	O$_2$ supply (ml/min)	O$_2$ consump. (ml/min)
1	745	540	205	8.0	0.191	0.052
2	750	573	177	7.8	0.187	0.044
3	770	580	190	3.9	0.096	0.024
4	753	593	160	7.0	0.169	0.036
5	733	623	110	10.0	0.234	0.035
6	728	520	208	8.0	0.186	0.053
7	728	583	145	6.7	0.156	0.031
aver.	744	573	171	7.3	0.174	0.039

Table 1. Oxygen consumption in eyes perfused with oxygen saturated Krebs solution with a control stage ERG.

320

this stage was 596 mmHg. As the average arteriovenous Po_2 difference was 114 mmHg and the average flow rate was 4.1 ml/min, the average oxygen consumption in this stage was calculated to be 0.015 ml/min/eye.

Furthermore, to produce the stage where both a- and b-waves vanished due to cellular damage, perfusion of 0.1N-KCN solution was carried out. The average venous Po_2 value was 598 mmHg. The average arterio-venous difference of oxygen volume was calculated as 0.009 ml/min/eye from the arterio-venous Po_2 difference of 95 mmHg and the flow rate of 3.0 ml/min.

IV.   DISCUSSION

For an investigation of the influence of the oxygen upon the retina, it is

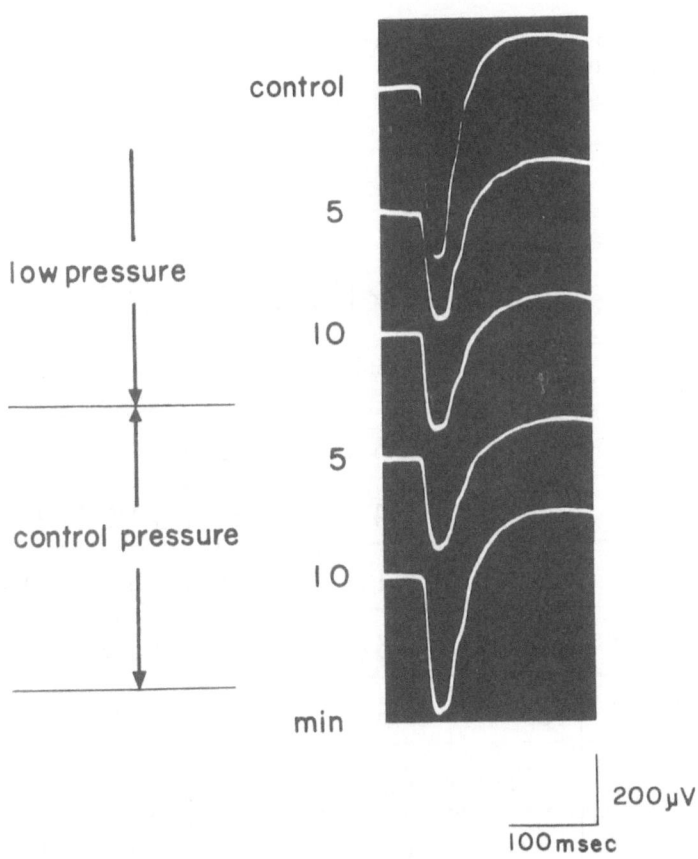

Fig. 6.   ERGs recorded in the living extracorporeal bovine eye perfused by the low pressure of 500 mmH$_2$0.

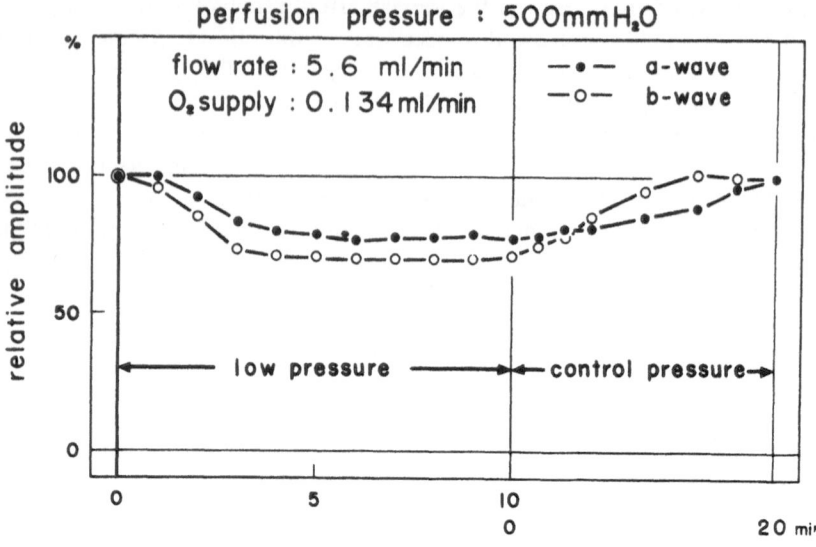

Fig. 7. Variations in amplitude of a- and b-waves recorded from eyes perfused by the low pressure of 500 mmH$_2$O.

a-wave isolated stage

eye No.	PA$_{O_2}$ (mmHg)	PV$_{O_2}$ (mmHg)	A-V diff. (mmHg)	flow rate (ml/min)	O$_2$ supply (ml/min)	O$_2$ consump. (ml/min)
1	773	540	233	5.3	0.131	0.040
2	500	355	145	5.9	0.094	0.027
3	733	617	116	5.9	0.138	0.022
4	693	555	138	6.2	0.137	0.027
5	728	577	151	7.1	0.163	0.034
6	810	690	120	3.9	0.101	0.015
aver.	706	556	151	5.7	0.127	0.028

Table 2. Oxygen consumption in eyes perfused with oxygen saturated Krebs solution in the a-wave isolated stage of the ERG.

desirable that the volume of the oxygen supply can be controled and calculated easily from Po_2 value. In the present experiment, Krebs solution which has linear relationship between oxygen content and Po_2 value was adopted as a perfusate.

Upon perfusion with Krebs solution, the a- and b-waves showed an increase in amplitude and maintained the level for 120 minutes. From these results it was evident that sufficient oxygen volume could be physically dissolved in Krebs solution and that the ERG could be maintained for a long period by using this solution as a perfusate instead of bovine blood.

There seems to be two methods for determining the necessary oxygen supply by observing ERG wave form as an indicator of the metabolic state

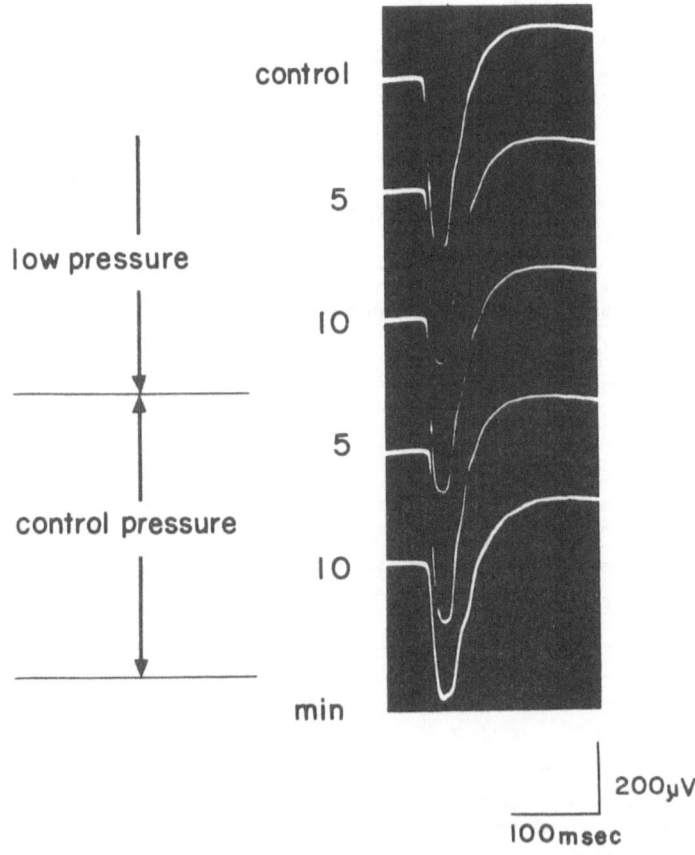

Fig. 8. ERGs recorded in the living extracorporeal bovine eye perfused by the low pressure of 650 mmH$_2$O.

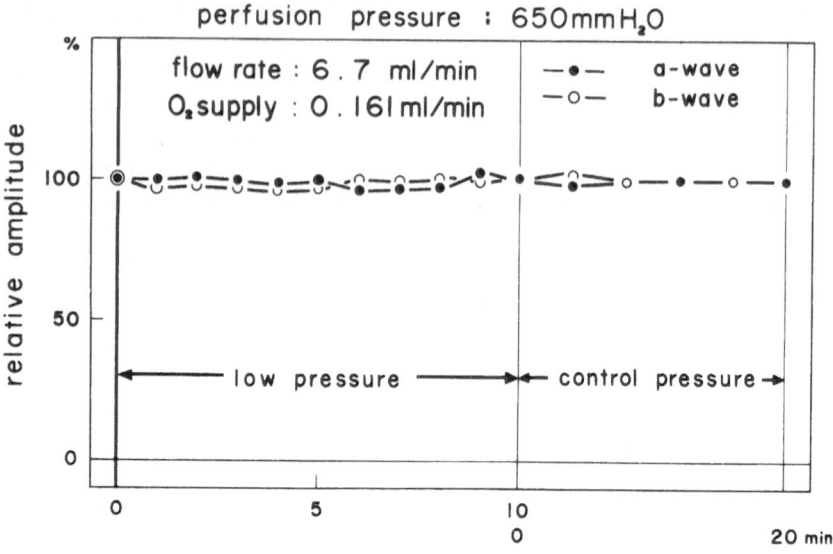

Fig. 9. Variations in amplitude of a- and b-waves recorded from eyes perfused by the low pressure of 650 mmH₂0.

no response stage

eye No.		P_{AO_2} (mmHg)	P_{VO_2} (mmHg)	A-Vdiff. (mmHg)	flow rate (ml/min)	O_2 supply (ml/min)	O_2 consump. (ml/min)
spontaneous deterioration	1	810	690	120	3.9	0.101	0.015
	2	753	632	121	4.3	0.104	0.017
	3	540	430	110	4.0	0.069	0.014
	4	733	630	103	4.1	0.096	0.014
	aver.	709	596	114	4.1	0.093	0.015
KCN perfusion	1	693	585	108	2.4	0.053	0.008
	2	693	613	80	3.7	0.082	0.009
	3	693	595	98	3.0	0.066	0.009
	aver.	693	598	95	3.0	0.067	0.009

Table 3. Oxygen consumption in eyes perfused with oxygen saturated Krebs solution in the no response stage of the ERG.

324

of the retina; one is by reducing the flow rate and the other by reducing the Po_2 value of the perfusate. The former was adopted in the present experiment. The minimum necessary oxygen supply of 0.134 ml/min to 0.161 ml/min corresponds to about 34 to 40 per cent of the oxygen supply in normal blood perfusion (o.4 ml/min; Imaizumi et al., 1974). Alm & Bill (1972) reported that oxygen extraction in the choroidea of the in-vivo cat's eye decreased abruptly by reducing the flow rate to 1/2-1/3 the normal one. There are many other reports that when the retinal oxygen supply was reduced to nearly 50 per cent of the normal, the amplitudes of b-wave began to show a decrease (Takahashi, 1962; Inomata & Tazawa, 1964; Imaizumi et al., 1974).

When measuring the oxygen consumption of the isolated eye, the most attention must be paid to the viability of the eye since the isolated eye is destined to lose its viability sooner or later. The metabolic state of the eye was classified into the four stages on the basis of differences in the ERG wave form.

There are few reports measuring oxygen consumption of the eye with simultaneous observation of ERG wave form. O'Rourke & Berghoffer (1968) reported that the oxygen extraction in an isolated canine eye perfused with blood under the atmospheric pressure was 2.71 mm^3/min as average, which could be converted into 0.00271 ml/min. This value is far less than the present result of 0.0039 ml/min/eye which was obtained from the eyes demonstrating control ERG. Since the metabolic state of the eye in O'Rourke and Berghoffer's experiment was not evaluated on the basis of ERG, it is difficult to compare the authors' results with theirs. Furthermore, this difference of the values might be considered due to the dimensional differences of the experimental animal's eye or due to the difference of Po_2 value in each perfusate. Bauereisen (1958) reported that the oxygen consumption in an isolated frog eye under the high pressure of oxygen (Po_2; 760 mmHg) was 100 mm^3/h/g, which can be converted into 0.00166 ml/min/g. This value is close to 0.00114 ml/min/g, which is the converted value from the present result of 0.039 ml/min/eye, since a bovine eye weighed 35g on the average.

Provided that 0.028 ml/min can be regarded as the oxygen consumption in the stage where the retinal cells contributing to b-wave generation are damaged, the difference of 0.011 ml/min (0.039 minus 0.028 ml/min/eye) might be presumed to indicate the oxygen volume necessary for activity of the generating site of the b-wave. In the same way, the difference of 0.013 ml/min/eye (0.028 minus 0.015 ml/min/eye) might be presumed to indicate the oxygen volume necessary for generation of an a-wave (Table 4).

However, since the generating mechanism of each wave in the ERG has not been clarified completely at present, it is difficult to estimate the oxygen consumption in the specific layer of retina on the basis of the changes of ERG wave form.

The arterio-venous difference of the oxygen volume in the stage where the viability of the eye was entirely damaged due to KCN perfusion was 0.009 ml/min/eye, which should be zero theoretically. This is the value measured immediately after returning from KCN perfusion under the atmos-

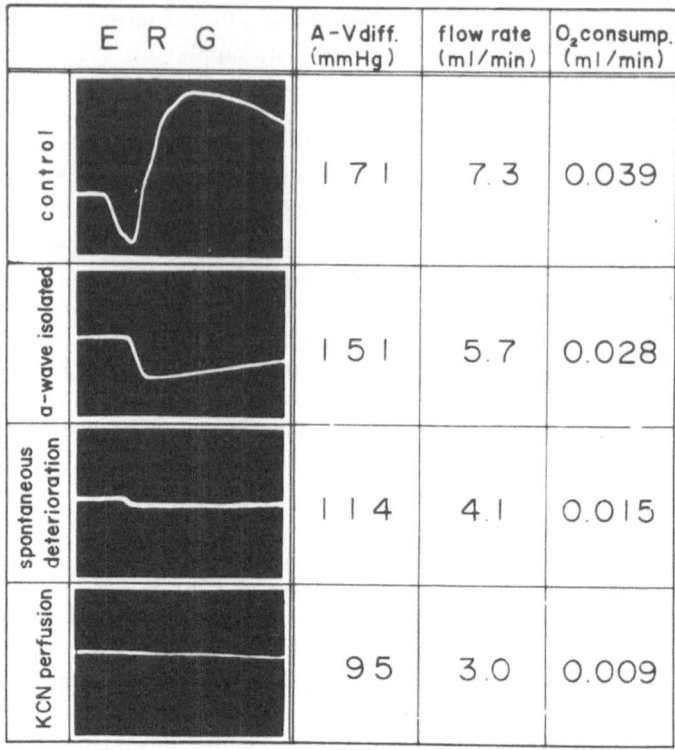

ERG		A–V diff. (mmHg)	flow rate (ml/min)	O₂ consump. (ml/min)
control		171	7.3	0.039
a-wave isolated		151	5.7	0.028
spontaneous deterioration		114	4.1	0.015
KCN perfusion		95	3.0	0.009

Table 4.   ERG wave form and oxygen consumption.

pheric pressure to oxygen saturated Krebs perfusion (Po_2; about 750 mmHg). Since the oxygen in Krebs solution with higher Po_2 value transfer to the ocular tissue until the intraocular Po_2 equilibrates with 750 mmHg, it can be explained that this transferred oxygen volume appeared as if it were consumed in the eye even after KCN perfusion.

V. SUMMARY

An attempt was made to know what oxygen supply was necessary for maintaining the ERG and oxygen consumption of an isolated perfusing bovine eye. The results were as follows:

1) The perfusion with the oxygen saturated Krebs solution could preserve the ERG wave form of the isolated perfusing eye.

2) The minimum oxygen supply necessary for maintaining the ERG of the perfused eye was in the range of 0.134 to 0.161 ml/min/eye.

3) The average oxygen consumption in the stage where the control ERG was produced was 0.039 ml/min/eye.

4) The average oxygen consumption in the stage where the b-wave

vanished was 0.028 ml/min, which was 0.011 ml/min less than that of the perfused eye producing a control ERG.

5) The average oxygen consumption in the stage where both a- and b-waves vanished was in the range of 0.009 to 0.015 ml/min. These values were 0.024 to 0.030 ml/min and 0.013 to 0.019 ml/min less than that of the eye producing control ERG, and of the a-wave isolated eye respectively.

REFERENCES

Alm, A. & Bill, A. *Acta Physiol. Scand.*, 84, *306* (1972).

Bauereisen, E. et al. *Pflügers Arch.*, 367, *636* (1958).

Brno, V.K. The Clinical Value of Electroretinography, ISCERG Symp., 60, Ghent Karger, Basel (1966).

Brown, J.L. et al. *Am. J. Ophthalmol.*, 44, *57* (1957).

Granit, R. Sensory Mechanism of the Retina, Oxford University Press, London and New York (1947).

Imaizumi, K. et al. *Jap. J. Ophthalmol.*, 18, *177* (1974).

Inomata, K. & Tazawa, Y. *J. Iwate Med. Ass.*, 16, *323* (1964).

Mera, H. *Acta Soc. Ophthalmol. Jap.*, 76, *921* (1972).

Noell, W.K. *Am. J. Ophthalmol.*, 35, *126* (1952).

O'Rourke, J. & Berghoffer, B. *Ophthalmologica*, 155, *205* (1968).

Otsuka, T. *Acta Soc. Ophthalmol. Jap.*, 77, *1102* (1973).

Takahashi, F. *Acta Soc. Ophthalmol. Jap.*, 66, *1437* (1962).

Tazawa, T. & Seaman, A.J. *Invest. Ophthalmol.*, 11, *691* (1972).

Authors' address:
Dept of Ophthalmology
Iwate Medical University
Uchimaru 19-1
Morioka, Iwate 020
Japan

CHANGES OF ERG DUE TO HIGH AND LOW SODIUM CONCENTRATION IN THE PERFUSING BLOOD OF THE ISOLATED EYE

Y. TAZAWA, H. MERA, H. IMAIZUMI, H. KURIHARA & K. IMAIZUMI

(Morioka, Japan)

I. INTRODUCTION

Most of the electrophysiological studies of the retina *in vitro* have been made by methods in which the retina is taken out of the eye and preserved in a circulating bathing solution. This method, however, places the retinas of warm-blooded animals in a condition quite unlike their physiologic conditions, and it may therefore be estimated that the information so obtained differs considerably from that obtained in the *in situ* condition. Ever since one of the present authors, Tazawa (Tazawa et al., 1969, Tazawa et al., 1972), in his study with Seaman et al., was successful in keeping the isolated whole bovine eye alive in a condition close to the physiologic one by perfusing it with bovine blood for a long period of time, the authors have made a series of studies upon relations of retinal metabolism to the ERG by this method, and the results have been published (Imaizumi, K. et al., 1971; Imaizumi, K. et al., 1972; Mera, 1972; Otsuka, 1973; Imaizumi, H. 1974; Takahashi, 1975; Imaizumi, K. et al., 1974).

In order to investigate what effect the sodium ion (Na⁺) (which plays an important role in the transmission of retinal excitation) would exert on the ERG, we have studied alterations in the ERG with variations in the concentration of Na⁺ in the perfusate. The changes of ERG due to high and low concentration of Na⁺ were reported from our laboratory, separately by Mera (1972) and Imaizumi, H. (1974). In the present paper, these results were reviewed and the effects of the Na⁺ concentrations from high to low upon the ERG were discussed.

II. MATERIALS AND METHODS

For details of the methods of perfusing an isolated eye, 'The Living Extra-corporeal Bovine Eye', the reader is referred to previous papers (Tazawa, et al., 1969; Tazawa, et al., 1972). But, a brief description of the method is given below. The eyeball is enucleated immediately after a cow is slaughtered; a 20-gauge polyethylene tube is inserted into the ciliary artery that courses along the optic nerve, and the blood vessels of the eye are perfused with heparinized fresh bovine blood saturated with 100 per cent oxygen via the polyethylene tube. The ciliary artery supplies all of the tissue of the bovine eye.

For experimental purposes, the perfused bovine eye was placed in a shielded box and adapted to the dark for about 20 minutes. This was used as the control condition.

For recording the ERG, a pair of non-polarized Zn-$ZnSO_4$ electrodes were used; one on the cornea and the other on the sclera near the optic nerve, connected with a cathode-ray oscilloscope (Nihon Kohden Kogyo Co, VC-7). The xenon stroboscope (Nihon Kohden Kogyo Co, MSP-2R flash light for retinography) was used as the flash light stimulator, and the light stimulus was conducted to the retina by glass fibers 10 mm in diameter and 60 cm in length (American Optics Co. LG-5-24) which had been fixed about 1 cm above the cornea. The intensity of the stimulus was set at 1,730 candelas, and the time constant at 0.3 seconds.

In order to check the effects of different concentrations of Na^+ on the ERG, perfusion of the bovine eye with normal bovine blood was switched to blood with a high or low concentration of Na^+. The perfusion with the latter was continued for ten minutes. The eye was then switched back to perfusion with normal blood. The ERG was taken every 30 seconds during this procedure. The low- and high-Na^+ bloods were prepared by the methods of Mera (1972) and Imaizumi, H. (1974). A Na-free pH-7.4 Krebs' solution in which Na^+ had been replaced with Tris (hydroxymethyl aminomethane) and Tris (hydroxymethyl aminomethane) hydrochloride was made available. This solution was mixed with fresh bovine blood in suitable ratios for preparing the low-Na^+ perfusing bloods containing 30 mM to 110 mM of Na^+. NaCl was further added to the bovine blood in suitable ratios for preparing the high-Na^+ perfusing bloods containing 190 mM to 540 mM of Na^+. The osmotic pressures of the bovine bloods containing various concentrations of Na^+ were not considered in the present experiments. All of the experiments were made under scotopic conditions at 32° C.

III. RESULTS AND DISCUSSION

1.   Effects of Na^+ concentration on the a-wave of the ERG

Under perfusion with the low-Na^+ bloods, containing Na^+ in the range of 70 mM to 110 mM, the amplitude of a-wave was markedly reduced with a decrease in Na^+ concentration. Under the perfusion with the bloods containing less than 70 mM of Na^+, the amplitude continued to be reduced but in a less sharp gradient than when the perfusing blood contained more than 70 of Na^+.

Under perfusion with the high-Na^+ bloods containing 180 mM to 540 mM of Na^+, the higher the Na^+ concentration, the more marked the increase in a-wave amplitude. When the perfusion with the low-Na^+ and with the high-Na^+ bloods were reviewed as a whole, it was disclosed as given in Fig. 1 that there was a relationship between the Na^+ concentration and the amplitude of a-wave which could be presented as a sigmoid curve having a plateau between 140 mM and 180 mM of Na^+. In his previous study in which perfusion with low-Na^+ bloods for 5 minutes was performed with the same apparatus, one of the authors (Imaizumi, H.) observed that the amplitude of the a-wave of the ERG was reduced only slightly with Na^+ concentrations in the range of normal to 110 mEq/liter. He also found that the amplitude was reduced at a higher rate with a decrease in Na⁺ concentration in the range of 110 to 70 mEq/liter, and that the perfusion with the bloods having even lower Na⁺ concentrations caused a smaller rate of reduction in the amplitude with decrease in Na⁺ concentration. This result was consistent with that of the present experiment of 10 minutes perfusion. In their study in which the effects of low Na⁺ concentrations on the preparation of the pigeon retina were investigated, Arden & Ernst (1970) showed that the sodium ion concentration of the perfusate and PIII amplitude were linearly related, except for the extremely low range of Na⁺ concentration. On the other hand, it was described by Hamasaki (1963), Hanawa (1967) and Silman et al. (1969) that in the experiments on the isolated frog retina the action potential was linearly related with the logarithm of low-Na⁺ concentration. This difference between the findings of these authors and those of the present authors may be considered to reflect the difference in the species of the animals used as predicted by Imaizumi, H. (1974) and by Arden et al. (1970), as well as due to differences in the experimental methods. It has been reported by Arden et al. (1969) that alterations in the permeability of receptor cells with low-Na⁺ concentrations are responsible for the reduction in the a-wave amplitude with low-Na⁺ concentrations.

Of the findings in the present study, it was of particular interest that the increase in the a-wave amplitude was intensified by the elevation of Na⁺

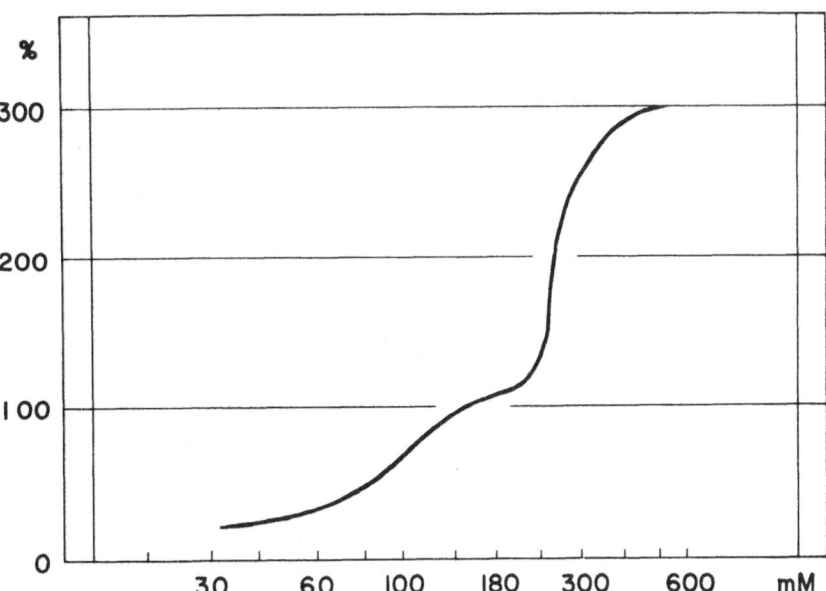

Fig. 1. Variations in the relative amplitudes of the ERG a-waves recorded from isolated bovine eyes perfused with low or high sodium ion concentration blood. The ordinate shows the percentage of a-wave amplitude against that of the control. The abscissa is a logarithmic scale of sodium ion concentration in the blood.

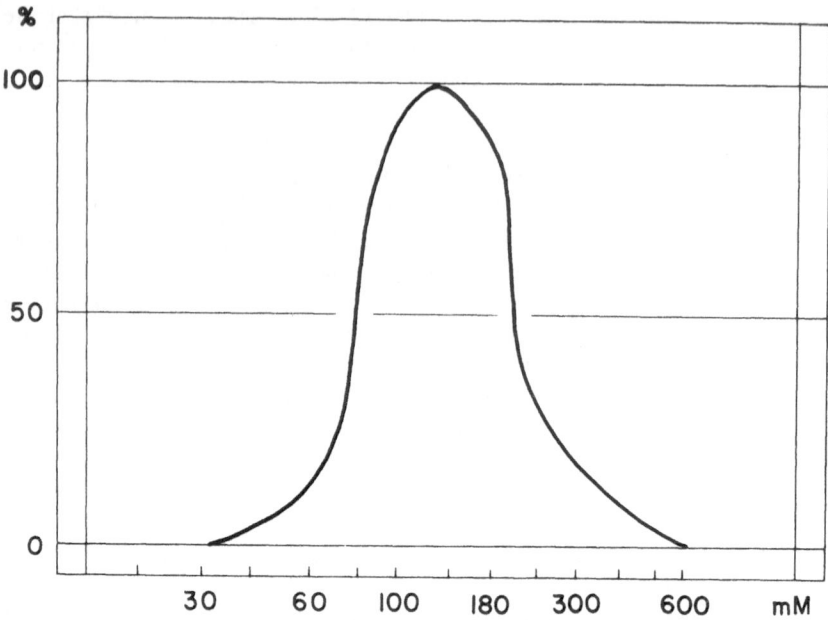

Fig. 2. Variation in the relative amplitudes of the ERG b-waves recorded from isolated bovine eyes perfused with low or high sodium ion concentration blood.

concentration. There are few papers on high-Na⁺ concentrations and the amplitudes of ERG parameters. Mera (1972) had postulated that this phenomenon would have resulted from the action of some acceleratory factors on the origin of the a-wave. The increase in the a-wave amplitude may also considered to have resulted from a transient change in the function of the sodium pump in the receptor cells (the origin of the a-wave) with the elevation of Na⁺ concentration in the extra-cellular fluid. From the findings in the present study, it still remains no more than a surmise what is responsible for the increase in the amplitude of a-wave with high Na⁺ concentrations, and this is a theme of future studies.

2. Effects of Na⁺ concentration on the b-wave of the ERG

The b-wave amplitude of the ERG was reduced when the Na⁺ concentration of the perfusing blood was elevated above or dropped below a level of about 140 mM. Therefore, when the relationship of the Na⁺ concentration to the b-wave amplitude was reviewed as a whole, the relationship presented a mountainshape curve as shown in Fig. 2. Furukawa & Hanawa (1955) showed in their study in which they perfused the isolated retina of turtles with a sodium-free perfusate, that the b-wave responded with a reduction in its amplitude to low Na⁺ concentrations. There are only a few published studies of the effects of high Na⁺ concentrations on the b-wave. In the present study, it was observed that the lower or higher the Na⁺ concentration, the more delayed was the recovery of the reduced b-wave amplitude to the control by perfusion with normal blood. It may therefore be reasonable to consider that the course of alterations in the b-wave amplitude may be a phenomenon which is provided by the process in which the equilibrium of the membrane potential changes by rapid alterations in the Na^+ concentration of the extracellular fluid.

IV. SUMMARY

Alterations in the ERG with variations in the Na^+ concentration of the perfusate were studied by the method of perfusing the isolated bovine eye.

The amplitude of the a-wave decreased with a decrease in the sodium concentration of the perfusate below normal, and increased with an increase in the sodium concentration above normal. The relationship of the amplitude of the a-wave to the Na^+ concentration presents as a sigmoid curve.

The amplitude of the b-wave was reduced either with a decrease in the Na^+ concentration below normal or an increase above normal. The relationship of the b-wave amplitude to the Na^+ concentration presented a : 1ountain-shape curve.

BIBLIOGRAPHY

Arden, G.B. & Ernst, W. I. Physiol., London, 204: Proceedings of the Physiological Society., June, 35 p. (1969).

Arden, G.B. & Ernst, W. J. Physiol., 211, 311 (1970).

Furukawa, T. & Hanawa, I. Jap. J. Physiol., 5, 289 (1955).

Hamasaki, D.I. Physiol., 167, 156 (1963).

Hanawa, I., Kuge, K. & Matsumura, K. Jap. J. Physiol., 17, 1 (1967).

Imaizumi, K., Tazawa, Y., Ogawa, K., Mera, H. & Otsuka, T. The Visual System: Neurophysiology, Biophysics and Their Clinical Applications, 24: Proceedings of the 9th ISCERG Symposium, p. 119, Plenum Press, New York, London (1972).

Imaizumi, K., Tazawa, Y., Mera, H. & Otsuka, T. Fifth Afro-Asian Congress of Ophthalmology: Acta, 420, Tokyo (1972).

Imaizumi, H. Acta Soc. Ophthalmol. Jap., 78, 831 (1974).

Imaizumi, K., Tazawa, Y., Mera, H., Imaizumi, H. & Takahashi, Y. Folia Ophthalmol. Jap., 25, 1134 (1974).

Mera, H. Acta Soc. Ophthalmol., Jap., 76, 921 (1972).

Otsuka, T. Acta Soc. Ophthalmol., Jap., 77, 1102 (1973).

Silman, A.J., Ito, H. & Tomita, T. Vision Ress., 9, 1443 (1969).

Tazawa, Y. & Seaman, A.J. Invest. Ophthalmol., (Abst.), 8, 238 (1969).

Tazawa, Y. & Seaman, A.J. Invest. Ophthalmol., 11, 691 (1972).

Takahashi, Y. Acta Soc. Ophthalmol., Jap., 79, 1167 (1975).

Authors' address:
Dept of Ophthalmology
Iwate Medical University
Uchimaru 19-1
Morioka, Iwato 020
Japan

RETINOTROPIC ACTIVITY OF ω-HYDROXYHEXYLPYRIDONE-2 IN METHANOL AND ALLYLALCOHOL INJURY*

K.K. GAURI*, K.A. HELLNER, R. SIEWERS & P. HEIN

(Hamburg)

Before we go into details of the data on the retinotropic activity of ω-hydroxyhexylpyridone-2 (OH-AAD), I would like first to describe what we understand under the term retinotropic, especially because this expression so far has not beem employed in the literature.

We know that quite a few compounds, drugs as well as non drugs, exhibit deleterious effects on specific retinal functions. Methanol for example, which is not a drug, causes blindness in man; chloroquine and other allied antriheumatics bring about changes which lead to loss of visual fields. These substances are classified as retinal poisons. Accordingly, I believe that it is justified to apply the term retinotropic to those compounds which: partially or fully antagonize the delterious effects of the retinal poisons, improve loss of retinal functions originating from sources such as old age, heriditary complications, or those resulting from disturbances in Vitamin A-household.

We have developed pyridones (Gauri, 1973) which from ERG-studies (Gauri et al., 1972/73; 1973) and rhodopsin measurements (Gauri & Scheppach, 1974) have been shown to replace Vitamin A activity in experimental A deficiency and which are capable of improving loss of ERG-functions resulting from senility in mice (Hellner & Gauri, 1974). We will now present evidence for these pyridones to potentially antagonize injurious effects of methanol and of allylalcohol, based on ERG experiments. Results with individual alcohols will be described separately.

A. Antagonization of methanol effect by ω-hydroxyhexylpyridone-2 (OH-AAD) in Mice

According to figure 1 methanol at 40 mg/kg intraperitoneally produces significant inhibition of the ERG. This effect is well pronounced starting from 20 min. up to elapse of 120 min. after the injection. A pretreatment of animals, 17hrs before the injection with 175 mg/kg of the OH-AAD by the same i.p. route, potentially antagonizes the effect of methanol. Under its effect the b-wave amplitudes are almost double that under methanol alone.

OH-AAD also improves the loss of retinal sensitivity due to methanol damage by one to two log. units (fig. 2).

---

* Dedicated to Prof. Dr. Joachim Kuhnau on the anniversary of his 75th birthday.

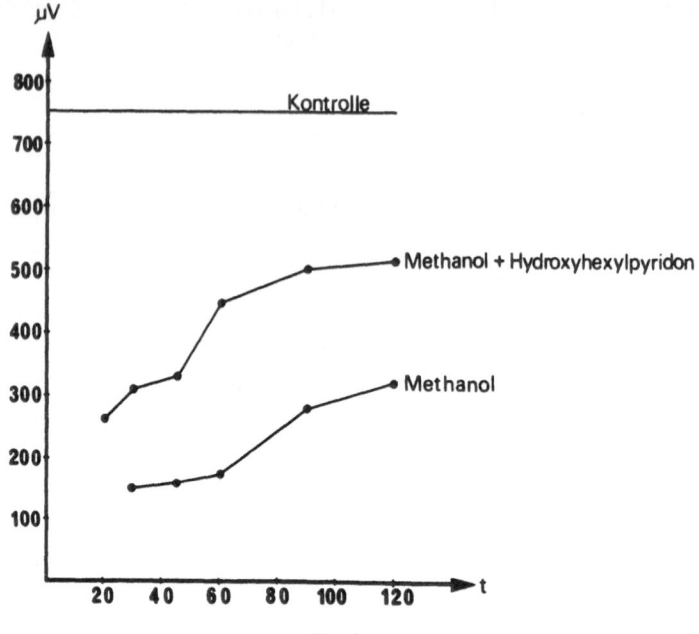

Fig. 1.

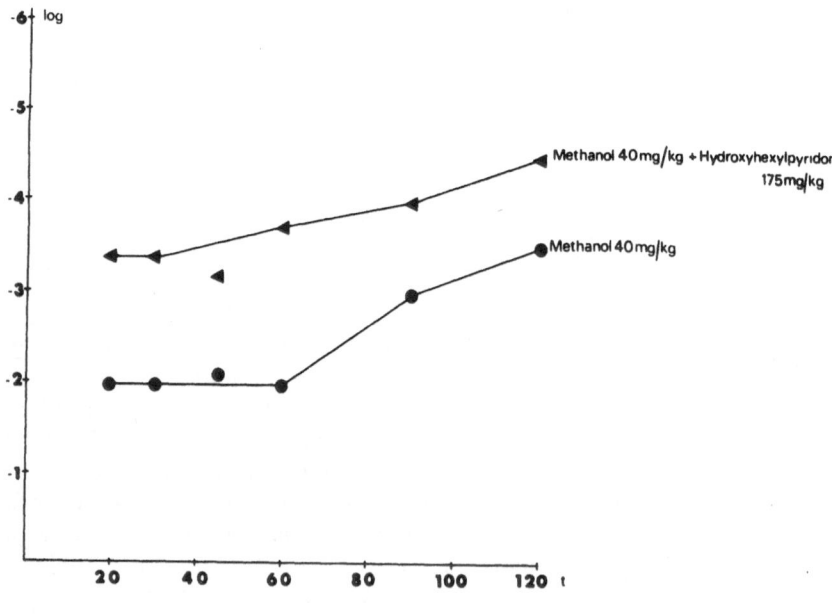

Fig. 2.

In a further experiment in mice the dose activity relationship for OH-AAD in methanol injury to retina was studied (fig. 3): Keeping the methanol dose of 40 mg/kg intraperitoneally constant a very clear dose response curve for OH-AAD is obtained. Maximum effect of the OH-AAD is present at 175 mg/kg. At this dose level the b-wave amplitudes are practically the same as for the control animals without treatment.

A far better effect of OH-AAD against the methanol injury in this series than in the preceeding (cf. Fig. 1) seems to be due to the higher starting potentials of the normal animals in this group. Whereas for the untreated controls in the previous group amplitudes of 750 µV were obtained in the present animals the mean of these amplitudes is 900 µV.

B. Retinotropic effect of ω-hydroxyhexylpyridone-2 against allylalcohol damage

Effect of allylalcohol on ERG has so far not been described. The reasons for this are that allylalcohol is not a drug and the likelihood of its accidental ingestion is low.

The reason for our selection of this compound as a retinal poison in an evaluation of retinotropic activity was the report of RANDO (1974) according to which its metabolic product acrolein inhibits only the yeast-ADH irreversibly and not the ADH from animal sources. Therefore it was expected that application of allylalcohol should not inhibit the ERG irrevers-

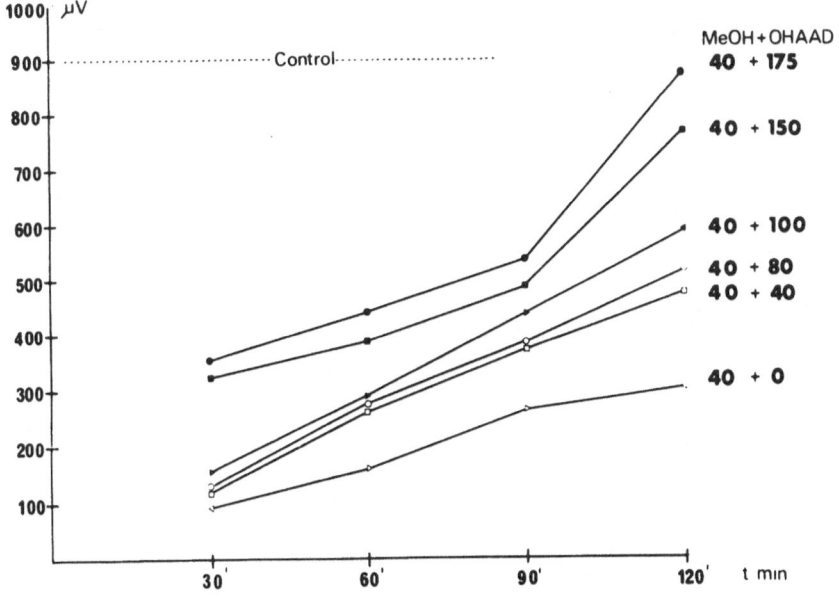

Fig. 3.

337

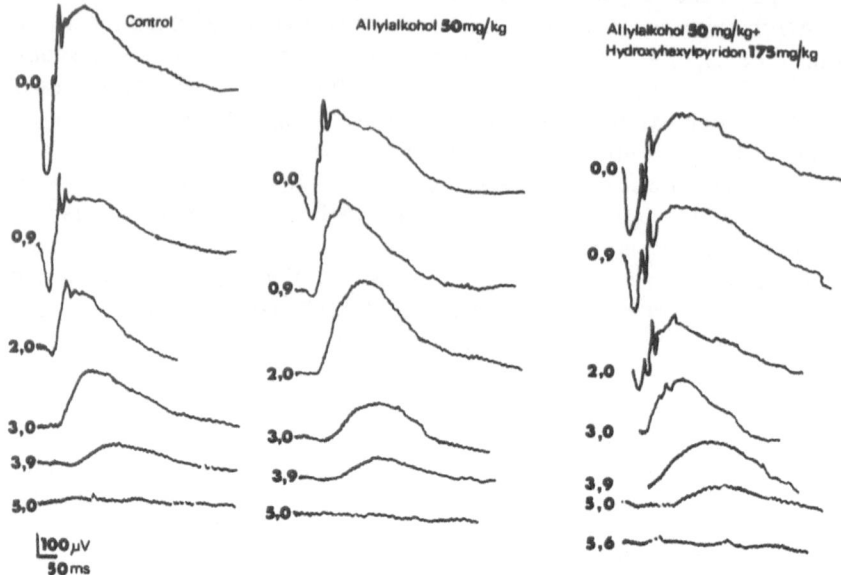

Fig. 4.

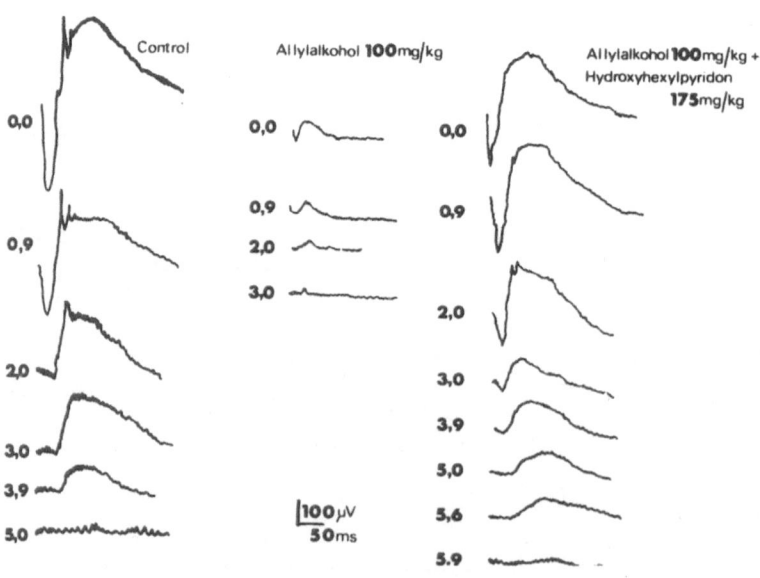

Fig. 5.

ibly; this is an important requisite for evaluation of the retinotropic activity.

Figure 4 shows the effect of 50 mg/kg allylalcohol. At this dose level allylalcohol is only slightly inhibitory when compared with the normal controls. As expected, also there is no considerable difference between the ERG under the allylalcohol alone and the animals which received allylalcohol and 175 mg/kg OH-AAD 17hr prior to the alcohol injection.

However, doubling the allylalcohol dose results in profound inhibition (fig. 5). As given before, ERG's were recorded 3 hours after the alcohol injection.

The b-wave just appears at light intensities lying 3 log. units higher than in the controls and the amplitudes are extremely low. For testing the retinotropic activity of OH-AAD the model of damage by allylalcohol is most interesting because the almost completely abolished ERG is highly compensated by treatment with 175 mg/kg intraperitoneally.

These results are expressed schematically in Figure 6.

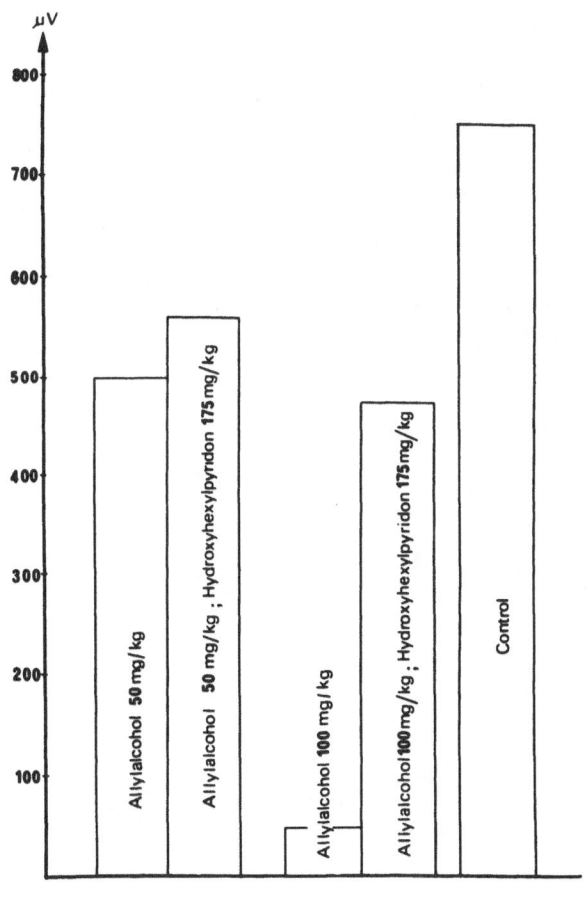

Fig. 6.

DISCUSSION AND SUMMARY

The compounds hexylpyridone-2 and the ω-hydroxyhexylpyridone-2, as had been shown earlier, possess protective effect on the loss of retinal functions resulting either from senility or from disturbances in the Vitamin A household. Now we show that these compounds are also protective against chemical injuries caused by methanol and allylalcohol treatment. Therefore it is justified to classify these pyridon derivatives as retinotropic compounds.

Another special feature of the present investigation is to offer experimental models to evaluate the retinotropic effect; here the use of methanol (40 mg/kg i.p.) and more especially that of the allylalcohol (100 mg/kg i.p.) to damage the retinal functions stands in the foregrounds.

REFERENCES

K.K. Gauri: N-alkylpyridonee-2 als Aktivatoren der Alkoholdehydrogenase aus Pferdeleber. *Arch. Pharm.* 306, *529* (1972a).

K.K. Gauri: 1. -Hydroxyalkylpyridone als funktionelle Analoga des Retinols. *Arch. Pharm.* 306, 765 (1972b).

K.K. Gauri K.A. Hellner, J.Rickers & I. Watanabe: Effect of N-Hexylpyridone-2 on the mouse electroretinogram. *Ophthal. Res.* 4, *265* (1972/73).

K.K. Gauri, K.A. Hellner, J. Rickers & I. Watanabe: Effect of alcohol-dehydrogenase activators on mouse ERG. Xth I.S.C.E.R.G. Symposium Los Angeles 1972, Documenta Ophthal. Den HEGUE 1973 K.K. Gauri and P. Scheppach, unpublished.

K.A. Hellner & K.K. Gauri: Mechanism of action of ω-Hydroxyhexylpyridon-2 on the ERG. XIth I.S.C.E.R.G. Symposium, 1973 Documenta Ophthal. Den HAGUE 1974.

R.R. Rando: Allylalcohol-induced irreversible inhibition of yeast alcoholdehydrogenase. *Biochem. Pharmacol.* 23, *2328* (1974).

Authors' address:
U.K.E. Augenklinik
D 2000 Hamburg 20
FRG

340

A CHROMATICITY DIAGRAM FOR DEFECTS IN COLOR VISION

RALPH D. GUNKEL & FRANK J. KOLLARITS

(Bethesda, Maryland)

ABSTRACT

An instrument is described for the measuring and plotting of color thresholds. A chromaticity circle is proposed as being more suitable and convenient than the conventional modified triangle for color designation, and particularly useful for describing defects in color vision, both as a function of degree and of spectral range.

A minute area of the color circle is enlarged and projected as a uniform field on a ground glass screen. The neutral area is first located and saturation is slowly increased in a given direction until the subject can establish a noticeable difference and name the color. Multiple color thresholds are determined to delineate the neutral area or defect.

Advantages of this method of color testing are: 1) Both hue and saturation are depicted on a card outlining the entire defect; 2) Central vision and good acuity are not required; and 3) The test is easily administered by non-skilled personnel.

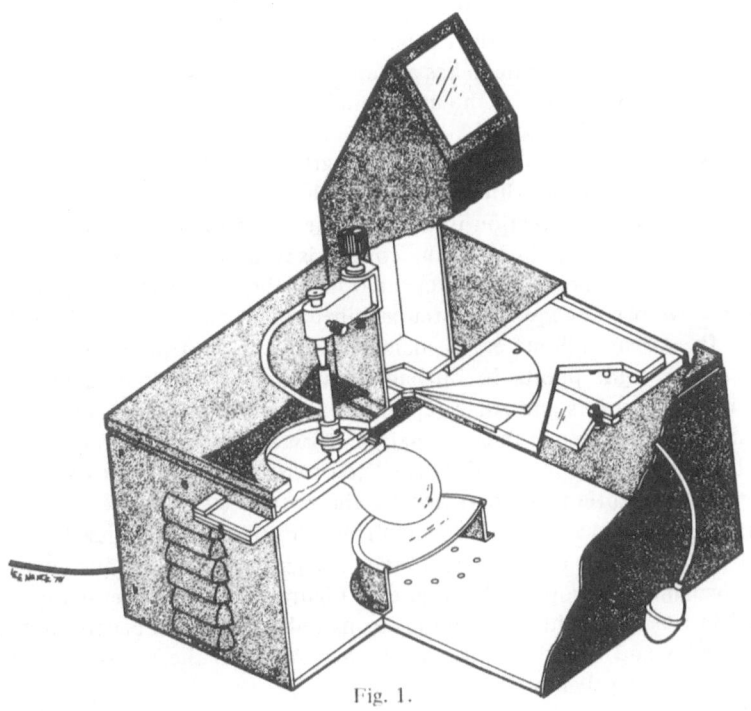

Fig. 1.

Most of you who are involved in psychophysical testing are familiar with the commonly used tests for defective color vision and the extensive literature which has proliferated on the subject (Wright, 1968; Armington & Biersdorf, 1963; Fishman, 1971; Neubauer, 1972; Sloan & Wollach, 1948; Linksz, 1971). Furthermore, most of you would probably agree with the Englishman who recently stated that '... no clinical test reliably measures the extent of a color vision defect'. (Dain, 1973)

The instrument being presented offers a new approach to the problem in that it creates a chromaticity circle (instead of a triangle) on which it plots any conceivable color defect simply as an enlargement or extension of the normal neutral area. The essentials consist of a means for producing a uniform viewing field of any hue or saturation and a convenient method for marking color thresholds on a chart. The heart of the instrument is a three-sector arrangement of red, blue and green filters instead of the rectilinear arrangement used in some earlier instruments (Geddie, 1974; Burnham, 1952) and an efficient diffusing block or prism.

A partially cut-away schematic view, (Fig. 1), will help in explaining how the instrument works. Starting at the source we have a 75 watt GE enlarger bulb PH211, which is stated to have a color temperature of about 2850 degrees Kelvin at 115 volts. A concave mirror is placed below the bulb to increase its effectiveness. A 6 mm plate of heat-absorbing glass helps protect the gelatin filters. The filters are mounted between sheets of transparent plastic in a 115 mm round aperture in a 23 cm square aluminium plate, which rolls around freely on ball bearings at each corner. The filter has equal sectors of Wratten Number 29, 47, and 61 balanced with neutral density to give white at the center of the circle. A marking device moves with the filter plate and pressing the bulb makes a punchmark in the record card. A 50 mm viewing screen is situated at the upper end of the mixing prism, directly over the center of the filters.

In using the instrument we always start in the central area which the subject concedes to be white or neutral. The control handle is then moved peripherally in any direction until the subject can see and name a trace of color. The point is marked and the control is returned to the neutral area to find another threshold. This is repeated until the investigator considers the area to have been adequately circumscribed. Most normal neutral areas are about five or six millimeters in diameter with this plotting scale, requiring only six or eight points to outline them conclusively, but large defects require many points and some repetition for confirmation. Figure 2 shows the small neutral area in the chromaticity diagram or 'chromagram' for right and left eyes of a subject with normal color vision. Figure 3 shows a bilateral defect too subtle to be detected by the routine tests. Figure 4 shows the neutral area in a 15 year old boy with ocular albinism. He missed the first HRR plate with his right eye and made a slightly protanomalous setting on the Nagel anomaloscope with either eye. Figure 5 shows a larger neutral area found in a boy who had a medium strong red-green defect according to the HRR plates and was deuteranomalous according to the Farnsworth Panel D-15 and the Nagel anomaloscope.

Figure 6 shows a larger neutral area found in a young doctor who was

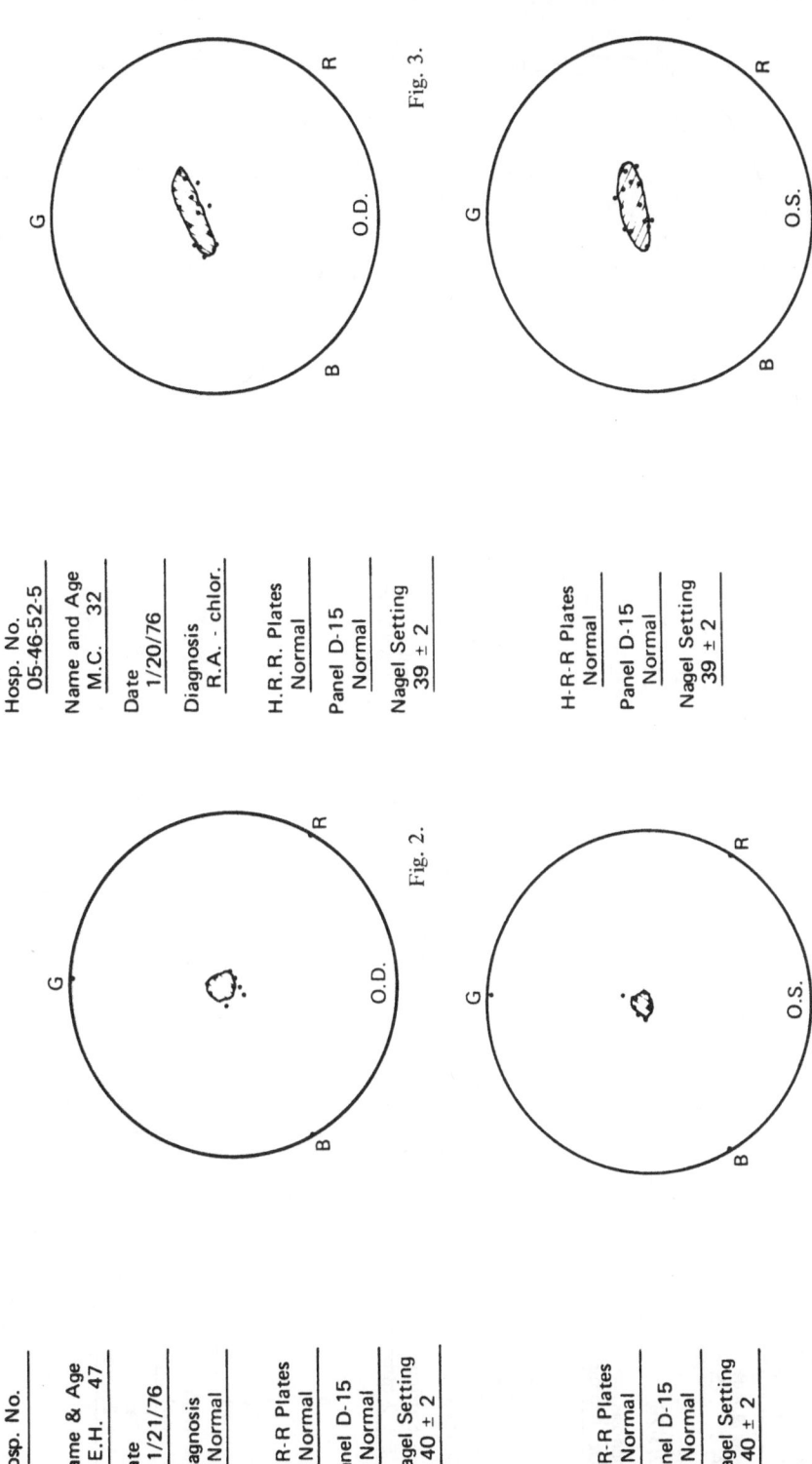

Fig. 3.

Hosp. No.
05-46-52-5

Name and Age
M.C.   32

Date
1/20/76

Diagnosis
R.A. - chlor.

H.R.R. Plates
Normal

Panel D-15
Normal

Nagel Setting
39 ± 2

O.D.

O.S.

H-R-R Plates
Normal

Panel D-15
Normal

Nagel Setting
39 ± 2

Fig. 2.

Hosp. No.

Name & Age
E.H.   47

Date
1/21/76

Diagnosis
Normal

H-R-R Plates
Normal

Panel D-15
Normal

Nagel Setting
40 ± 2

O.D.

O.S.

H-R-R Plates
Normal

Panel D-15
Normal

Nagel Setting
40 ± 2

343

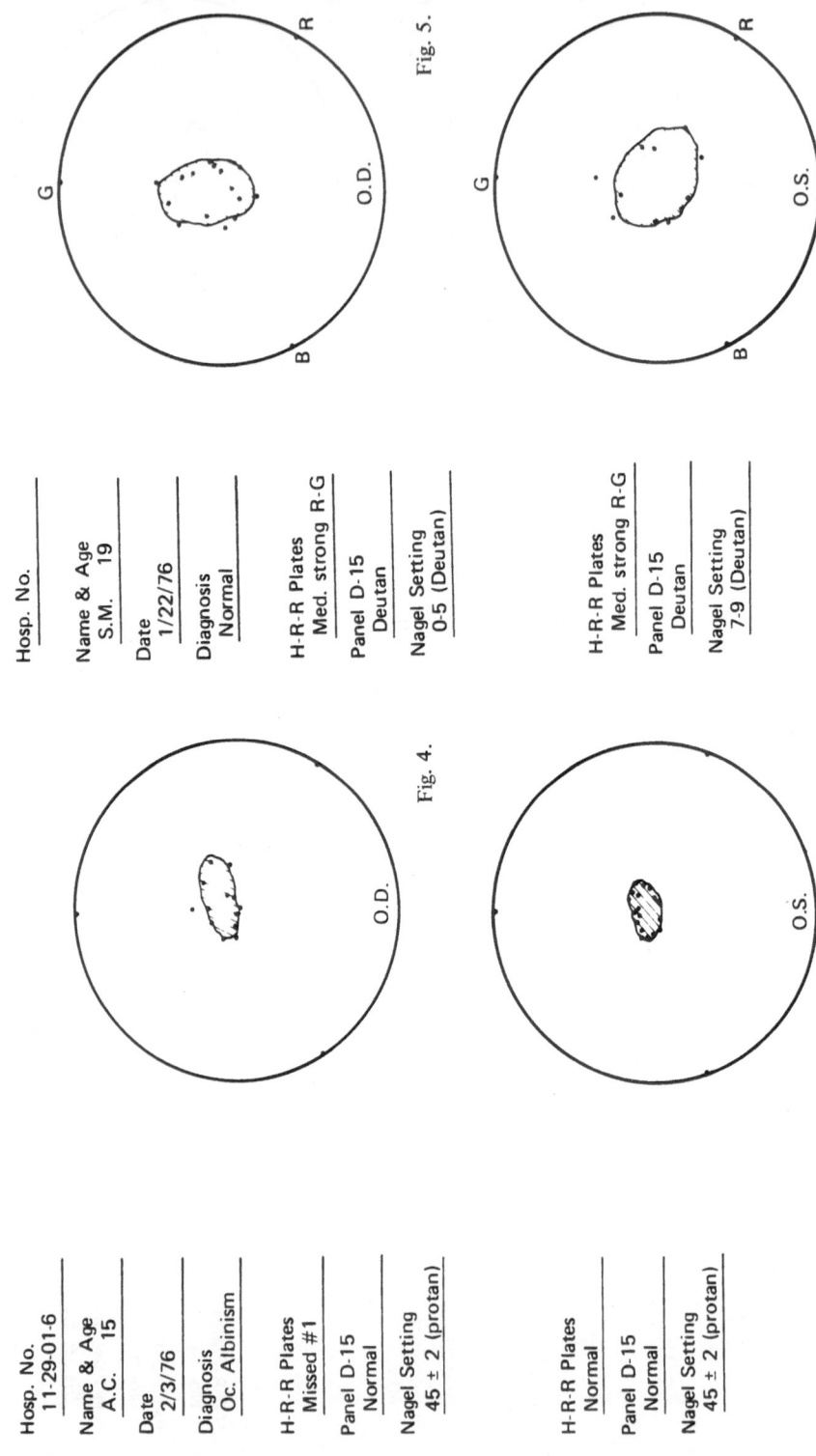

Fig. 5.

Hosp. No.

Name & Age
S.M.   19

Date
1/22/76

Diagnosis
Normal

H-R-R Plates
Med. strong R-G

Panel D-15
Deutan

Nagel Setting
0-5 (Deutan)

H-R-R Plates
Med. strong R-G

Panel D-15
Deutan

Nagel Setting
7-9 (Deutan)

O.D.

O.S.

Fig. 4.

Hosp. No.
11-29-01-6

Name & Age
A.C.   15

Date
2/3/76

Diagnosis
Oc. Albinism

H-R-R Plates
Missed #1

Panel D-15
Normal

Nagel Setting
45 ± 2 (protan)

H-R-R Plates
Normal

Panel D-15
Normal

Nagel Setting
45 ± 2 (protan)

O.D.

O.S.

344

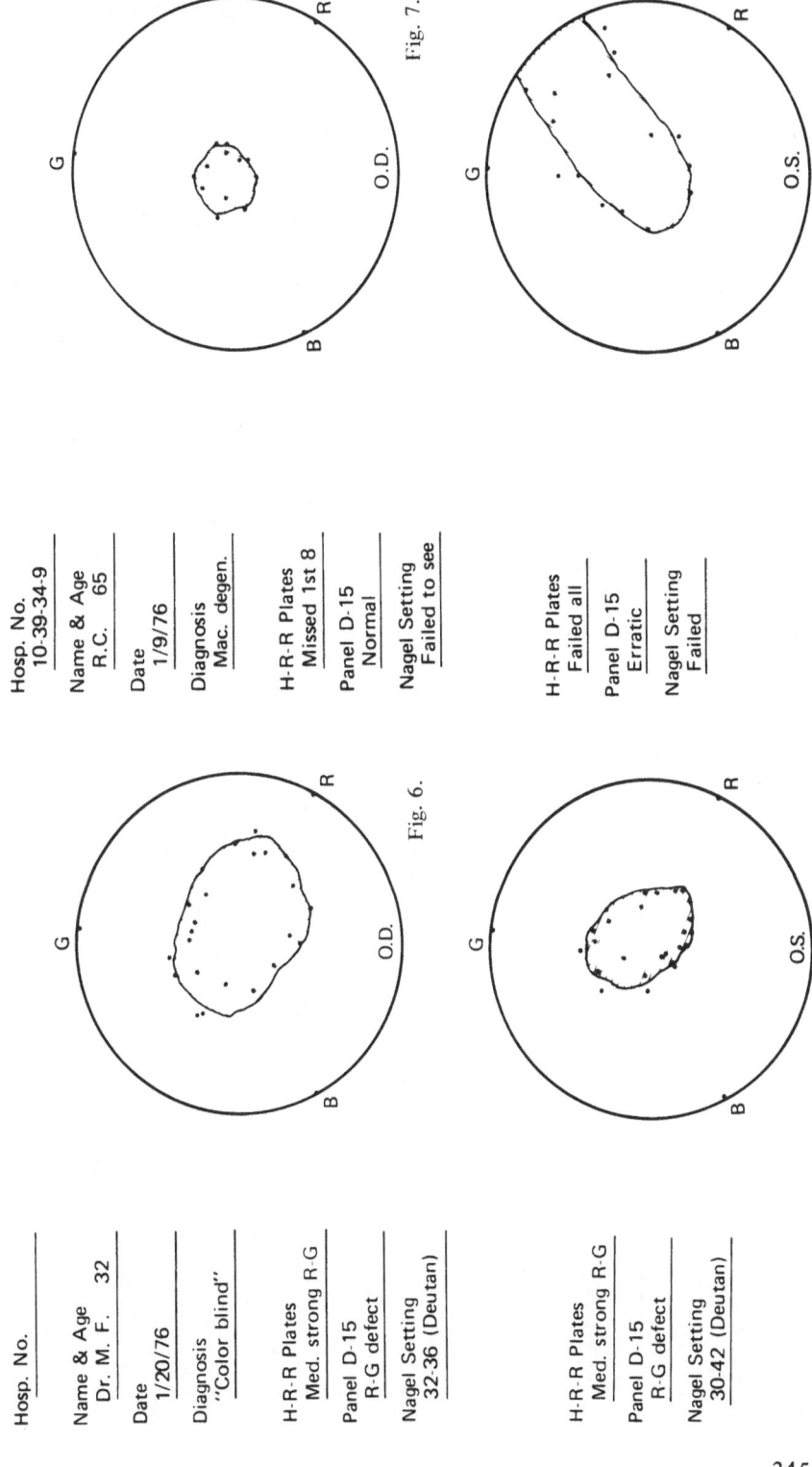

Hosp. No.

Name & Age
Dr. M. F.   32

Date
1/20/76

Diagnosis
"Color blind"

H-R-R Plates
Med. strong R-G

Panel D-15
R-G defect

Nagel Setting
32-36 (Deutan)

O.D.

H-R-R Plates
Med. strong R-G

Panel D-15
R-G defect

Nagel Setting
30-42 (Deutan)

O.S.

Fig. 6.

Hosp. No.
10-39-34-9

Name & Age
R.C.   65

Date
1/9/76

Diagnosis
Mac. degen.

H-R-R Plates
Missed 1st 8

Panel D-15
Normal

Nagel Setting
Failed to see

O.D.

H-R-R Plates
Failed all

Panel D-15
Erratic

Nagel Setting
Failed

O.S.

Fig. 7.

345

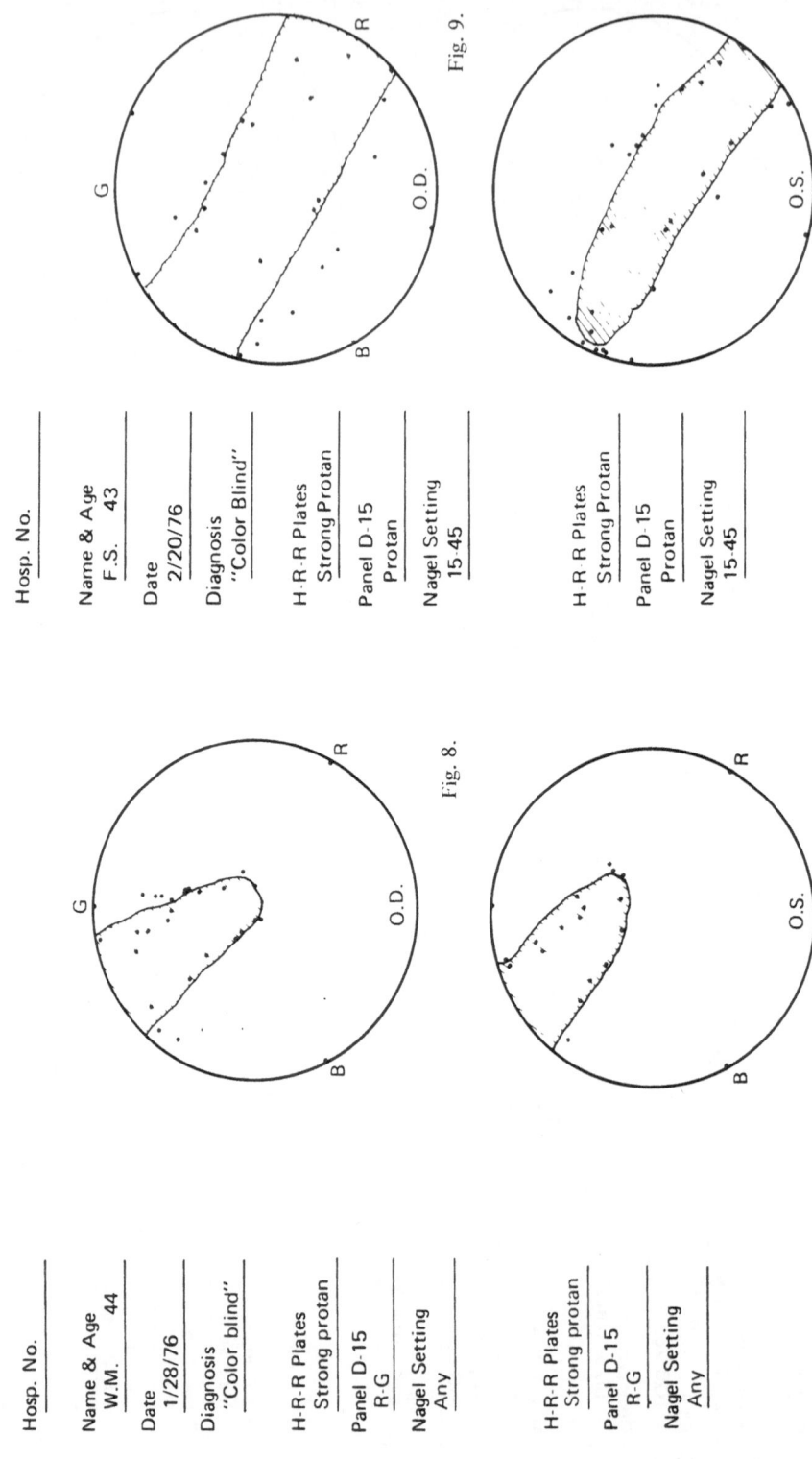

Hosp. No. _____

Name & Age
F.S.   43

Date
2/20/76

Diagnosis
"Color Blind"

H·R·R Plates
Strong Protan

Panel D-15
Protan

Nagel Setting
15-45

H·R·R Plates
Strong Protan

Panel D-15
Protan

Nagel Setting
15-45

Fig. 9.

G   R

O.D.   B

O.S.

Hosp. No. _____

Name & Age
W.M.   44

Date
1/28/76

Diagnosis
"Color blind"

H·R·R Plates
Strong protan

Panel D-15
R·G

Nagel Setting
Any

H·R·R Plates
Strong protan

Panel D-15
R·G

Nagel Setting
Any

Fig. 8.

G   R

O.D.   B

R

O.S.   B

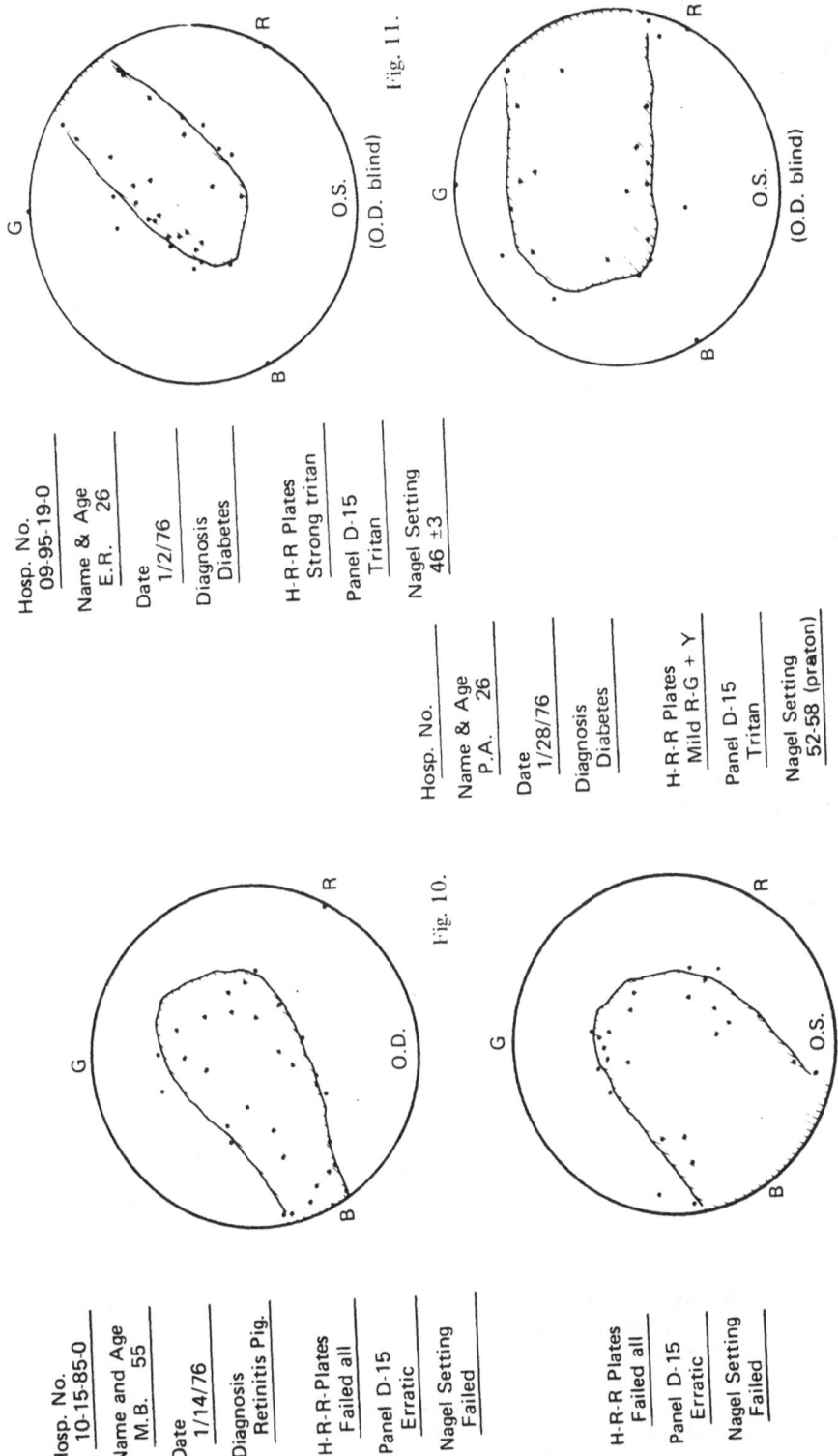

Hosp. No.
09-95-19-0

Name & Age
E.R.   26

Date
1/2/76

Diagnosis
Diabetes

H-R-R Plates
Strong tritan

Panel D-15
Tritan

Nagel Setting
46 ±3

(O.D. blind)

O.S.

Fig. 11.

Hosp. No.

Name & Age
P.A.   26

Date
1/28/76

Diagnosis
Diabetes

H-R-R Plates
Mild R-G + Y

Panel D-15
Tritan

Nagel Setting
52-58 (protan)

(O.D. blind)

O.S.

Fig. 10.

Hosp. No.
10-15-85-0

Name and Age
M.B.   55

Date
1/14/76

Diagnosis
Retinitis Pig.

H-R-R-Plates
Failed all

Panel D-15
Erratic

Nagel Setting
Failed

O.D.

H-R-R Plates
Failed all

Panel D-15
Erratic

Nagel Setting
Failed

O.S.

347

classified as having a medium strong red-green defect by the HRR plates, an indeterminate red-green defect by the Panel D-15, and mild deuteranomaly by the Nagel anomaloscope. It begins to look as if some color defects which have been typed might better be designated as simply poor color discrimination. Figure 7 is from an older man with macular degeneration who missed the first eight HRR plates with his better eye, arranged the Panel D-15 correctly and could not find the test spot in the Nagel anomaloscope. His left eye being much worse, failed all three conventional color tests, but clearly shows a yellow defect on the chromagram. Figure 8 shows results on a man who was considered normal except for his 'color blindness.' According to the HRR plates he had a strong protanomaly; the Panel D-15 could not distinguish between protanomaly and deuteranomaly, and the anomaloscope matched anywhere on the scale. His deficiency appears to lie entirely in the blue-green sector. This man (Fig. 9) is classified as protanomalous with the HRR plates, and Panel D-15, indeterminate with the Nagel anomaloscope, and shows a wide neutral band extending from the blue-green to the red where he sees no color at any saturation level. This patient (Fig. 10) has retinitis pigmentosa in an advanced stage and was unable to respond to the usual tests. However, he could see and name most of the more saturated colors except for blue, where he shows a large neutral area.

Figure 11 shows the left eyes of two young diabetics who showed tritanomaly with the Panel D-15 and one of them was definitely tritanomalous with the HRR plates. Both made protanomalous settings on the anomaloscope and both had large neutral areas mainly in the yellow and orange region.

As you can see, this system appears to answer some of our most troublesome questions, but it poses others which may also be interesting.

REFERENCES

Armington, J.C. & Biersdorf, W.R. Color vision, *Ann. Rev. of Psychol.* 14, *93-114*, (1963).

Burnham, R.W. A colorimeter for research in color perception. *Am. J. Psychol.* 65, *603-608* (1952).

Dain, S.J. The lovibond color vision analyzer. (Defic. II) Int. Symp. Edinburgh, (1973). *Mod. Probl. Ophthalmol.* 13, *79-82* (Karger, Basel, 1974) (1973).

Fishman, G. Techniques, merits and limitations of basic tests for color defects. *Surv. Ophthalmol.* 15, *370-373* (1971).

Geddie, J.C. An inexpensive additive tricolor mixer capable of continuous variations in hue and saturation. *Psychophysiology* 11, No. 3, 388-390 (1974).

Linksz, A. Color vision tests in clinical practice. *Trans. Am. Acad. Ophthalmol. Otolaryngol.* 75, *1078-1080* (1971).

Neubauer, O. Comparing methods of examination in acquired color vision deficiencies. *Mod. Probl. Ophthalmol.* 11, *19-21* (1972).

Sloan, L.L. & Wollach, L. Comparison of tests for red-green color deficiency. *J. Aviation Med.* 19, *447-455* (1948).

Wright, W.D. The measurement of Color, Adam Hilger Ltd., London (1968).

Authors' address: Dept of Health, Education and Welfare
National Eye Institute   Bethesda, Md 20014
                           USA

UNSEDATED CORNEAL ELECTRORETINOGRAMS FROM CHILDREN

MICHAEL F. MARMOR

(Stanford, California)

ABSTRACT

General anesthesia or sedation has often been used for recording corneal electroretinograms (ERG's) on children. For this reason, testing is sometimes deferred or less accurate recording methods are used. To avoid these problems, routine contact-lens ERG's were attempted on 40 consecutively referred children (aged 2 months to 6 years) using topical anesthesia only. Mild restraint was occasionally needed, but satisfactory oscilloscopic records were obtained from all children tested. The records were less stable than those from adults, but the response amplitude, the waveform and the timing could always be evaluated, and the cone and rod systems could be clearly differentiated. Thus, ERG's may be obtained routinely on most children without systemic medication or special techniques.

INTRODUCTION

The electroretinogram (ERG) is an important diagnostic test for evaluating retinal and visual dysfunction in children, but many ERG laboratories seem wary of performing unsedated contact-lens recordings on young children. Furthermore, many ophthalmologists are reluctant to refer children for an ERG because of fear that anesthesia or sedation (cf. Krill, 1972; Ogden & Van Dyk, 1973; Frens & Horsten, 1975) would be necessary to perform the test or that the method of testing (cf. Ogden & Van Dijk, 1973; Frens & Horsten, 1975; Harden, 1974) would compromise the results.

I have been attempting routine contact-lens ERG's with topical anesthesia only on consecutive pediatric ERG referrals (Marmor, 1976). My results suggest that with appropriate care, and with no special equipment or protocols (beyond child-size lenses), one may reliably obtain unsedated oscilloscopic cone and rod ERG's on children of all ages.

METHODS

The recording equipment and protocols normally used for adults were used for children, and have been described in more detail elsewhere (Marmor, 1976).

A full-field (Ganzfeld) stimulator (Berson, Gouras & Gunkel, 1968) incorporating a Grass flash lamp (Figure 1) was used routinely, either upright or hung over a supine patient. The flash lamp could be removed and hand-held for the rare hyperactive child who might be injured by the dome.

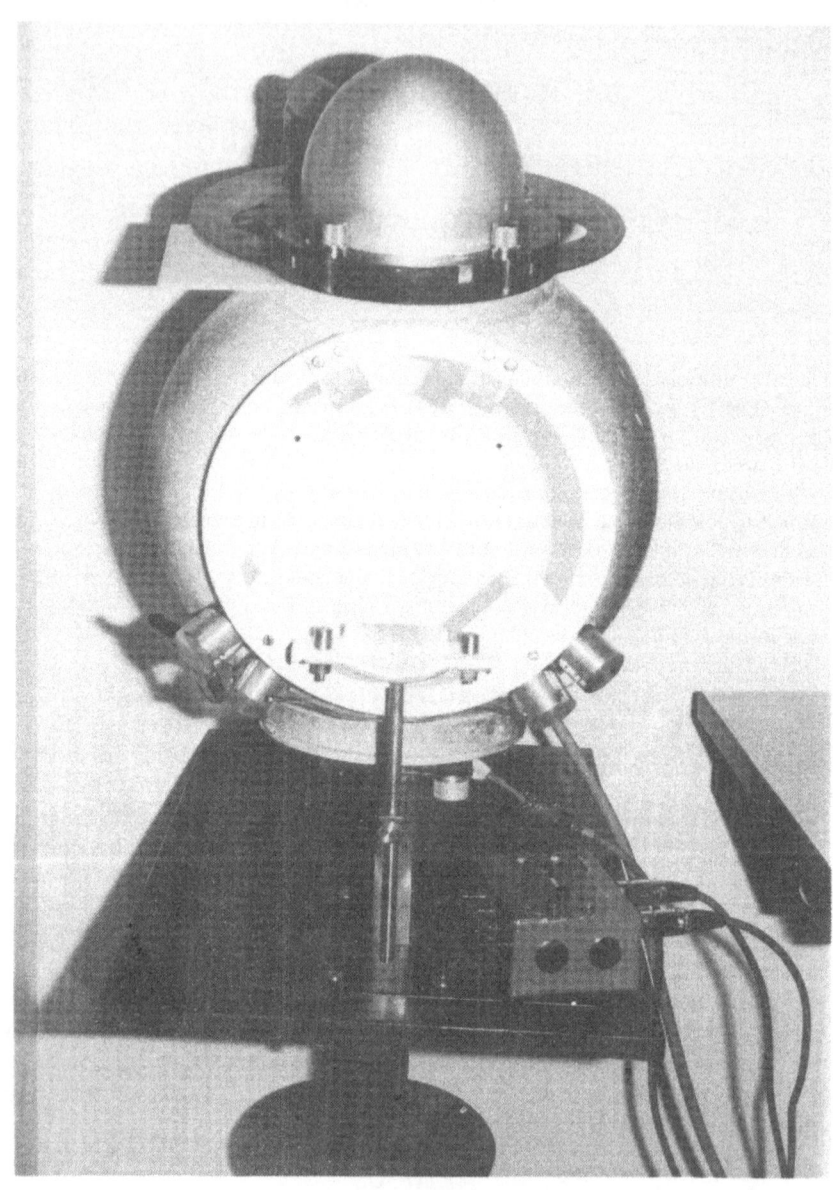

Fig. 1. Full-field stimulator. The flash-lamp is held by a retaining ring, and overlies a rotating filter plate and a plastic diffuser. Fixation lights are inside the dome to serve both ERG's and EOG's. The background lights are hidden by baffles. A connector box on the table contains fuses.

Both eyes were dilated, and bipolar Burian-Allen contact-lens electrodes (Lawwill & Burian, 1966) of the appropriate pediatric size were used. Topical anesthesia was obtained with 0.5% proparacaine. The bipolar signals were fed without pre-amplification into a differential oscilloscope amplifier (Tektronix 5A22) with 1 MΩ input impedance and 100,000:1 common mode rejection. The signals were displayed on a storage oscilloscope and photographed.

The recording protocol was designed to separate cone and rod responses (Berson, Gouras & Gunkel, 1968; Brunette, 1973; Marmor, 1976). Cone function was isolated by a 15 foot-lambert background, or by 30 Hz flicker. After 10-15 minutes dark adaptation, a weak white flash produced a predominantly rod response, and a flash 2 log units brighter (W-8) produced a typical mixed response.

Referrals were not selected in any way. Parents were encouraged to participate and help restrain younger children who were fearful of strangers. Most youngsters were tested upright in front of the stimulator, often using a parent's lap for security or height. Restraint was used primarily during lens insertion, to prevent the child from pulling out the electrode. Thereafter, gentle restriction (or none at all) usually sufficed, since the lens was not painful (Figure 2). The contact lens was chosen on the small side since difficulty with insertion was the greatest problem. Usually only one eye was tested at a time.

At least two flashes (roughly 10 seconds apart) were given under each

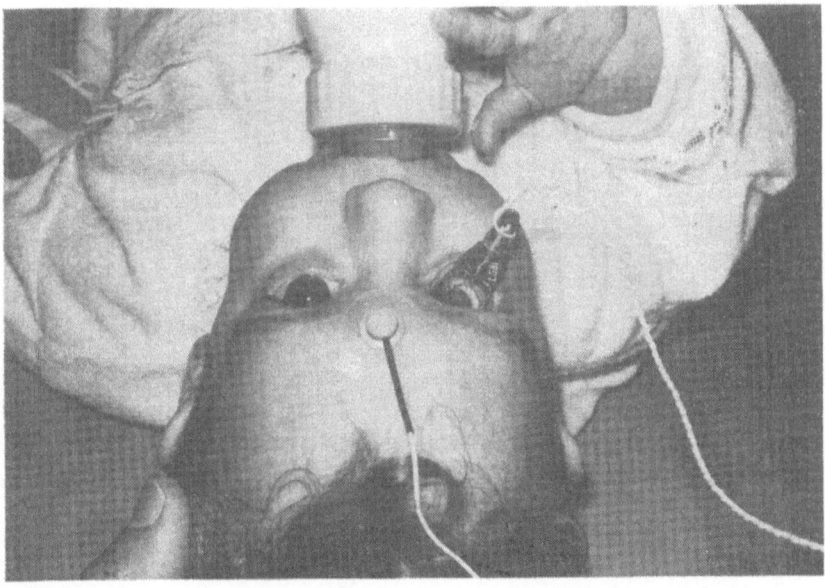

Fig. 2.   An unsedated 5-month-old infant, with a contact lens electrode in place. The child was comfortable, and required little restraint, until the bottle ran out.

stimulus condition. The responses were retained for comparison on the storage oscilloscope, and were accepted and photographed only after two similar and identifiable signals were obtained. Dark adaptation was sometimes abbreviated if the signals were adequate to answer the clinical questions.

Table 1. Diagnostic Classification of the Children Tested.

Diagnosis	Number of Patients
Normal	4
Tapetoretinal dystrophy	9
Macular Disease	4
Achromatopsia	5
Optic Nerve and CNS Disease	14
Miscellaneous	4

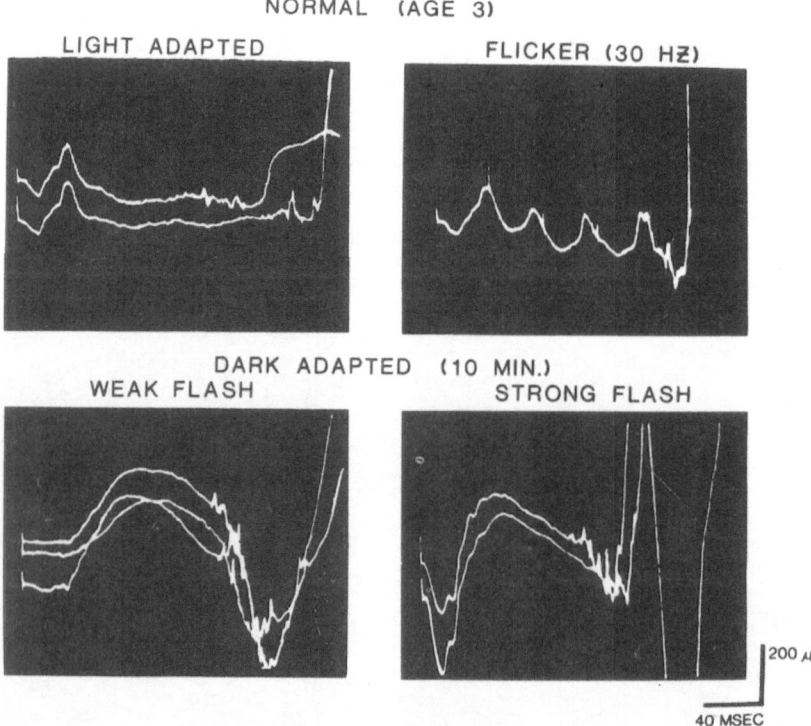

Fig. 3. ERG from a normal 3-year-old child. Each picture shows two or more flashes from the same eye to demonstrate reproducibility. Cone and rod signals can easily be recognized. (After Marmor, 1976).

RESULTS

This report only concerns children aged 6 and under, since older children will usually cooperate. ERG's were attempted, using topical anesthesia only, on 40 consecutive referrals aged 2 months to 6 years (15 patients less than 2 years, 25 patients between 2 and 6 years). None received systemic medication except one 3-year-old boy who had been given a Nembutal suppository prior to arrival (but did not appear very sedate). The children displayed a broad spectrum of visual disability, ocular disease (see Table 1) and behavioral cooperation (or lack thereof).

Recording was successful on the first attempt with all children except one 6-year-old girl who required a second visit. There were no ocular injuries or side effects from the tests, and no complaints of untoward psychological effects. The chilren younger than 2 needed continuous, but rarely severe,

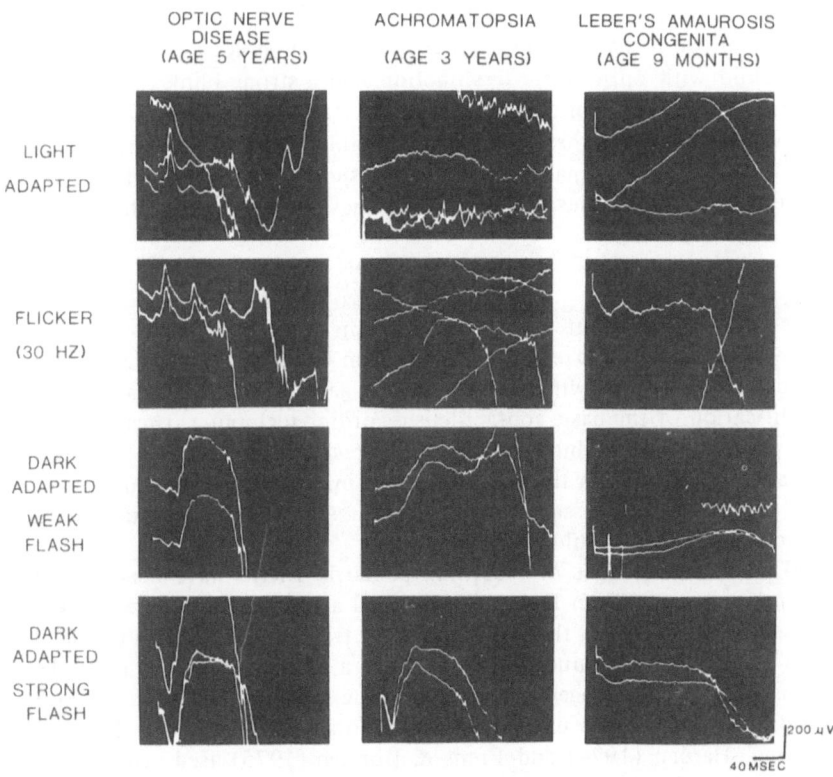

Fig. 4. ERG's from three unsedated children with clinically poor vision. Each picture shows two or more flashes from the same eye. Ragged baselines and artifactual responses have not been retouched. The first column shows an essentially normal ERG. The second column shows absent cone responses. The third column shows only a minimal signal to the strongest stimuli. (After Marmor, 1976).

restraint. Youngsters older than 2 often required hand restraint during placement of the lens. A miraculous calm usually followed, as the child realized that the lens did not hurt; and most cooperated voluntarily for the rest of the procedure. No special personnel were required for testing children, but patience was definitely an asset. The best sedatives for the children were a warm bottle (Figure 2), a warm parent, a favorite toy, and a promise of ice cream.

Eye movement was the greatest source of artifacts. These were minimized by storing successive responses on the oscilloscope screen until recognizable and reproducible waveforms were obtained. Figure 3 shows responses from a normal and cooperative 3-year-old to demonstrate the high quality of recording that was frequently possible. Youngsters who were more restless, of course, produced more artifacts on the screen but recognition of these posed no problem and did not prevent accurate reading of the ERG.

Figure 4 shows representative ERG's from children with three categories of disease. These records were purposely chosen from among the less cooperative patients because these tracings — rather than more perfect ones — must prove to be of clinical value if this methodology is to be accepted. The child with optic nerve dysfunction had a strong blink reflex, but the characteristics of a normal ERG are still clearly discernible. The achromat showed no cone responses but had reasonable dark adapted responses. The child with Leber's amaurosis congenita showed only minimal responses under any condition, despite the irregularities on the photographs.

DISCUSSION

This study demonstrates that oscilloscopic ERG's showing satisfactory waveform, timing, and cone/rod separation can be obtained reliably from children of all ages, without sedation or general anesthesia, and without modification of the basic contact-lens recording technique. These ERG's are not perfect quality — but artifacts can be recognized easily, and the records are adequate to obtain the needed clinical information. Some mild physical restraint is often necessary, but this requires no special preparation and is not damaging to the child.

Two other methods of recording pediatric ERG's have been described recently. Ogden & Van Dyk (1973) placed a fine platinum wire under the closed lid and recorded the ERG from light transmitted through the lid. The wire electrode is less uncomfortable than a contact lens, but multiple responses must be averaged (which limits the range of photopic or scotopic conditions than can be used) and the authors recommend that the child be sedated. Harden (1974) and Frens & Horsten (1975) used skin electrodes only and performed the test without any sedation or eye drops. However, averaging was again needed. These methods have their advantages, but they both require special technology (e.g. an averager) and they do not provide the same range or quality of cone and rod signals that can be obtained using the method described here.

Special equipment is not required for pediatric ERG's (except for pediatric size contact-lens electrodes), but certain items are particulary helpful. A storage oscilloscope is the most critical item since restlessness and eye movements invariably cause artifacts. These can be examined on the storage screen, and many can be erased before making a permanent record. An oscilloscope, as opposed to a paper recorder, is important if accurate measurements of waveform and timing are desired. A full-field stimulator greatly reduces artifacts from poor fixation (Berson, Gouras & Gunkel, 1968). The use of bipolar electrodes (Lawwill & Burian, 1966) and differential recording through amplifiers with high common mode rejection minimizes the need for special shielding.

If uncompromised ERG records can be obtained from children, without the risks, drug effects and cost of anesthesia, then pediatric ERG's may become more easily available and more widely utilized.

REFERENCES

Berson, E.L., Gouras, P. & Gunkel, R.D.: Rod responses in retinitis pigmentosa, dominantly inherited. *Arch. Ophth.* 80, *58-67*, (1968).

Brunette, J.R.: A standardizable method for separating rod and cone responses in clinical electroretinography. *Am. J. Opth.* 75, *833-845*, (1973).

Frens, A.M. and Horsten, G.P.M.: Letter to the editors. *Vision Research.* 15, *455,* (1975).

Harden, A.: Non-corneal electroretinogram. *Brit. J. Ophthal.* 58, *811-816,* (1974).

Krill, A.E.: Hereditary Retinal and Choroidal Diseases. Vol. I. Evaluation. Hagerstown: Harper & Row, 1972, p. 249.

Lawwill, T. & Burian, H.M.: A modification of the Burian-Allen contact-lens electrode for human electroretinography. *Am. J. Ophth.* 61, *1506-1509,* (1966).

Marmor, M.F.: Corneal electroretinograms in children without sedation. *J. Ped. Ophthal.* 13, *112-118,* (1976).

Ogden, T.E. & Van Dyk, H.J.L.: A technique for ERG recording in infants and young children. *Vision Research.* 14, *305,* (1973).

Authors' address:
Ophthalmology Section
Veterane Administration Hospital
Palo Alto, Cal. 94304
USA

EVALUATION OF MICROELECTRODES CHRONICALLY
IMPLANTED ON THE RETINA

WILLIAM W. DAWSON & NORMAN D. RADTKE

(Gainesville, Florida)

The methods available for the recording of both gross and unitary action potentials from the mammalian retina have been improved significantly in recent years (Werblin & Dowling, 1969; Dawson, Zimmerman & Houde, 1974). Both identification of cells producing unitary responses and safety of contact lenses have been improved. However, unit recording methods still require extensive surgery with anesthesia and/or neuromuscular blocking. Unit recording durations are limited under these circumstances (Rodieck, 1967; Kuffler, 1953). Corneal contact lenses provide the opportunity of recording potentials from unanesthetized animals and humans but such lenses may not be left in place indefinitely while their replacement on subsequent days may contribute to data variability (Lawwill, 1969). Experimentation with chronic electrode implantations upon the retinal surface has probably been impeded by the well known toxic response of the eye to foreign materials.

This report describes our experience with the consequences of the implantation of multiple microelectrodes upon the surface of the retina over a six month period.

SUBJECTS AND MATERIALS

Electrodes were fabricated from wires of 25 micron diameter quadruple insulated with enamel. The wires were of nickel-chromium alloy and were purchased from the Wilbur B. Driver Company (lot number 240231380) and had a resistance of 572 ohms/foot. The electrodes were uninsulated only at the tips and were bundled together in 8 centimeter lengths. The ends were free at one end of the bundle forming a 'mop-like' array. One array of six electrodes and a second array of nine electrodes was implanted on the surface of two cat retinas. One cat was surgically implanted in October, 1975, and the second in November, 1975. The details of the implantation, electrode placement and exteriorization are described in figure 1.

Adult cats were used. Under deep sodium pentobarbital anesthesia the lateral aspect of the left eye orbital area was dissected. The temporal portion of the globe was exposed with a 2 mm scleral incision at the level of the pars plana. Avoiding the lens, the 'mop' electrode was introduced through the scleral opening and passed through the vitreous so that the electrode tips

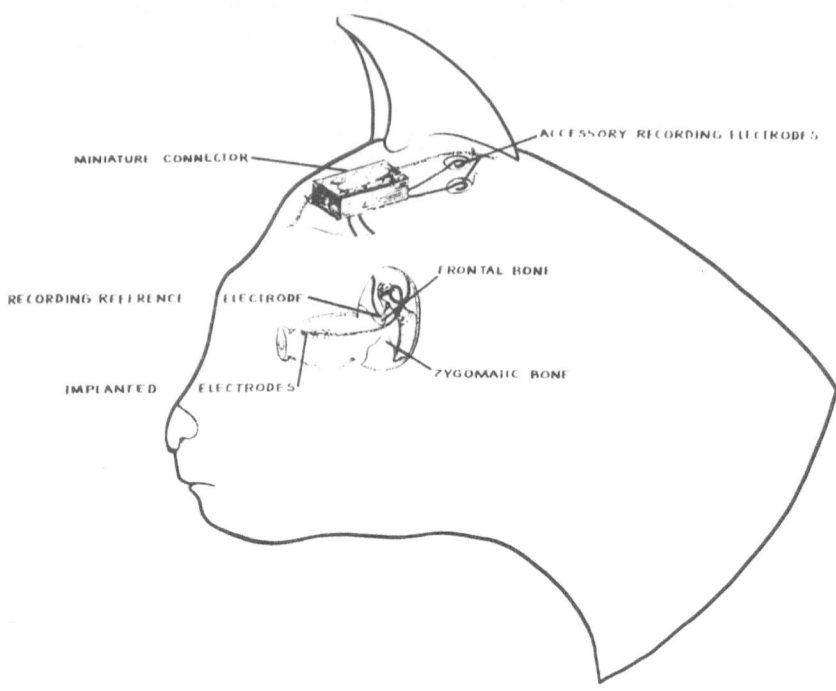

Fig. 1. (Dawson, Radtke) Diagram of electrode implant. Accessory electrodes are on the surface of the visual area.

rested upon the surface of the retina. The bundle was sutured externally to the sclera and carried to the rear to exit from the orbit just above the zygomatic bone. A reference electrode was attached by a stainless steel screw to the bone at the rear of the orbit. The electrode cable was then passed subcutaneously to the dorsal aspect of the cranium and connected to pins of a miniature integrated circuit connecter. A ground lead was also attached from the cranium to a connecter pin as were two accessory electrodes which were placed upon the surface of the visual area following reflection of the dura. The cranium was covered by a thin layer of methyl methacrylate which also served to firmly attach the miniature connecter. The skin incisions were then closed with silk. Sterile procedure was observed.

Recovery of the two animals was uneventful except for the development of a small area, exposure keratitis in the October animal. With topical, steroid and antibiotic treatment the keratitis disappeared within a period of a few weeks. The external appearance of the eye and the fundus was followed for six months. By the end of four weeks a fine grey membrane appeared to form on the surface of the retina adjacent to the region of the electrode contacts. The area included under the electrodes was approximately three disc diameters toward the temporal retinal aspect. Local hemorrhages were visible under four of the electrodes in animal #2 (November implant) but cleared in one week. The electrode tips in animal #1 could not be clearly visualized at their place of contact with the retina because of the far temporal placement. Externally, the eyes appeared normal and after a few weeks, appeared to have full movement capability. Pupillary responses were normal. Since no indications of toxic response or gross abnormality could be seen at the end of two months, electrophysiological measures (electroretinograms) were begun on a routine basis. Retinal potentials were measured simultaneously from implanted electrodes and from a corneal contact electrode. The reference electrode for the contact lens was placed on the skin above the orbit and was attached with EEG electrode paste. Measures were made every two weeks from December until late April. For the first four months the animals were given 10 mg of Thorazine, I.M., to reduce struggling during the test procedure which was carried out in a commercially constructed animal restraining box. After mid-March the Thorazine was discontinued and measures were made without any medication. During testing, the restraining box with the animals head free was placed in the center of a 60° ganzfeld whose surface luminance was −1.5 log fL. Above and behind the animal's head a Grass PS2 xenon flash lamp, with

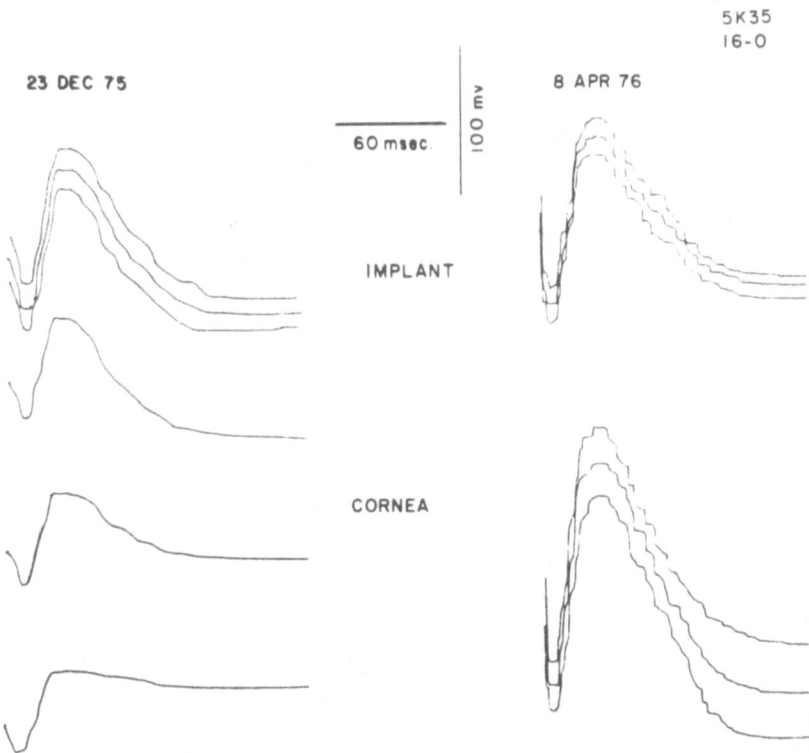

Fig. 2. (Dawson, Radtke) Averaged ERG's from corneal and implanted electrode (no. 6) measured in December and four months later. Scale is in milliseconds and microvolts. Signals are in sets of three. Central signal of each set is mean and others are ± 1 sd. Maximum flash intensity.

diffusing lens, served to illuminate the ganzfeld for the production of ERG potentials. The flash lamp intensity was set at maximum and was further attenuated with neural density filters. All signals were amplified (bandpass 3 db points, 0.02 - 1 KHz) and processed for average and variance calculation by a general purpose computer. Data was stored on discs and retrieved later for write out and computations. All signals are the average of twenty stimulations delivered at a rate of 1 per 20 seconds. Data will be presented on animal #1 (October implant). Results from animal #2 (November implant) were similar.

RESULTS

Averaged electroretinograms and variance (± 1 standard deviation) recorded in December and the subsequent April are presented in figure 2. Signals are presented in sets of three. The mid-signal of each is the mean. Those on either side are ± 1 sd. Figure 2 shows that the standard deviation of the corneal signals measured in December exceed the amplitude of the mean measured peak to peak. The variance of these signals from the corneal electrodes was reduced in the April measures but still remained larger than the variance from the implanted electrodes.

ERG b-wave amplitude (measured from a-wave to b-wave peak) was related to stimulus intensity. Figure 3 provides a comparison of b-wave amplitudes over a 5 log unit range of stimulus intensities. Both corneal and intraocular electrode (#6) results are shown. Measures of signals from both electrode sites were made in December and four months later. For clarity, the intraocular electrode signals are presented below the x axis. Signals derived from the intraocular electrodes in December were of larger amplitude than from the corneal electrodes. This situation is reversed in April. However, the overall change was less in the intraocular electrodes. Signals derived from the corneal electrodes exhibited more variance in December and in April then did the recordings from the implanted sites (Fig. 4). Although there was a noticeable decrease in variance of the corneal signal during the measures taken in April, it was still almost five times as great as the variance from the implanted electrodes. An overview of variance results at any recording session seems to offer no link between stimulus intensity and variance magnitude.

Electroretinograms were measured from corneal lenses placed upon the control and implanted eyes in late April 1976. These showed no difference in amplitude, waveform or size of standard deviation values. Recordings of spike potentials (probably of ganglion cell origin) were made over a period of two days in March 1976, five months after electrode implantation. These recordings showed the presence of three or fewer fibers isolated from the background. Spike potential discharges up to 300 uv in amplitude were recorded in response to the movement of light bars in the temporal region of the field. The unit potentials were recorded with frequencies below 100 Hz rejected. Implanted electrodes #3 and #4 showed this potential type.

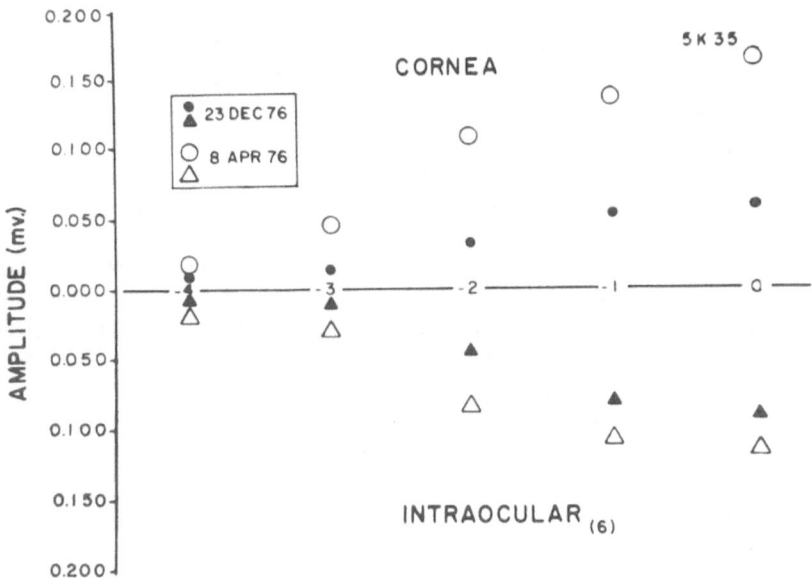

Fig. 3. (Dawson, Radtke) ERG b-wave amplitudes recorded in December and four months later from corneal and retinal electrode (no. 6). Amplitudes are in millivolts. X-axis scale is in log relative intensity. All signals are positive.

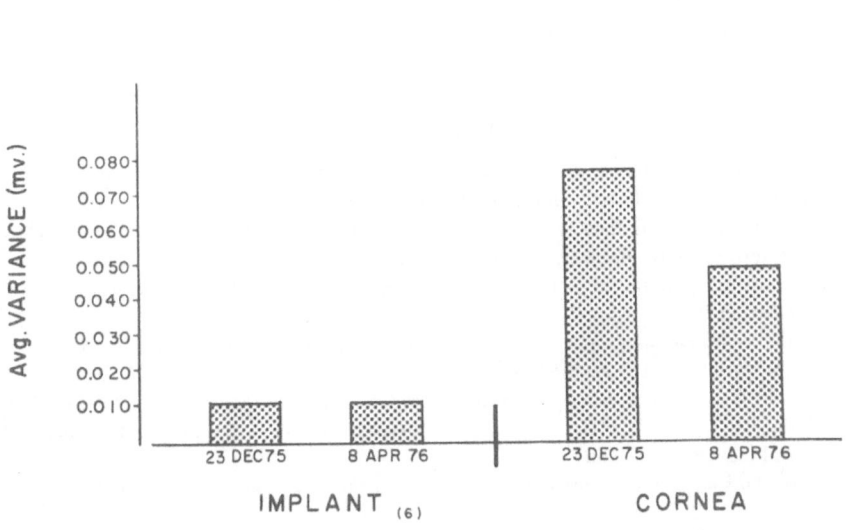

Fig. 4. (Dawson, Radtke) Variance of b-wave measured as ± 1 sd from two electrode sites in December and four months later. Implanted electrode was no. 6.

DISCUSSION

All of the electrodes implanted in either October or November 1975 continue to record gross or spike, action potentials from the retina after seven months, Thorough analysis of the spike potentials has not been attempted since the initial design considered only retinal toxicity and its implications. If a toxic response were present it would be expected to result in a sharply reduced electroretinogram amplitude (Karpe, 1957). In fact, there is evidence from Figure 3 that response amplitudes grew over a period of four months of testing. This growth was not gradual. From December until March 10, 1976, the average corneal electrode b-wave amplitude did not exceed 50 uv when the maximum stimulus intensity was delivered. After March 10, the tranquilizer medication was discontinued. Subsequent average b-wave amplitudes ranged from 85 to 100 uv.

Examination of the eyes of both animals, six months after implantation continues to show the presence of a localized fibrous membrane slightly larger than the area covered by the 'mop' electrode array. Uninformed visitors are unable to detect which eye received the implant in either animal when allowed to judge only external appearance and eye mobility.

SUMMARY

Multiple microelectrodes were implanted upon the retinal surface of two cats and followed over a six month period. There have been no signs of general eye toxicity. The eyes remain clear and mobile. All implanted electrodes record gross and/or unit retinal potentials. Measures of electroretinogram response over the six month period indicate that signals derived from the cornea with contact electrodes are of higher variability then those derived from indwelling intraocular electrodes. Discontinuation of the use of Thorazine as a tranquilizing medication caused a 100% increase in the amplitude of the corneally derived signal and a smaller increase in signals from the microelectrode.

REFERENCES

Werblin, F. & Dowling, J. Organization of the retina of the mudpuppy, Necturus maculosus: II. Intracellular staining. *J. Neurophysiol.*, 32, *339*, (1969).

Dawson, W., Zimmerman, T. & Houde, W.: A method for more comfortable electroretinography. *Arch. Ophthalmol.* 91, *1*, (1974).

Rodieck, R.: Maintained activity of cat retinal ganglion cells. *J. Neurophysiol.*, 30, *1043*, (1967).

Kuffler, S.W. Discharge patterns and functional organization of mammalian retina. *J. Neurophysiol.*, 16, *37*, (1953).

Lawwill, T.: Practical rabbit electroretinography. *Amer. J. Ophthal.*, 74, *135*, (1972).

Walsh, F.B. & Hoyt, F.H.: Clinical Neuro-Ophthalmology, Baltimore, Williams and Wilkins, 1969, p. 2560.

Karpe, G. Das Elektroretinogramm bei siderosis. *Bibl. Ophthal.*, 48, *182*, (1957).

Authors' address:
Dept of Ophthalmology, Box J 285   Gainesville, Florida 32610
JHM Health Centre   USA

RETINAL ACTION POTENTIAL OF RABBITS RECORDED
BY A PAIR OF ELECTRODES ON THE SCLERA

Y. HONDA & E. ADACHI-USAMI

(Kyoto/Hamamatsu)

INTRODUCTION

The electroretinogram (ERG) is routinely recorded through a pair of electrodes; an active electrode on the cornea and a reference electrode on tissue bio-electrically near the sclera (forehead, chin, orbital margin...). Based on this recording system, a normal pattern of clinical ERGs has been established (Standardization Committees of ISCERG, 1962). However, the horizontal distribution of the receptor cells in the retina is not uniform, and the retina is attached to the posterior wall of the eyeball. The 'normal' pattern can be said to be temporarily established in this situational relationship between the electrodes and the eyeball (Noonan, Wilkus, Chatrian & Lettich, 1973).

In this study, a pair of electrodes was freely moved on the sclera, unlike the routine electrode-position of the ERG; and the mass action potential of the retina *in situ* was recorded.

METHODS

Albino rabbits weighing 3.5 kgs. were used. Under general anesthesia with urethane (1.0 g/kg body weight into the abdominal cavity), the upper and lower lids, the conjuctiva and other surrounding tissue were removed. The skull was partially cut off at the orbital margin. A pair of stainless steel electrodes (0.25 mm in diameter) was held by microelectrode-manipulators (Narishige Instrument Lab.), and was placed on the sclera. The position of the electrodes was measured by the distance in longitude directly measured from the corneal limbus (0 mm) (negative distance to the corneal center, positive distance to the optic nerve). The electrode on the nasal side was connected to an active input (positive) of the amplifying system. In Fig. 2, the electrode near the corneal limbus was connected to the active input. The positivity of the active electrode was recorded as an upward deflection. Responses were written about 10 times on the oscilloscope by Dawson's superimposition technique (1954). The time constant of the amplifying system was 0.003, 0.01 and 0.3 sec.

A diffuse white light of xenon discharge was used as the stimulus. The discharged energy was 0.6 joules, and the distance between the light source and the eye was 30 cm. The frequency of the stimulus was set at 1 f/sec throughout the experiments. The duration of the stimulus was about

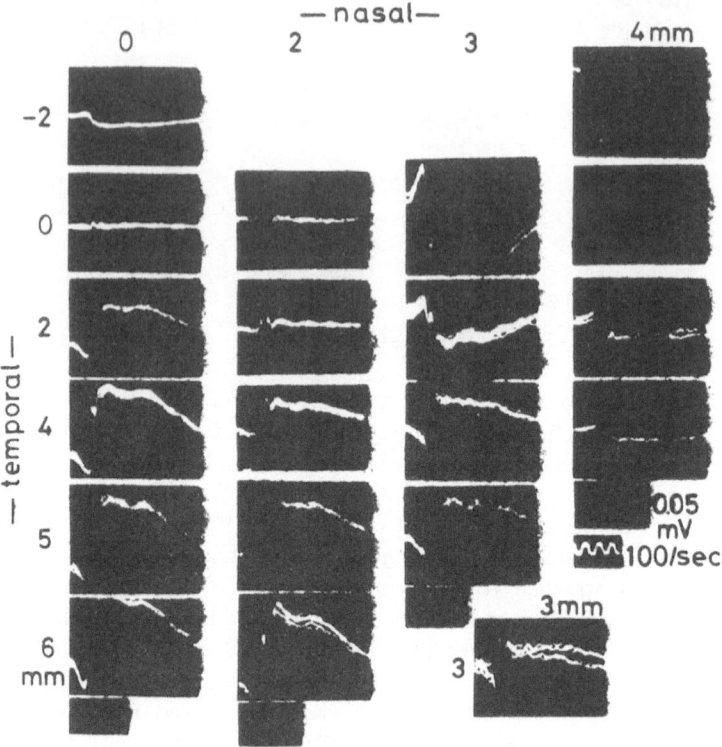

Fig. 1. Two electrodes are moved on the sclera. The positive electrode is moved from the corneal limbus to the optic nerve on the longitudinal line of the nasal side and the other (negative) electrode is moved on the longitudinal line of the temporal side. The position of the electrodes is shown by the distance from the corneal limbus (negative to the corneal center, positive to the optic nerve). The calibration marks on the bottom of the columns indicate 0.05 mV. The time constant of the amplifying system is 0.3 sec.

10 microsec. The pupil of the stimulated eye was dilated to the maximum by a mydriatic. The non-stimulated eye was shielded from the stimulus light by a black eye-patch, but was not enucleated. Before the beginning of the experiments, the eye was dark-adapted for 30 minutes with intermittent flashes of xenon light.

RESULTS AND DISCUSSION

Light-evoked responses were recorded between the electrode on the nasal side (n) and the electrode on the temporal side (t) (Fig. 1). The electrodes were attached onto the sclera at points along the same longitudinal line on the nasal and temporal sides. Responses between nO-t2, t4, t5, t6, and n2-t5, t6,

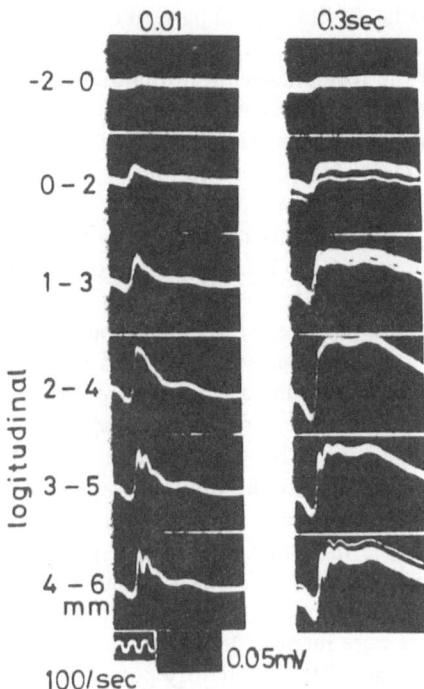

Fig. 2. A pair of electrodes are moved along a longitudinal line keeping a constant distance (2 mm) between them longitudinally. Two kinds of time constants are employed: 0.01 sec in the left column and 0.3 sec in the right column. The position of the electrodes is shown by the distance from the corneal limbus on the left side of the recordings.

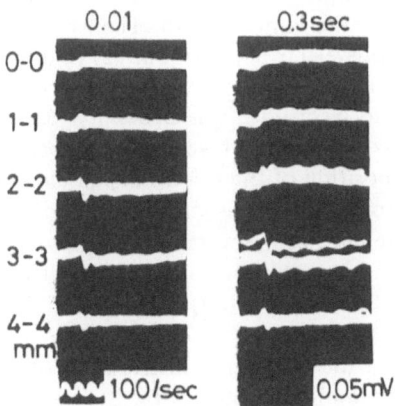

Fig. 3. The electrodes are moved keeping a constant distance (2 mm) between them in parallel with the corneal limbus (crossing the longitudinal line). The position of the electrodes is shown by the distance from the corneal limbus on the left side of the recordings.

365

and n3-t5 were similar to the normal pattern of clinical ERGs. On the other hand, responses between n3-tO, t2, t4, and n4- t-2, tO seemed to be the inverted pattern of the former. An interesting finding in this experiment was that oscillatory potentials appeared to be isolated from the a- and the b-wave of the ERG when the meridional depth of the two electrodes was almost equal (nO-tO, n2-tO, t2,, n3-t3,, n4-t4, t5). When responses in the same column are compared, the wave form changes as follows: The a-wave is positive and the b-wave is negative when the temporal electrode is near the corneal center. The a- and the b-waves decrease in amplitude, isolating the oscillatory potentials, as the temporal electrode approaches the same meridional depth as the nasal one. When the temporal electrode is moved further toward the optic nerve, the b-wave is inverted to positive.

In Fig. 2, a pair of electrodes was moved from the corneal limbus to the optic nerve keeping a constant distance between the electrodes (2 mm) along the longitudinal line. The b-wave and the oscillatory potentials recorded by electrodes closer to the optic nerve were more prominent than those recorded by electrodes near the corneal limbus. In Fig. 3, the distance between electrodes was the same as in Fig. 2 (2 mm), but the electrodes were separated parallel with the corneal limbus (crossing the longitudinal line). In this recording system, the b-wave amplitude was quite small but the oscillatory potentials were recordable.

In Fig. 4, the change of the oscillatory potentials in the longitudinal line is shown by the recordings using high gain and a shorter time constant. The early phase of ERGs (mainly a-wave) seemed to be inverted similar to that shown for the b-wave. But the polarity of each peak of oscillations was not simply reversed. The peak times moved and some peaks seemed to be masked as humps on the ascending and descending phases of slow waves.

From this series of experiments, the following interesting findings were noted: (1) Oscillatory potentials seemed to be isolated from the a- and the b-waves of the ERGs employing a pair of electrodes on the opposite sides of an eyeball at the same meridional depth. The a- and the b-wave seemed to be cancelled out in this electrode-position. (2) In order to record the a- and the b-wave of the ERG as a mass response, a distance in the longitudinal direction between the electrodes was necessary. (3) The polarity of oscillatory potentials was not simply reversed. The peak time seemed to move with changes in the position of the electrode pair along the longitudinal line.

The oscillatory potentials are usually superimposed on the b-wave of the ERG. However, there have been several reports showing that the characteristics of the oscillatory potentials are considerably different from those of the b-wave (Brown, 1968; Honda, 1969). This paper also supports a possible different origin of the oscillatory potentials from that of the a- and the b-wave, after studying the horizontal distribution of the mass response of a retina attached on the wall of the eye-ball.

SUMMARY

The action potential of the rabbit retina *in situ* was recorded as a mass, moving a pair of electrodes on the sclera, and the following findings were noted: The polarity of the a-wave and the b-wave of the ERGs was easily changed by the movement of the electrodes in the longitudinal lines. The oscillatory potentials seemed to be isolated from the a- and b-wave by employing a pair of electrodes on the opposite sides of an eyeball in the same meridional depth. The a- and the b-wave was cancelled out in this

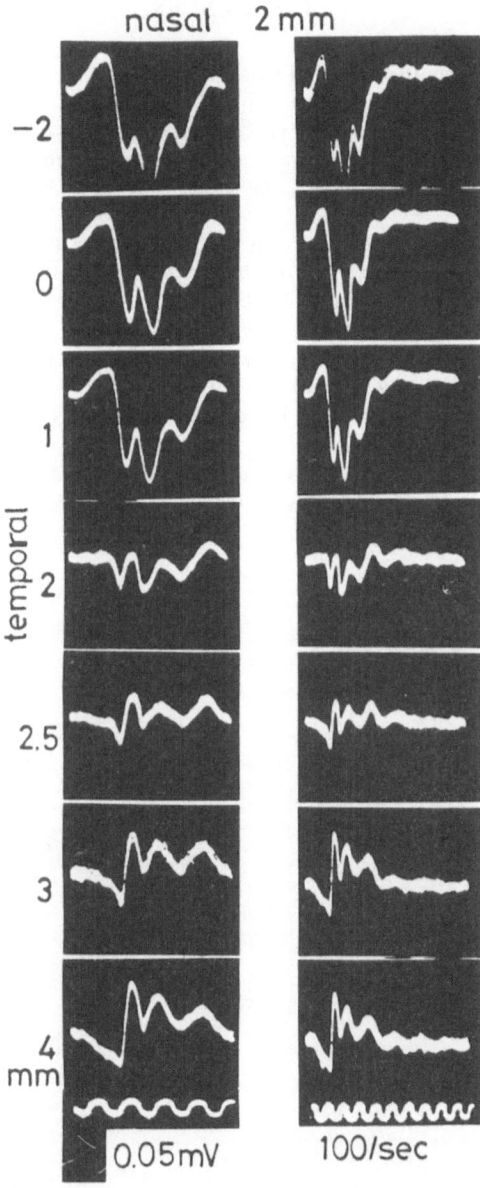

Fig. 4. The polarity change of the oscillatory potentials is shown by the recordings of a higher gain and a shorter time constant (0.003 sec).

electrode-position. For the detection of the a- and the b-wave of the ERG as a mass, a distance between electrodes in the longitudinal direction was necessary. The polarity of the oscillatory potentials was not simply reversed as the a- and the b-wave. The peak times of oscillations seemed to move with the movement of electrodes.

REFERENCES

Standardization Committees of ISCERG: ISCERG recommendations on June 4th, 1961, in Stockholm. Acta Ophthal. Suppl. 70: 97, (1962).

Noonan, B.D., Wilkus, R.J., Chatrian, G.E. & Lettich, E.: The influence of direction of gaze on the human electroretinogram recorded from periorbital electrodes: A study utilizing a summating technique, *Electroenceph. clin. Neurophysiol.*, 35, *537*, (1973).

Honda, Y.: Effects of eye movement on the ERG pattern followed by orbital skin electrodes (in Japanese), *Acta Soc. Ophthalm. Jap.*, 80, 7 (1976).

Honda, Y.: A few fundamental problem of ERGs followed by orbital skin electrodes (in Japanese), *Acta Soc. Ophthalm. Jap.*, 80, *117*, (1976).

Dawson, G.D.: A summation technique for the detection of small evoked potentials. *Electroenceph. clin. Neurophysiol.*, 6, *65*, (1954).

Brown, K.T.: The electroretinogram: Its components and their origins, *Vision Res.*, 8, *633*, (1968).

Honda, Y.: Studies on electrical activity of the mammalian retina and optic nerve in vitro, I. Factors affecting activity of the retina., *Acta Soc. Ophthalm. Jap.*, 73, *1865*, (1969).

Authors' address:
Dept of Physiology
Hamamatsu University School of Medicine
Handa-cho 3600, Hamamatsu-shi
Japan 431-31

LASER GENERATED PATTERNED STIMULI FOR VISUAL EVOKED RESPONSES

KARL J. FRITZ, CAROL S. FRITZ, ELEANOR HOMENA & STEVEN M. MEYER

(Chicago)

ABSTRACT

The coherent radiation produced by a laser may be used to produce a variety of interference patterns. These patterns may be projected on a screen or projected directly onto the retina. Several methods exist whereby these patterns may be changed rapidly. Use of changing laser generated interference patterns as a stimulus for visual evoked responses is described. Use for clinical evaluation of visual acuity in anesthetized, comatose or infantile patients or those unable to recognize a stable interference pattern is proposed.

INTRODUCTION

The light emitted from an 0.7 milliwatt neon laboratory laser has frequency spread of approximately 10^{-10} times its basic frequency and therefore has a coherence length of many meters. This makes the generation of interference patterns easy and, in fact, almost impossible to avoid. Laser generated interference patterns have been used to measure the potential visual acuity of patients with cataract (Green & Cohen, 1970; 1971; Gstalder & Green, 1971, 1972; Rassow & Wolf, 1973). The technique is based on the penetrance of enough of the coherent light to allow production of interference patterns while the rest of the light is scattered so that it simply decreases the contrast of the image. Once such interference patterns are present on the retina, they may be rapidly modified through mechanical or optical means. This provides the basis for their use as a stimulus for visual evoked responses. Use of laser generated patterns is not restricted to direct projection on the retina; patterns may also be produced in a variety of shapes and textures and projected onto a screen. Several of the methods available for varying patterns do so at nearly constant average illuminance so that the evoked responses produced are due to variation in the pattern itself.

METHODS AND MATERIALS

A Metrologic model 660 laser is used as a light source. This laser emits in the transverse electric transverse magnetic mode (TEM 00) at approximately 632.8 nanometers wavelength. The power output is 0.7 milliwatts. Because the light emanating from the laser is nearly unidirectional, it is necessary to introduce spreading lenses to make the beam wider. We use a −20 diopter lens from a clinical trial set to do this. The light then impinges on a 200 line

369

per inch replica Ronchi grating with the lines vertical. A second Ronchi grating with 100 lines per inch is attached to a motor drive and provides the next optical element. The angle of this grating is variable but we usually use it with the lines horizontal. A −30 diopter lens is used to spread the beam further causing an effective magnification of the interference pattern. The beam emerging from the magnifying lens is then either projected on a screen or viewed through an eyepiece and a neutral density filter. Direct viewing produces a much brighter image and is the way in which we use the apparatus to produce evoked responses. The observer's eye is placed in Maxwellian view position and held in place with a combination head and chin rest. The signal is obtained from the scalp with Beckman miniature skin electrodes placed in positions O_z, P_z with respect to a linked earlobe ground. For amplification, a Grass model P511E AC coupled preamplifier is used with a gain of 100,000 and bandwidth of 1 Hz. to 100 Hz. (−6 DB points). Filtering is done to eliminate 60 Hz. noise. The amplified signal together with impulses coincident with the stimulus change are recorded on a FM cassette tape recorder, TEAC Model-70A. After data have been obtained, the signal is replayed with an additional amplification of 5 to a digital equipment corporation PDP-15 computer using a 12 bit analog to digital converter. Signal averaging and analysis of the resultant waveform are done digitally on the computer. During the analog to digital conversion, points are taken 4 milliseconds apart from 50 milliseconds before the stimulus marker to 500 milliseconds after the stimulus marker. After conversion to digital form, all computer calculations are made with more than 7 significant figures. Variance of the data is computed for each point of the averaged signal. A graph of the averaged signal and the variance is presented on a Tektronix storage cathode ray tube driven by the computer. Intermittent motion of the 100 line per inch Ronchi grating is provided by an eccentric arm mounted on a small electric motor. The repetition rate is approximately 1 change in pattern per second. A micro switch provides the stimulus marker and is switched coincident with the beginning of motion of the Ronchi grating. The pattern with the Ronchi grating at rest is a pattern of bright squares on a dark background. When the Ronchi grating moves, the pattern dissolves into alternate bright and dark vertical lines. The eyepiece provides a field stop for the optical system, such that the observer sees a 3 degree pattern. The spatial frequency of the pattern is approximately 0.3 degrees per cycle. The optical portion of the apparatus is shown in Figure 1 and the pattern used is shown in Figure 2. During recording of an evoked response, 250 changes in pattern are used. An opaque screen is then substituted for the neutral density filter with the rest of the apparatus left unchanged and another 250 events are recorded for a control response.

RESULTS AND DISCUSSION

An evoked response, its variance, a control response and its variance are shown in Figure 3. A minimum in the evoked response occurs at about 150 milliseconds and a maximum at about 225 milliseconds. The overall amplitude of the response is approximately 3.5 microvolts. This response is of somewhat longer latency and smaller amplitude than that usually obtained from checkerboard patterned stimuli (Harter & Salmon, 1971). The pattern of squares is not directly comparable to a checkerboard and the change in pattern is quite different from the total reversal of a checkerboard so that some differences in the response are expected.

Laser generated interference patterns may be used in many ways to produce evoked responses. They may be projected directly on the retina as we describe here, or they may be used by projecting the pattern on a screen. The pattern size is easily changed by moving the position of the eyepiece.

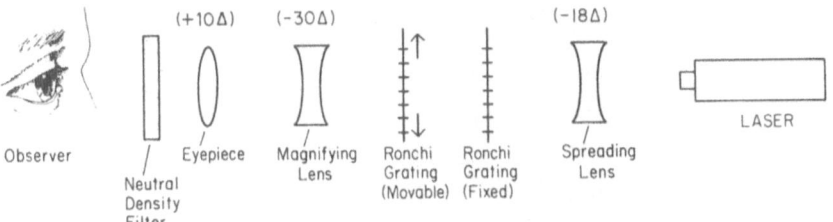

Fig. 1. Optical portion of the interference pattern generating apparatus. A wide variety of patterns can be produced by varying the spacing of the optical elements.

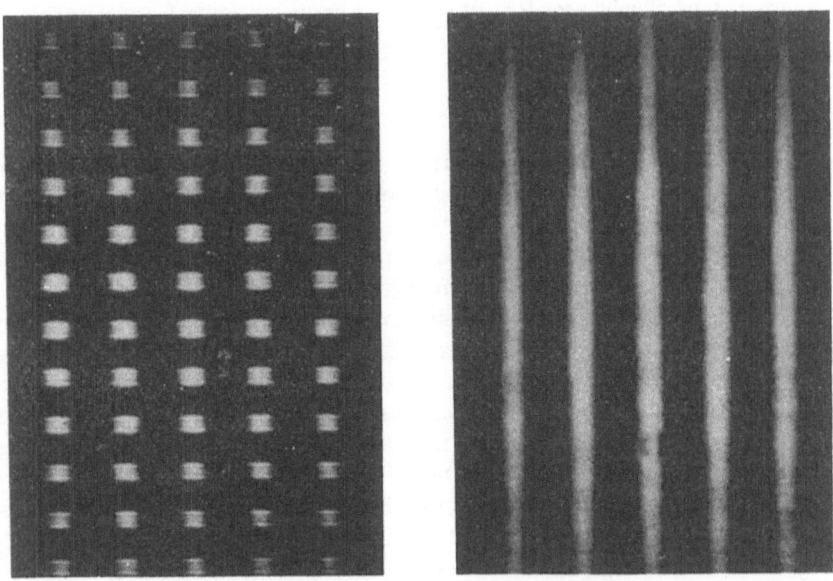

Fig. 2. Interference patterns used to produce a visual evoked response. The square pattern is seen when the movable Ronchi grating is at rest. When the grating moves the square pattern dissolves into the linear one.

371

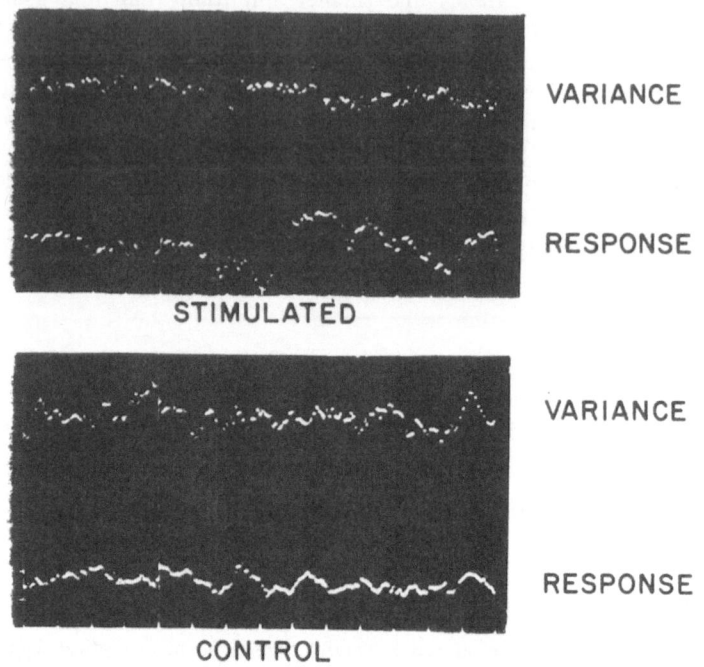

VARIANCE

RESPONSE

STIMULATED

VARIANCE

RESPONSE

CONTROL

Fig. 3.   A sample of the evoked response produced by the apparatus. The response and a control together with the variance of each waveform is plotted. Marks on the horizontal axis are 50 milliseconds apart and marks on the vertical axis are one microvolt apart.

Pattern texture can be changed from the simple array of squares we have used to an exceedingly complex structure. Some examples of possible patterns are shown in Figure 4. Patterns may be changed mechanically by moving the second Ronchi grating perpendicular to the optical axis as we did, or by rotating the second Ronchi grating.

Visual acuity measurements using evoked responses have been described (Sokol & Bloom, 1973; Millodot & Riggs, 1970; Regan, 1972). We propose to use laser interference patterns generating evoked responses to measure visual acuity of patients with opacities in the media who are either uncooperative or unable to recognize stable interference patterns on the retina. Many patients with cataracts are not able to recognize such patterns (Green & Cohen, 1971). This, however, should not prevent the evoked response from occurring whenever the pattern size is within the resolution capability of the retina. Therefore, even in the absence of objective recognition of a pattern, we hope to be able to evaluate patients before cataract surgery using laser interferometry.

Interference patterns may be created using Ronchi gratings with the method described by Green in which the first order interference regions are

372

recombined with suppression of the zero order and all higher order regions. This technique produces approximately sinusoidal intensity variation in the interference bands. With division of the light into two optical paths (the two first order regions), many possible recombining methods exist. We plan to explore two of these in the immediate future. The first method produces sinusoidal intensity lines which fade from vertical to horizontal. To do this the two first order regions are separated, one is polarized vertically and the other horizontally. After the beam in each region is spread by passing through negative lenses, the beam passes through vertical and horizontal Ronchi gratings and then through a rotating polarizing filter before recombination.

The second method produces rapid reversal in the interference pattern by phase shifting the two beams by a total of 1/2 cycle. This is done by passing the separated first order regions through an electro-optical switch such that 1/4 wavelength of optical path is added to one beam and subtracted from the other. The activation time for changing the optical path is about one microsecond so there should be no observable motion in the patterns. The orientation of the patterns and spatial frequency can be varied without changing the path length switching apparatus which should make this stimulation apparatus quite versatile for evaluating visual acuity as well as linear directional sensitivity of the retina for evoked responses.

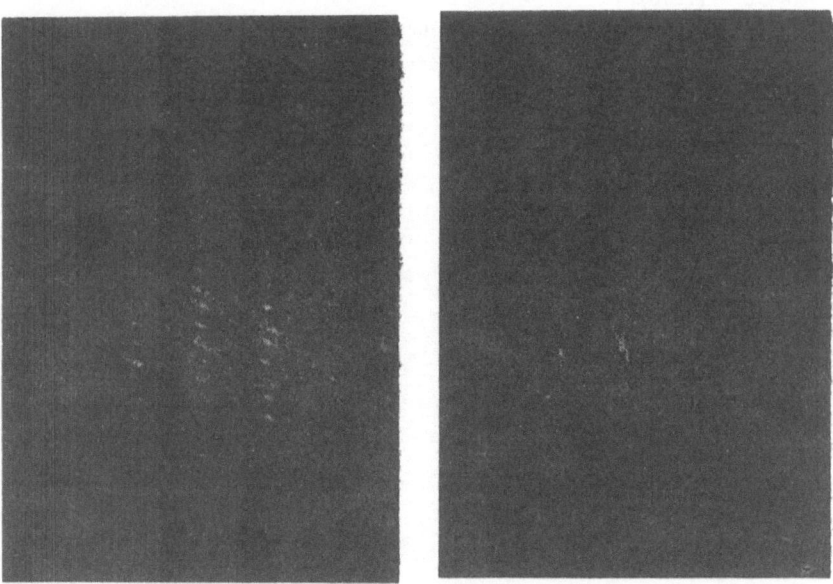

Fig. 4. Examples of possible interference patterns. A rich variety of structures and ranges of contrast can be obtained with laser interferometry.

ACKNOWLEDGMENT

The authors wish to thank Dr. Joel Pokorny for many valuable discussions and for the use of some crucial equipment. Dr. John Trimble provided essential help in generating the evoked responses and allowed us to use his specially equipped laboratory as well as his many talents.

REFERENCES

Green, D.G. & Cohen, M.M.: Testing the vision of cataract patients by means of laser generated interference fringes. *Science* 168, *1240*, (1970).

Green, D.G. & Cohen, M.M.: Laser interferometry in the evaluation of potential macular function in the presence of opacities in the ocular media. *Trans. Am. Acad. Ophthalmol. Otolaryngol.* 75, *629*, (1971).

Gstalder, R.J. & Green, D.G.: Laser interferometric acuity in amblyopia. *J. Ped. Ophthalmol.* 8, *251*, (1971).

Gstalder, R.J. & Green, D.G.: Laser interferometry in corneal opacification. Preoperative visual potential estimation. *Arch. Ophthalmol.* 87, *269*, (1972).

Rassow, B. & Wolf, D.: Erfahrungen mit dem Laser-Interferenz-streifen-Test bei der Messung des retinalen Auflösungsvermögens. *Graefes Arch. klin. exp. Ophthalmol.* 187, *61*, (1973).

Harter, M. & Salmon, L.E.: Evoked cortical responses to patterned light flashes: effects of ocular convergence and accommodation. *Electroenceph. clin. Neurophysiol.* 30, *527*, (1971).

Sokol, S. & Bloom, B.: Visually evoked cortical responses of amblyopes to a spatially alternating stimulus. *Invest. Ophthalmol.* 12, *936*, (1973).

Millodot, M. & Riggs, L.A.: Refraction determined electrophysiologically. *Arch. Oph.* 84, *272*, (1970).

Regan, D.: Evoked Potentials in Psychology, Sensory Physiology and Clinical Medicine. Chapman and Hall, London, 1972, p. 167.

Authors' address:
Dept of Ophthalmology
University of Chicago
950 East 59th Street
Chicago, Ill. 60637
USA

REMOTE MEASUREMENTS OF THE VISUALLY EVOKED CORTICAL POTENTIAL BY TELEPHONE LINES

E. ADACHI-USAMI, T. ADACHI & Y. ISHIKAWA

(Hamamatsu, Japan)

ABSTRACT

It is reported that trial transmission experiments of the visually evoked cortical potential through telephone lines both for local and long distance (about 450 km) connections demonstrated the feasibility of VECP transmission.

Our major concerns are how to transmit the synchronization pulse stably and without any adverse influence on the VECP.

The transmitted VECP waveforms (VECPs to flash stimuli and those to pattern reversal stimuli) are proved to be good duplicates of the original ones. The synchronization pulse of the stimuli is transmitted by combining it with the VECP using a mixing amplifier.

Several properties of a transmission link used in this study are examined. This system may be of use for data-exchanges between different laboratories, transmission to a large computer room and for remote diagnosis of diseases.

Studies of the visually evoked cortical potential (VECP) have depended strongly upon the aid of the kind of a computer which has only some fixed programmes including averaging. However, there will arise, in the near future, requirements for more sophisticated analysis methods than what a so-called 'averager' can do.

To extend the possibilities of VECP analysis, real time entry of VECP data to a larger computer is desirable.

Remote measurements of the electrocardiogram (Rahm et al., 1953) is nowadays widely put in practice, and those of the electroencephalogram are also becoming progressively utilized (Bickford et al., 1969). In 1965 Ray and others made demonstrative telemetry experiments of the auditory and visually evoked cortical potential.

As primary step for this purpose we made trial VECP transmissions by telephone lines using an inexpensive ready-made modem with some added simple circuitry.

METHODS

The block diagram for our experimental transmission of the VECP by telephone lines is shown in figure 1a. The synchronization pulse of a stimulus trigger and a VECP signal are combined by the mixing circuit shown in figure 1b. The combined signal is fed to the input terminal of the sending part of an acoustic coupler. The first stage of the mixing circuit mixes two

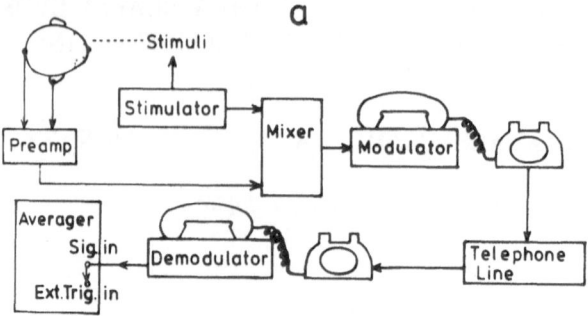

Fig. 1a. Schematic representation of the experimental arrangement for transmission of the visually evoked cortical potential (VECP) by telephone lines.

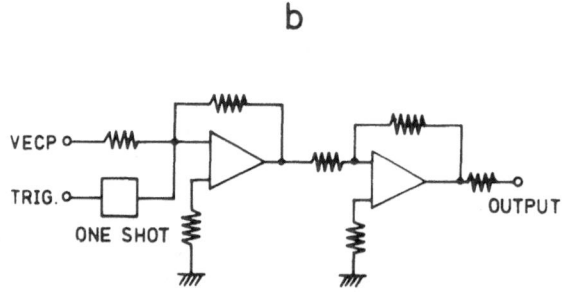

Fig. 1b. Basic circuit diagram of the mixer for mixing the VECP signal and the synchronization pulse.

inputs with high impedances to avoid mutual interference, and the second stage amplifies the combined signal to the necessary level. The acoustic signal, modulated with a VECP-synchronization-pulse-signal, is then received by the receiving part of a coupler at the remote site through telephone lines.

The output from a coupler can be connected directly to the signal and external trigger input terminals, in parallel without separating the VECP and the synchronization pulse, since most averaging computers have high impedance input.

Since TTL (transistor-transistor logic component) is used in the trigger circuits of both of our kinds of stimulators (for plain stimuli and pattern reversal stimuli), the mixing circuit is designed to match the level of TTL.

Recording methods of the VECP are the same as in a previous paper (Adachi-Usami et al., 1972/73). In the present experiment, the VECP to light pulses of 100 ms duration with two beams (Adachi-Usami et al., 1974) and to pattern reversal stimuli (Adachi-Usami et al., 1975) have been transmitted by telephone lines. The transmitted VECPs are compared with the VECPs recorded before transmission, and several properties of the transmission system in this study are investigated.

Figure 2a represents the VECPs to light pulses of 100 ms duration. Trace A is the VECP to be transmitted, and B is the one after transmission by local telephone lines at 13.00 o'clock.

Figure 2b is the same experiment on the VECP to pattern reversal stimuli. The traces of transmitted VECPs are a little noisier than the ones to be transmitted, but no distortion is seen in the waveform.

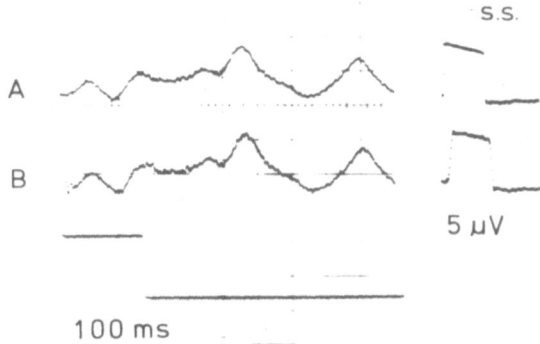

Fig. 2a. Summed VECPs (n = 200) in response to light pulses of 100 ms duration (indicated below records) of green (λ = 522 nm) light flickering at a rate of 2.0 Hz with luminance of –2.0 log ft-Lt. Size of the test field is 15°, central fixation. Subject, S.S., a 19-year-old man. Trace A represents the VECP recorded before transmission and trace B, the VECP recorded after transmission by local telephone lines at 13.00 o'clock.

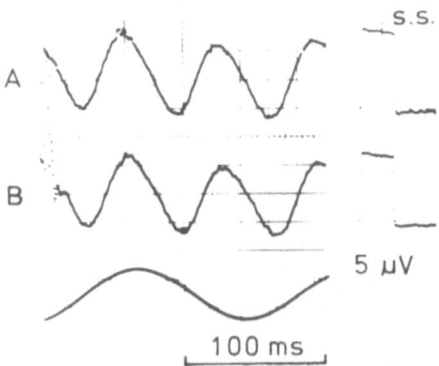

Fig. 2b. Summed pattern specific VECPs (n = 200) in response to checkerboard pattern reversal stimuli. Visual angle of each check is 22′ and that of total plane 4°. Pattern luminance is kept at 1.2 log ft-Lt and frequency of pattern reversal is at 12.0 Hz, equal to four times the rotation of the polaroid disc as indicated below the records. Subject, S.S., a 19-year-old man. Trace A is the VECPs before transmission and B, the record after transmission by local telephone lines at 13.00 o'clock.

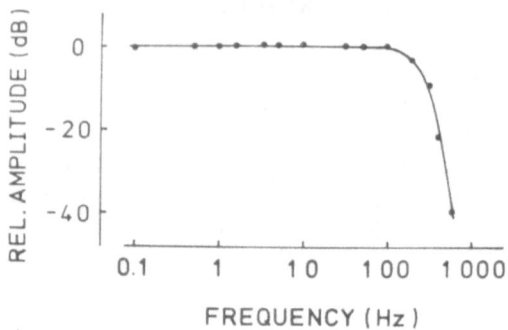

Fig. 3a. Relative amplitude in dB vs. frequency curve of transmission by local telephone lines, 0 dB at 10 Hz. A sinusoidal test signal of 0.8 V is sent to the mixer input and the transmitted output signal is measured on the scope of an averager.

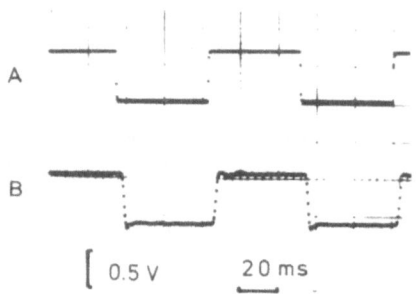

Fig. 3b. Square wave of 10 Hz before (trace A) and after (trace B) transmission by local telephone lines at 13.00 o'clock.

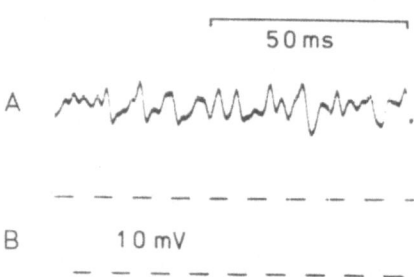

Fig. 3c. Trace A; instantaneous noise level at the output of the receiving coupler after transmission by local telephone lines at 13.00 o'clock. Trace B; reference, 100 Hz, 10 mV.

378

The general characteristics measured on the transmission line (from the input terminal of the pre-amplifier to the output of the receiving coupler) are shown in figure 3. Figure 3a is the amplitude vs. frequency curve, 3b is the transmitted waveform of 10 Hz square wave and 3c shows typical instantaneous noise.

Since the signal level is generally very low, unsatisfactory transmission characteristics such as poor linearity and drift may not affect transmission quality seriously.

Accordingly, a remaining unknown factor is the noise from telephone

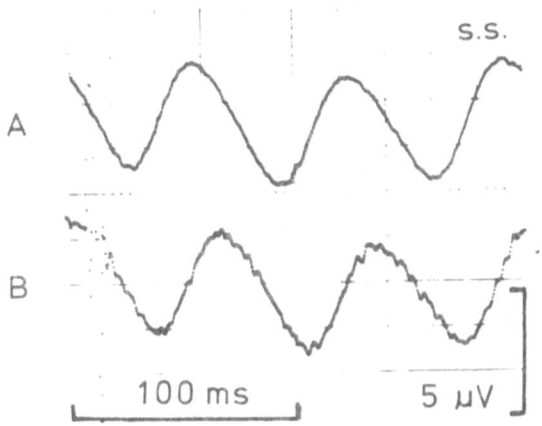

Fig. 4a. Summed pattern specific VECPs (n = 200) before (trace A) and after (trace B) transmission by telephone lines over long distance (450 km) at 11.00 o'clock. Stimulus condition for evoking the VECP is the same as the one explained in Fig. 2b.

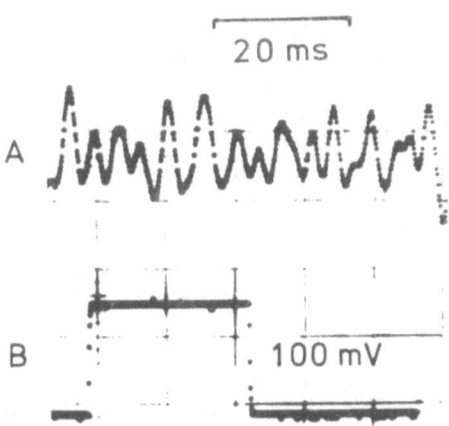

Fig. 4b. Trace A; typical instantaneous noise level at the output of the receiving coupler after transmission by telephone lines over long distance (450 km) at 11.00 o'clock. Trace B; reference, 20 Hz, 100 mV.

lines which will vary with distance, time, selected channels etc.

Therefore, transmission of the VECP has been done by telephone lines over about 450 km which is rather long, at 11.00 o'clock when the line is most crowded (figure 4a). As a test signal source, the data which were previously recorded on a data recorder are used. A typical instantaneous noise level (figure 4b) is much larger than the one transmitted with local telephone lines (see figure 3c). It can be seen in figure 4a that the transmitted VECP trace suffers little from distortion. The detectable deterioration is that the transmitted VECP becomes a little noisier than before transmission.

Next, the transmission stability of the synchronization pulse is examined. A synchronization pulse has a width of 2.3 ms and an amplitude of 0.5 V at the input of the coupler. Since a coupler link has no level difference between sending and receiving terminals, the received synchronization pulse can be compared directly on the scope as demonstrated in figure 5a and c.

In order to check the degree of jitter produced by the trial transmission link with local telephone lines and by the long distance lines of about 450 km, the synchronization pulse after transmission is stored for 80 seconds

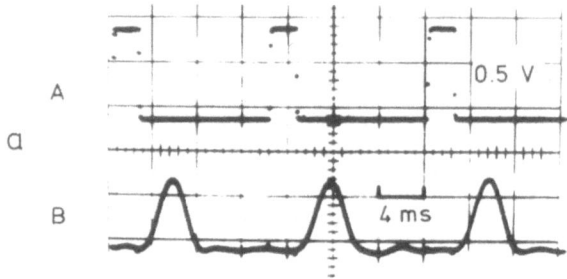

Fig. 5a. Synchronization pulse (2.3 ms, 0.5 V) at the input of the mixer (trace A) and at the output of the receiving coupler after transmission by local telephone lines recorded at 13.00 o'clock (trace B).

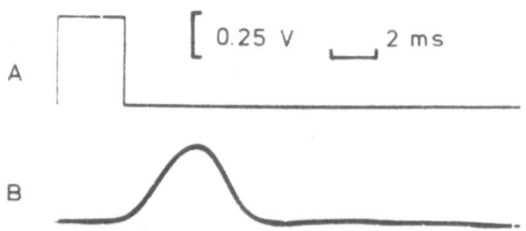

Fig. 5b Trace A; synchronization pulse at the input of the mixer, Trace B; synchronization pulse at the output of the receiving coupler after transmission by local telephone lines at 13.00 o'clock stores for 80 seconds by a storage oscilloscope in order to check the jitter of the pulse.

380

by a storage oscilloscope (figure b and d). Little jitter is found in either set of data. Moreover, a square wave synchronization pulse with duration of 2.3 ms changes to a symmetrical sine square wave after transmission and no ringing occurs. This means that the phase-characteristics of the transmission link must be uniform and the amplitude vs. frequency curve at high frequencies must have smooth roll off characteristics.

These results seem to coincide well with the general characteristics of the transmission lines studied before (figure 3a and 3b).

DISCUSSION

Both analog and digital methods of transmission of the VECP by telephone lines are possible.

Since the data should be processed by a digital computer, it might be better to transmit in digital form after AD convertion. In this study, an analog method utilizing an acoustic coupler has been tried, because the coupler could be obtained easily on the market as ECG telemetry equipment. The another reason is that simple analog transmission would be the

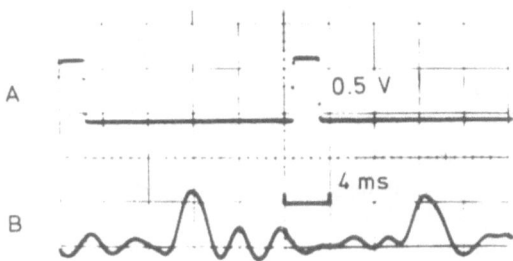

Fig. 5c. Synchronization pulse at the input of the mixer (trace A) and at the output of the receiving coupler after transmission by telephone lines over long distance (450 km) at 11.00 o'clock (trace B).

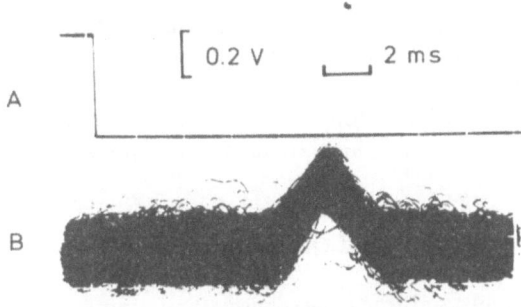

Fig. 5d. Trace A; synchronization pulse at the input of the mixer, Trace B; synchronization pulse at the output of the receiving coupler after transmission by telephone lines over long distance (450 km) at 11.00 o'clock stored for 80 seconds by a storage oscilloscope.

best choice when an averager was available as a peripheral of the central computer. Digital transmission would require a high speed modem, a complex control device and a high quality line for the averaging procedure.

There are two problems which must be cleared for the analog transmission of the VECP. The first is the circuit noise. Since the signal level of the VECP is extremely low, comparable to the noise level of a good pre-amplifier, and the signal to noise ratio is already around zero at the output of a pre-amplifier, the added noise from the transmission circuit is considered to be, in most cases, not fatal. Improvement of S/N can be achieved by averaging more responses.

Generally speaking, the higher the level of S + N signal at the input of a coupler is, the less the relative added noise from the link is. However, the signal level at the input of a coupler should be limited when superimposition of the synchronization pulse is made. Secondly, the timing information of stimuli should be transmitted together with the VECP.

There are two different systems to measure VECPs depending on whether the control point is at the sending place or the receiving place where the data are to be processed.

In the former case like in this report, the synchronization pulse of stimuli can be superimposed on the evoked potential, transmitted together with it and if necessary, separated at the receiving place. In order to get stable triggering for averaging, the relative level of the signal to the synchronization pulse at the mixing inputs should be limited.

When the control point is at the data processing end, a trigger pulse must be sent out to start the stimulus. As there are transmission delays for sending a trigger pulse and sending back the VECPs, it must be noted that the data obtained at the receiving place contain the doubled delay.

In this case one merit is that the modulation level of the VECP at a coupler is not limited to accomodate the synchronization pulse. Judging only from the fact that transmission of the ECG by telephone lines has been widely used, there should be no problem with the acoustic coupler link through telephone lines as a waveform transmission system for the VECP.

Our major concerns were how to transmit a synchronization pulse stably without an adverse influence on the VECP. As far as our several trials are concerned, there was no serious problem on this matter.

Since the frequency response of the transmission system is limited, it is preferable that the synchronization pulse to be sent be shaped into a sine-square wave by filtration before transmission in order to avoid interference caused by reflexion of the high frequency components of a square wave pulse.

CONCLUSION

The present study confirmed inexpensive and simple transmission of the VECP by telephone lines.

This system will be of use for data-exchanges between different laboratories, transmissions to a larger computer room and remote diagnosis of diseases, possibly using an averager as peripheral.

ACKNOWLEDGEMENT

This work was supported by grant No. 187013 from the Japanese Education Ministry.

REFERENCES

Adachi-Usami, E., F.J. Kellermann & R. Makabe: VER threshold in different stages of optic neuritis. *Ophthal. Res.* 4, *284-297*, (1972/73).

Adachi-Usami, E., V. Gavriysky, J. Heck, E. Schenkel & H. Scheibner: Psychophysical and VECP examination of a rod monochromat and a cone monochromat. Documenta Ophthal. Proc. series XIth ISCERG symp. in Bad Nauheim, 1973. *176-186*, (1974).

Adachi-Usami, E., T. Adachi, D. Kanaizuka & Y. Chiba: New stimulating devices for the cherckerboard pattern reversal evoked cortical potentials. *Folia Ophthal. Jap.* 26. *516-518*, (1975).

Bickford R.G., G. Merby, W. Karnes & R. Groover: Teleprocessing of the EEG from the patient's residence. *Electroenceph. clin. neurophysiol.* 26, *117-118*, (1969).

Rahm, Jr., W.E., J.L. Barmore, I.M. Ellestad & F. Lowell Dunn: Local and long distance transmission and storage of electrocardiograms and other low frequency signals. *Circulat. Res.* 1, *518-522*, (1953).

Ray, C.D., R.G. Bickford, W.G. Walter & A. Rémond: Experiences with telemetry of biomedical data by telephone, cable and satellite: domestic and international. *Med. Electron. Biol. Engng.* 3, *169-177*, (1965).

Authors' address:
Hamamatsu University School of Medicine
3600 Manda-cho
Hamamatsu
431-31 Japan

A NEW CONTACT LENS ELECTRODE

COLIN BARBER, D.J. COTTERILL & J.R. LARKE

(Nottingham/Birmingham)

ABSTRACT

A new kind of contact lens electrode is described which has superior electrical charac-teristics to the traditional type and overcomes many of its disadvantages. In addition it can permit unimpaired vision by the subject for the simultaneous recording of ERG and pattern VER

Of all electrophysiological signals the electroretinogram (ERG) provides the investigator with a site which is at once the best and the worst for recording. No other signal can be recorded from the surface with such a direct elec-trical pathway to its source; no other surface electrode site is as sensitive as the cornea. Hence, although the ERG can be recorded using skin electrodes, some means of making electrical contact with the cornea is invariably used.

Fundamentally, the method of making this contact has not changed since it was described by Dewar (1877). Isotonic saline solution is held in contact with the cornea by means of a container of some kind and this also supports an electrode (generally metallic) with its end in the saline. The design of the saline container has been greatly improved since Dewar used a ring of clay and Hartline (1925) used goggles. The major step forward was the introduction of the contact glass electrode independently by Riggs (1941) and Karpe (1945). Electrodes of this type, including the many varia-tions subsequently introduced by other workers, are commonly in use today. The contact glass is made of moulded plastic and the most favoured material for the electrode is silver, although stainless steel and, occasionally, gold or platinum are used. The main disadvantages of the contact glass electrode are discomfort, difficulty in avoiding air bubbles, which spoil the electrical contact, and difficulty in fitting. On the other hand they can be fenestrated if clear vision is required (Jacobson et al. 1958) and the photo-voltaic artefact may generally be avoided by the use of sufficient black paint (Best, 1953).

A different approach to containing the saline is to make it effectively viscous. Jacobson (1955) used saline in methyl cellulose. Bornschein et al. (1966) described an electrode for animal work consisting of a hydrophilic gel soaked in saline. Subsequently Dawson et al. (1974) used a hydrophilic gel lens as a cushion (and saline carrier) under a Burian-Allen electrode. Schoessler & Jones (1975) have described an electrode consisting of two hydrophilic gel lenses embracing a fine platinum or gold wire which emerges through a hole in the outermost lens. These lenses, too, are soaked in saline. The soft lens electrode overcomes the mechanical difficulties of the contact glass type but unimpaired vision is generally not attainable and it is particularly susceptible to the production of a photo-voltaic artefact when a metal connection is used. A hydrophilic gel electrode with a carbon rod connec-

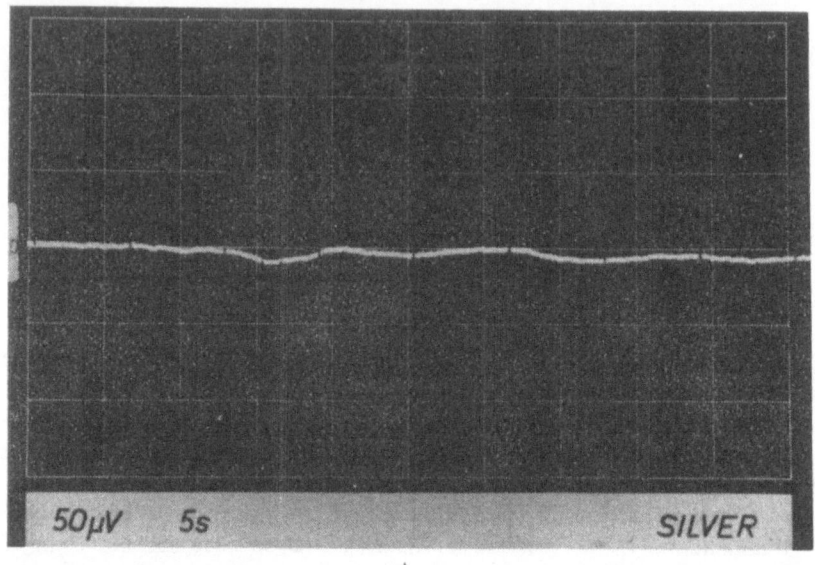

A

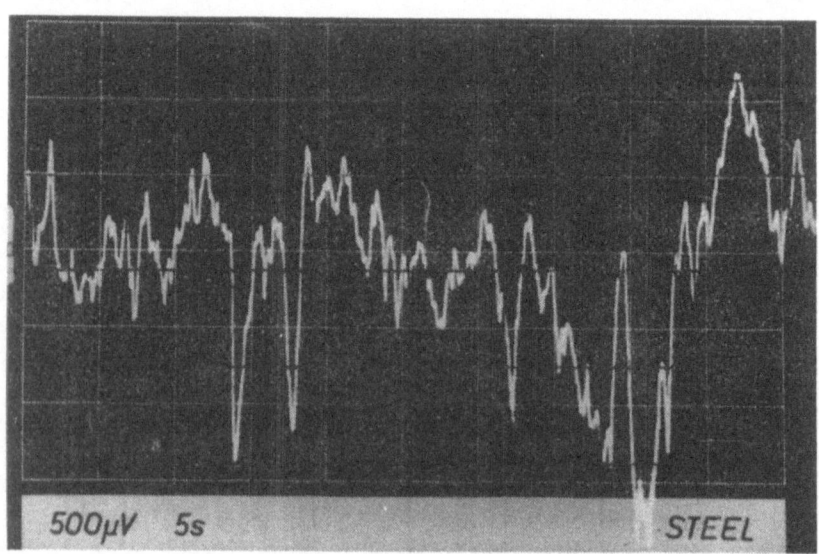

Fig. 1. Electrode noise for different materials. Calibrations are per division, note different scale for steel.

tion has been described by Wündsch & Lützow (1969) which produces no photo-voltaic artefact but is only suitable for animal work. It is very fragile due to the brittleness of the material.

We have constructed a contact lens electrode, based on a fitting lens for ophthalmic measurement (FLOM) using carbon and saline-equilibrated

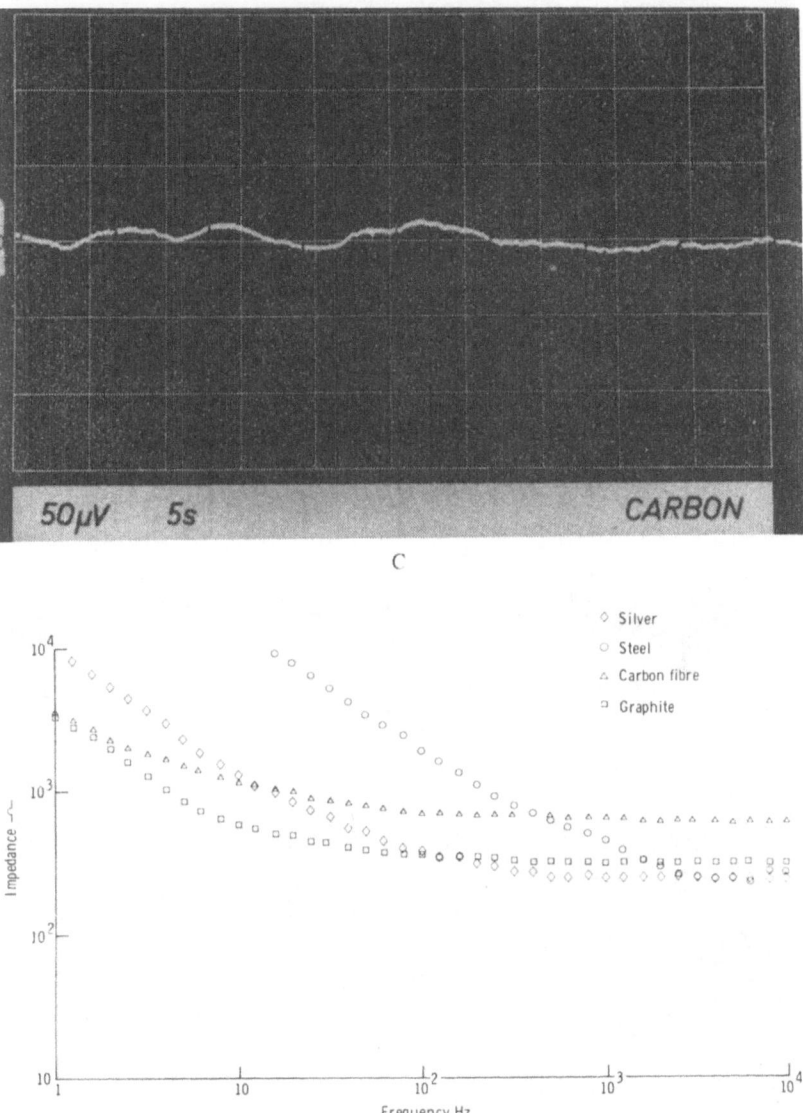

Fig. 2. The variation of impedance with frequency for different materials in saline-equilibrated hydrophilic gel. The measurements were made with a signal amplitude of 400 µV.

hydrophilic gel as the conducting materials. The electrical characteristics of the carbon/hydrogel combination compare favourably with those of commonly used materials. The electrode noise is low (fig. 1). The frequency response is good (fig. 2). The offset potential is negligible (carbon is essentially non-polar) and there is no photo-voltaic response (fig. 3).

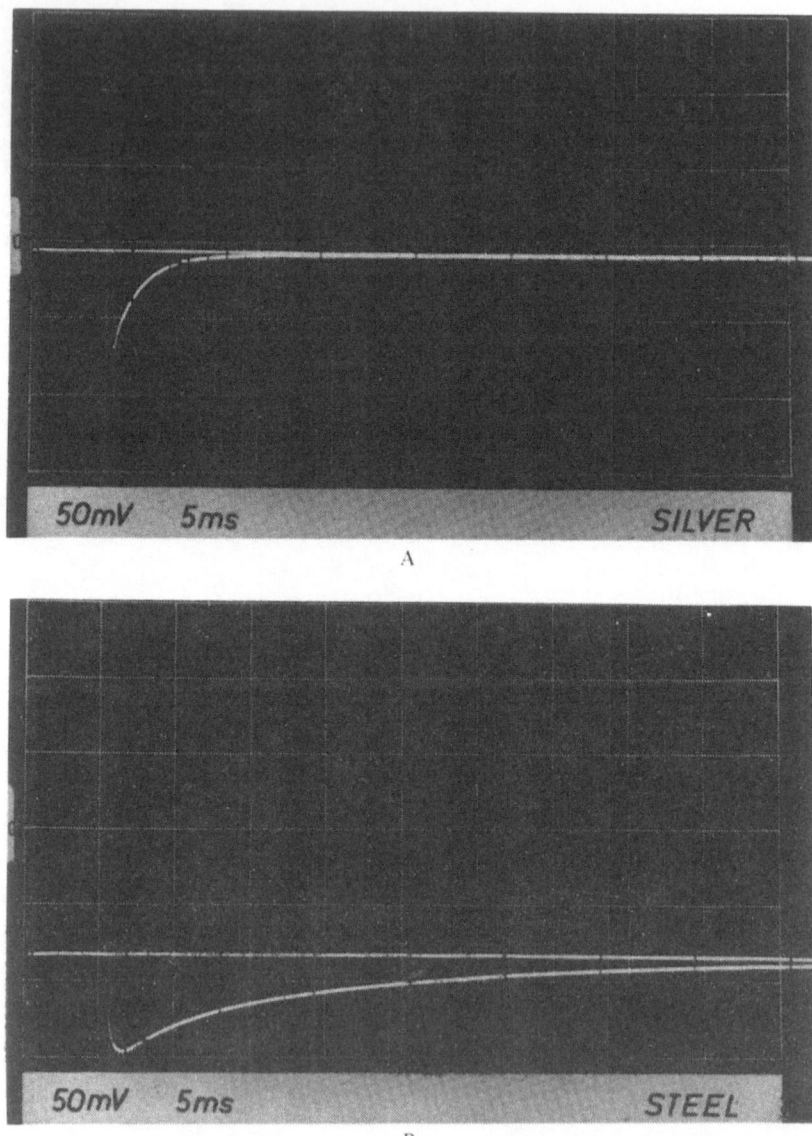

Fig. 3. The standing offset potential and response to ERG stimulus flash for different materials. Calibrations are per division, note different scale for carbon.

The mode of construction is shown in fig. 4. A graphite ring is fitted into a groove cut in the inner surface of the FLOM. The inner surface is then polished smooth and a layer of hydrogel monomer is spin-polymerised onto it. Trapped between the graphite ring and the FLOM is a braid of carbon fibres which emerges through a hole in the FLOM and terminates in a small

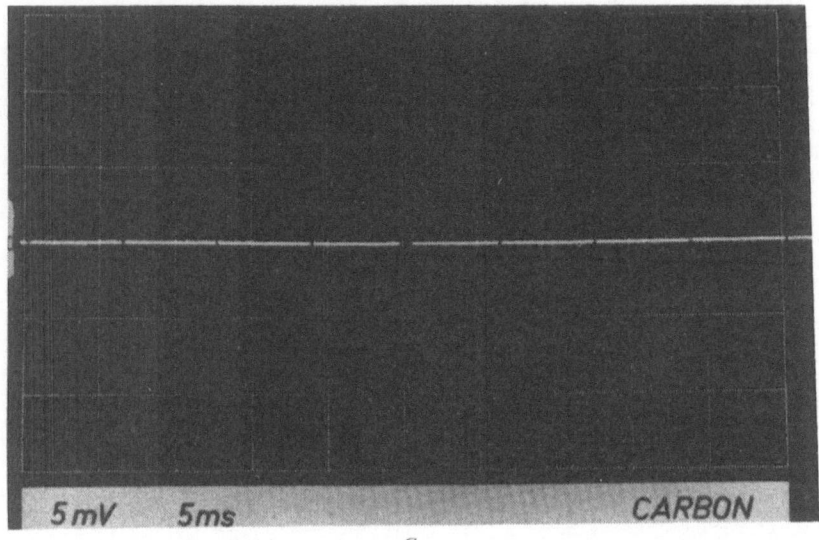

5 mV   5ms   CARBON

C

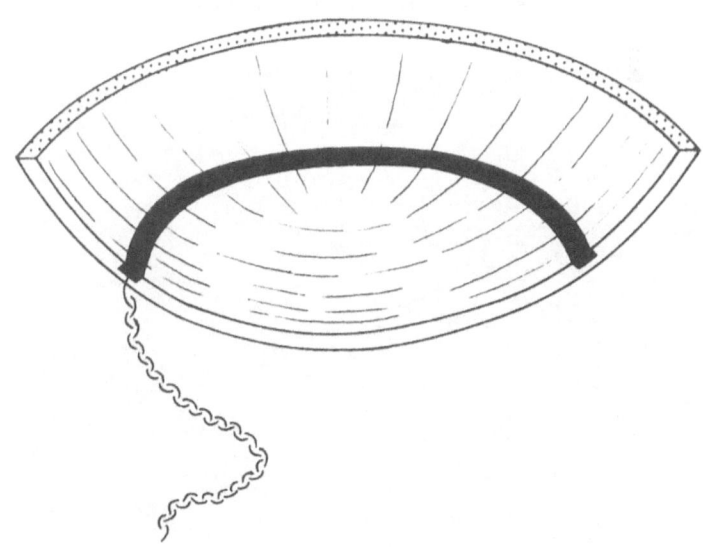

Fig. 4. Cut-away drawing of the electrode showing the method of construction. The inside surface is subsequently coated with hydrophilic gel.

plug. A layer of silicone rubber on the carbon braid provides electrical insulation and some degree of mechanical strength (fig. 5). The electrode is robust and comfortable in use, although it has been found advantageous to have a set of differing radii. Fenestrated versions have been made for simultaneous recording of ERG and pattern visual evoked response (VER), where

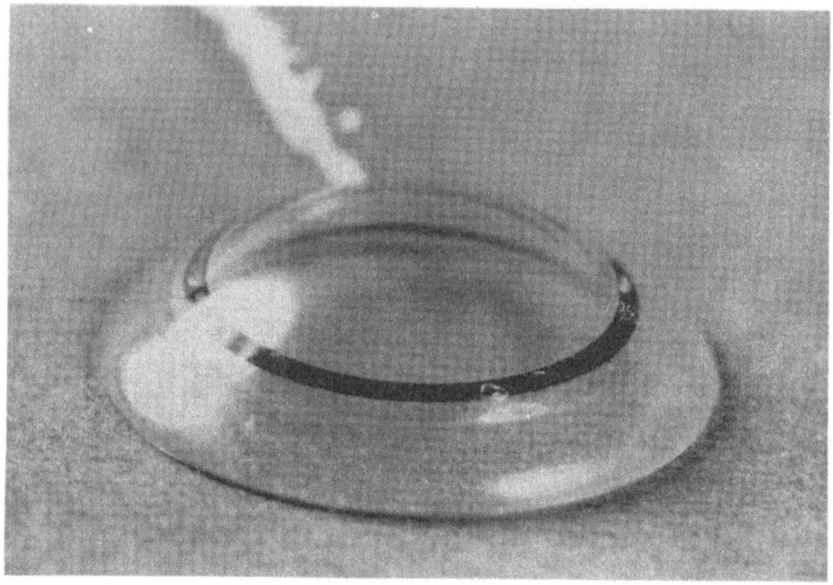

Fig. 5. The completed electrode.

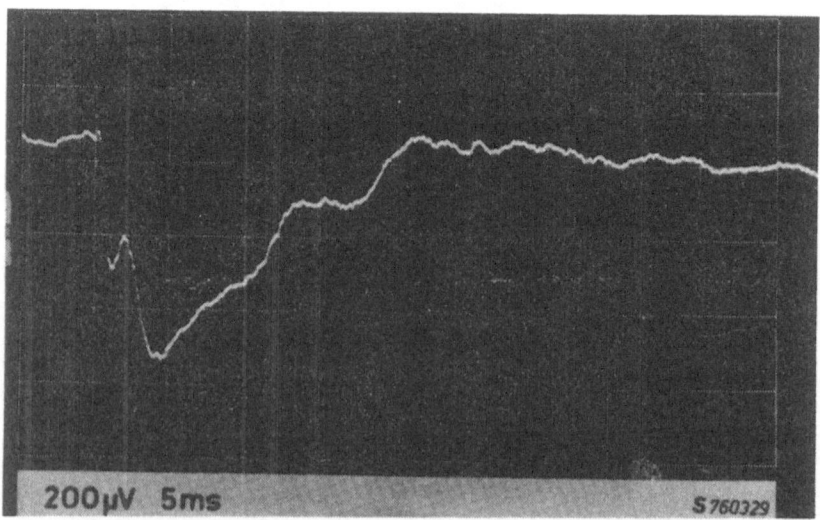

Fig. 6. ERG's recorded under identical conditions using (a) the traditional electrode and (b) the new electrode. Calibrations are per division.

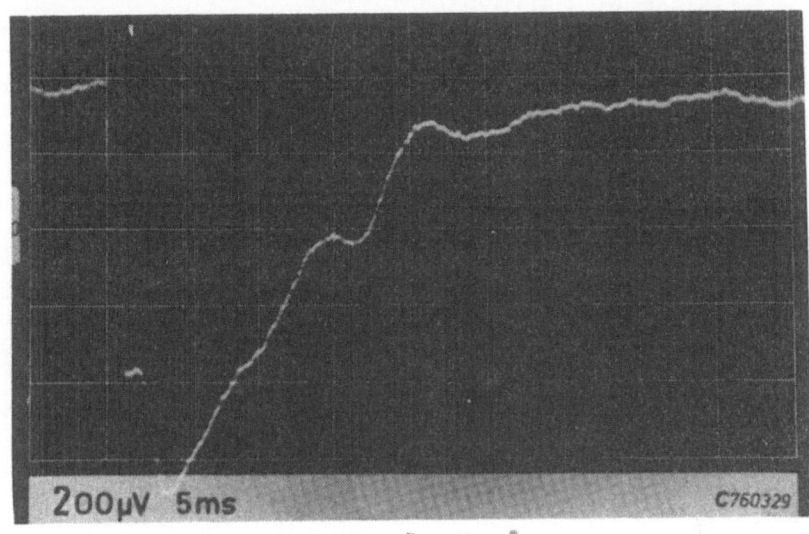

200µV 5ms   C760329

B

unimpaired vision is essential. ERG's recorded with this electrode, using an intense flash method to elicit the early receptor potential (ERP) and the oscillatory potentials, have the same form as those recorded with a traditional electrode but are slightly larger (fig. 6). There is no photo-voltaic artefact and, since the outer surface is non-conducting, there are no problems with eyelid artefacts.

To summarise, the electrode appears to satisfy the criteria for use in clinical electroretinography. It provides patient comfort and distorts neither the light entering the eye nor the electrical signal leaving it.

ACKNOWLEDGEMENTS

This work was supported in part by a grant from the Special Trustees for University Hospital, to whom we record our thanks.

REFERENCES

Best, W. Das menschliche Elektroretinogram während der Dunkeladaption. *Acta Ophthal.*, 31, *71-116*, (1953).

Bornschein, H., Wichterle, O. & Wündsch, L. A contact lens electrode for comparative ERG studies. *Vision Res.*, 6, *733-734*, (1966).

Dawson, W.W., Zimmerman, T.J. & Houde, W.L. A method for more comfortable electroretinography. *Arch. Ophthal.*, 91, *1-2*, (1974).

Dewar, J. The physiological action of light. *Nature*, 15, *433-435*, (1877).

Hartline, H.K. The electrical response to illumination of the eye in intact animals, including the human subject; and in decerebrate preparations. *A. J. Physiol.*, 73, *600-611*, (1925).

Jacobson, J. A new contact lens electrode for clinical electroretinography. *Arch. Ophthal.*, 54, *940-941*, (1955).

Jacobson, J., Romaine, H.H., Halberg, G.P. & Stephens, G. The electrical activity of the eye during accomodation.*Am. J. Ophthal.*, 46, *231-238*, (1958).

Karpe, G. The basis of clinical electroretinography. *Acta Opthal. Supplementum*, 24, *1-118*, (1945).

Riggs, L.A. Continuous and reproducible records of the electrical activity of the human retina. *Proc. Soc. exp. Biol. Med.*, 48, *204-207*, (1941).

Schoessler, J.P. & Jones, R. A new corneal electrode for electroretinography. *Vision Res.*, 15, *299-301*, (1975).

Wündsch, L. & Lützow, A.V. Zur Ausschaltung des becquereleffektes in der elektroretinographie. *Experientia*, 25, *1119-1120*, (1969).

Authors' address:
Middlebrook House
261 Alfreton Road, Underwood
Nottinghamshire NG16 5 GX
England

CALIBRATION OF THE ERG STIMULUS

LYMAN C. NORDEN & NORMAN E. LEACH

(Birmingham, Alabama)

INTRODUCTION

Calibration of the photostimulus has long been a problem in clinical electroretinography. Each investigator must normalize his own apparatus with a series of normal subjects, and he is then unable to accurately compare his clinical findings with those of other investigators. He is also unable to monitor changes in his own apparatus as the components age or become altered, thus making follow up patient examinations less accurate.

Krill (1970) and others have shown that ERG amplitude and temporal characteristics are dependent on flash intensity. Burian (1970) has shown that the ERG is dependent on stimulus duration up to 100 milliseconds. Tsuchida, Kawasaki & Jacobson (1971) have shown that ERG readings follow Bloch's law (threshold stimulus intensity is inversely proportional to stimulus duration) for stimulus durations up to 100 milliseconds. The Bunson-Roscoe law states that, in photochemistry, the product of stimulus intensity and duration is a constant, for short flashes of light. Therefore, in order to express the most meaningful relationship between stimulus and response, the ERG photostimulus should be measured in footlambert-seconds, i.e., integrated light value.

Photometric calibration of the ERG stimulus is preferable to radiometric because we are accustomed to assessing vision function in photometric terms. However, the radiometric energy output of the photostimulus can be easily recorded with a sensitive photodiode connected to an oscilloscope. Conversion of this measured energy output to photometric units will then provide the investigator with a simpler and more reliable basis for the comparison and evaluation of clinical data.

THE PHOTOSTIMULUS

The Grass PS 22 photostimulator adapted to an integrating sphere (ganzfeld) appears to be the preferred stimulus for clinical electroretinography. The photostimulus used in this study follows the basic design recommended by Gouras (1970), Rabin & Berson (1974), and Gunkel, et. al. (1976). It consists of a PS 22 flash tube mounted at the top of a 16 inch integrating sphere with provision for the use of wavelength and neutral density filters.

The PS 22 is capable of producing a consistent, intense, short flash of light. The PS 22 instruction book rates the peak flash intensity at

19,000,000 lumens and the flash duration at 10 microseconds. However the conditions of its use can add considerable variability to the amount of light actually presented to the electroretinography patient.

The PS 22 flash tube is described as having a useful life of from 50 to 1000 hours depending on how it is used. As the flash tube ages it produces less light; therefore, the instruction book recommends the use of a suitable light meter for maximum accuracy in critical experiments.

The flash intensity also varies with the third power of the line voltage variation. As the instruction book states, this is probably not a significant variable in most cases because the visual response varies with logarithmic changes in stimulus intensity. However, specifying even small variations in stimulus intensity may be useful in more highly refined testing techniques.

Probably the largest variable in the ERG recording system lies within the design of the ganzfeld. The amount of light actually presented to the patient depends on factors such as: 1) the location of the flash tube in relation to the integrating sphere, 2) the size of the light aperture, 3) the use of a diffusing plate between the flash tube and the integrating sphere, and 4) the reflecting properties of the integrating sphere.

STANDARD PHOTOMETER

Rabin & Berson (1974) recommended calibrating the ERG photostimulus by generating a 50 Hz flicker of the PS 22 flash tube at its lowest intensity setting. This makes the stimulus nearly appear as a constant light source so it can be measured with a standard photometer. However, when measuring a flashing light source, one should consider the Talbot-Plateau law. This law states that the apparent intensity of an intermittent light is equal to the absolute peak intensity times the ratio of light duration divided by the interval between flashes.

At a frequency of 50 Hz, the interval between flashes is 0.02 seconds, or 20,000 microseconds. If the flash duration is 10 microseconds, the apparent intensity is equal to 10/20,000 = 0.0005 times the peak intensity. Conversely, the actual peak intensity should equal the apparent, or measured, intensity divided by 0.0005.

We used a Tektronix J-16 digital photometer to measure our photostimulus set at 50 Hz flicker on its lowest intensity setting. The measured value was 2.5 footlamberts. According to the formula above, the actual light value is 2.5/0.0005 = 5,000 footlamberts. The instruction book states that the intensity settings on the PS 22 are multiples of the lowest setting; therefore, the actual light values for the remaining intensity settings can be easily calculated as shown in Table 1.

In order to specify the stimulus luminance as an integrated light value, we must consider the stimulus wave form shown in Figure 1. Brunette & Molotchnikoff (1970) stated that multiplying the peak amplitude by the 1/3 peak duration is a simple means of approximating the integrated value. The diagram of the stimulus waveform in Figure 1 shows the 1/3 peak duration to be approximately 15 microseconds. If the peak amplitude is considered to be the calculated luminance value for each of the five intensity settings we can calculate the integrated light values as shown in Table 2.

All of the calculations above are, of course, based on the following assumptions: 1) stimulus duration is actually 10 microseconds, 2) the 1/3 peak duration is actually 15 microseconds, 3) flash frequency is actually 50 Hz, 4) actual flash intensities are exact multiples of the lowest intensity setting, and 5) the J-16 photometer actually responds to flickering light according to the Talbot-Plateau law.

Table I. Calculated peak luminance values for each of the PS 22 intensity settings

PS 22 Intensity Setting	Luminance (Footlamberts)
1	5,000
2	10,000
4	20,000
8	40,000
16	80,000

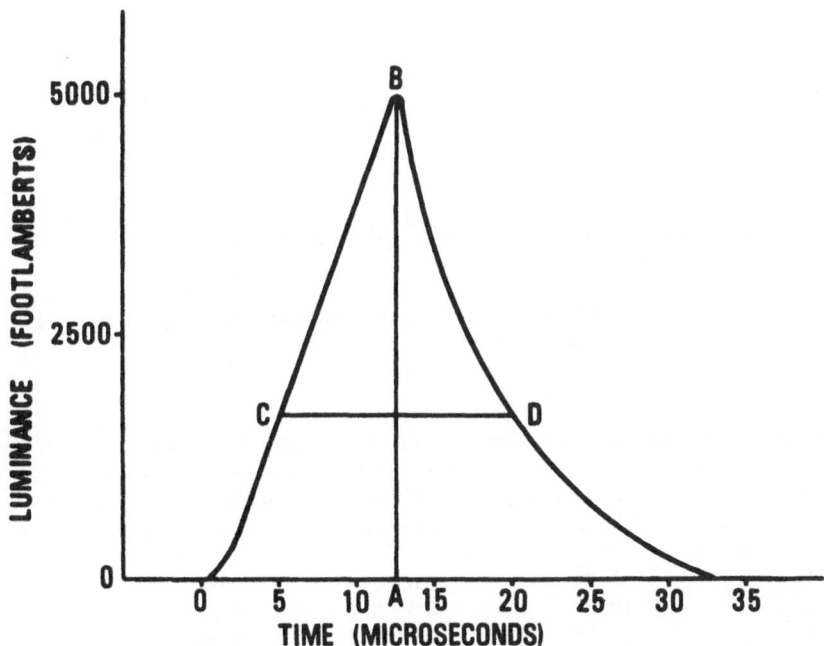

Fig. 1. PS 22 photostimulus waveform. Redrawn from the Grass PS 22 instruction book. AB = peak amplitude, CD = 1/3 peak duration.

PULSED LIGHT PHOTOMETER

We used a Pritchard 1980 PL (pulsed light) photometer to measure directly the single flash light output of our ERG photostimulus. The Pritchard is capable of measuring flash durations as short as 1 microsecond, and the integrated light values of single flashes as short as 10 microseconds. Its response may be calibrated according to either the standard photopic luminous efficiency curve or the standard scotopic luminous efficiency curve.

Our measurements were made with the Pritchard photometer placed one meter away from, and focused on, the posterior, inner surface of the ganzfeld. The PS 22 flash duration was recorded (Figure 2) and found to corres-

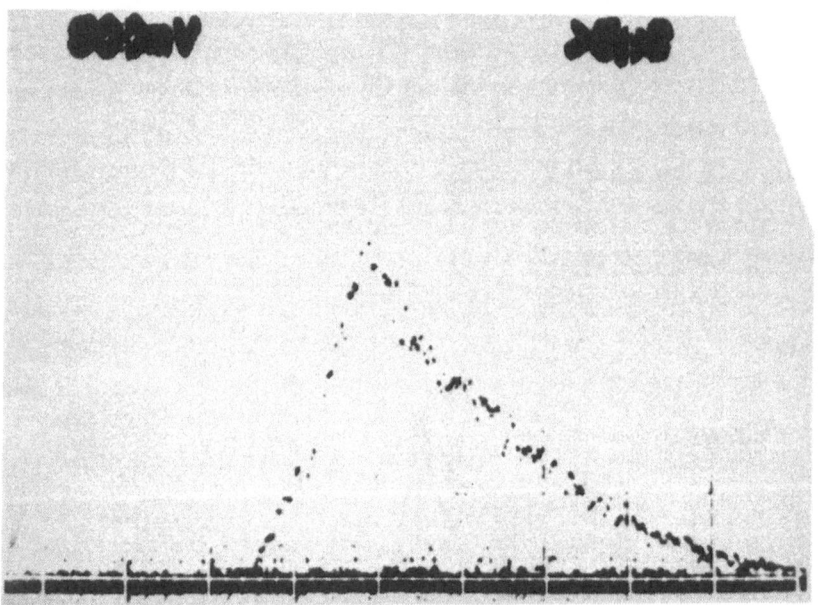

Fig. 2. PS 22 flash duration recorded with the Pritchard 1980 PL photometer. Horizontal scale, 5 μ S per division.

Table II. Calculated integrated light values for each of the PS 22 intensity settings

PS 22 Intensity Setting	Peak Luminance (Footlamberts)	1/3 Peak Duration (Seconds)	Integrated Light Value (Footlambert-Seconds)
1	5,000	0.000015	0.075
2	10,000	0.000015	0.150
4	20,000	0.000015	0.300
8	40,000	0.000015	0.600
16	80,000	0.000015	1.200

pond with the diagram of the stimulus flash in the PS 22 instruction book.

We then measured five single flash luminances for each of the five intensity settings on the PS 22 photostimulator. The means and standard deviations for these measurements are listed in Table 3.

We also measured the flash luminances for a series of neutral density

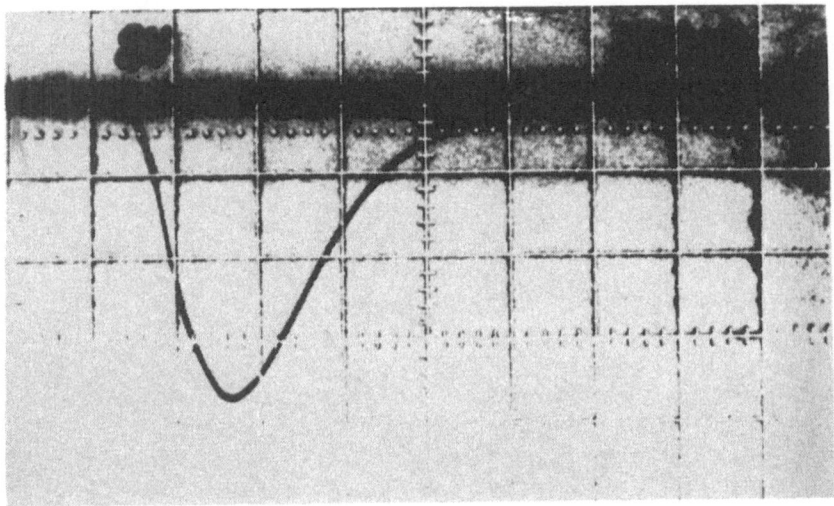

Fig. 3. SGD-100A photodiode response. Vertical scale, 2 V per division. Horizontal scale, 10 uS per division.

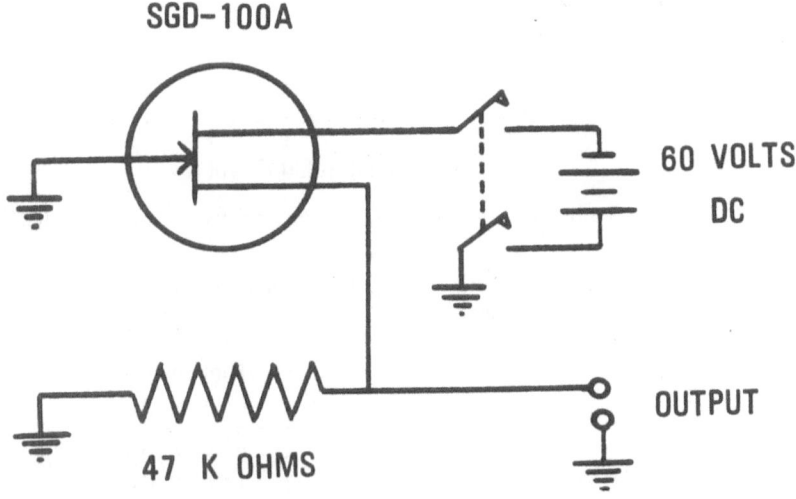

Fig. 4. Photodiode apparatus. SGD-100A photodiode from: EEG Elector-Optics Division, 35 Congress St., Salem, MA 01970.

filters interposed between the flash tube and the integrating sphere. The means and standard deviations for these measurements are listed in Table 4.

We then measured the flash luminances for the long and short wavelength filters used for both photopic and scotopic ERG recording. The flash luminances for the scotopic ERG filters were measured on the instrument's

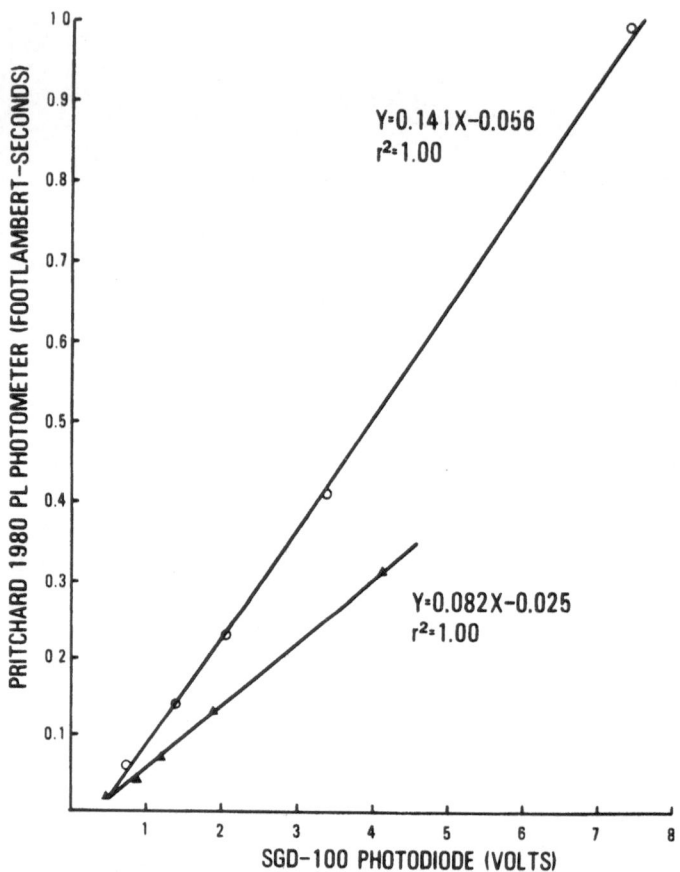

$$Y=0.141X-0.056$$
$$r^2=1.00$$

$$Y=0.082X-0.025$$
$$r^2=1.00$$

Fig. 5. SGD-100A photodiode vs. Pritchard photometer o white light; ▲ Wratten #21

Table III. Measured integrated light values and SGD-100A photodiode output for each of the PS 22 settings

PS 22 Intensity Setting	Integrated Light Value (Footlambert-Seconds)	Photodiode (Volts)
1	0.06 ± 0.004	0.74 ± 0.010
2	0.14 ± 0.010	1.41 ± 0.010
4	0.23 ± 0.020	2.05 ± 0
8	0.41 ± 0.010	3.37 ± 0.060
16	0.99 ± 0.060	7.36 ± 0.900

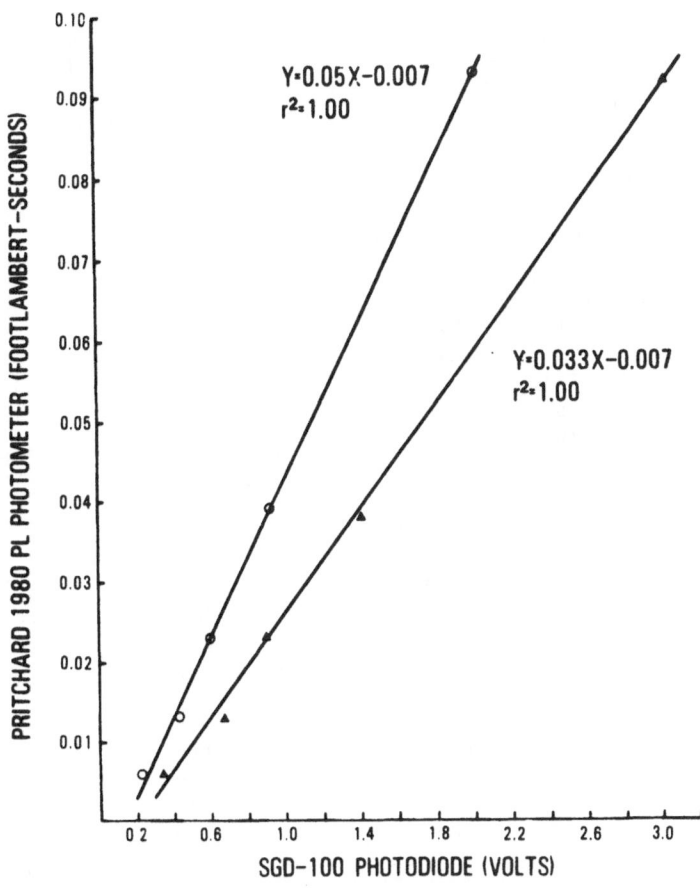

Fig. 6. SGD-100A photodiode vs. Pritchard photometer o Wratten #22, ND 0.4; ▲ Wratten #65A.

Table IV. Measured integrated light values and SGD-100A photodiode output for a series of ND filters. PS 22 intensity setting at 16

Filter	Integrated Light Value (Footlambert-Seconds)	Photodiode (Volts)
Clear Glass	0.85000 ± 0.04000	6.00 ± 0
ND 0.5	0.24000 ± 0.01000	2.49 ± 0.010
ND 1.0	0.07700 ± 0.00300	1.04 ± 0.010
ND 1.5	0.02700 ± 0.00100	0.53 ± 0.010
ND 2.0	0.00700 ± 0	0.25 ± 0.003
ND 2.5	0.00190 ± 0.00100	0.11 ± 0.010
ND 3.0	0.00054 ± 0.00003	0.06 ± 0

Table V. Integrated light values and photodiode output for each of the PS 22 intensity settings using long and short wavelength photopic ERG filters. #21 and #22, long wavelength. #65A, short wavelength. #22, ND 0.4 and #65A are photopically balanced.

PS 22 Intensity Setting	Integrated Light Value (Footlambert-Seconds)	Photodiode (Volts)
Wratten #21		
1	0.018	0.46
2	0.044	0.88
4	0.073	1.20
8	0.128	1.90
16	0.312	4.10
Wratten #22, ND 0.4		
1	0.006	0.23
2	0.013	0.43
4	0.022	0.60
8	0.039	0.92
16	0.093	2.00
Wratten #65A		
1	0.006	0.36
2	0.013	0.66
4	0.023	0.90
8	0.038	1.40
16	0.092	3.00

photopic luminous efficiency curve, and the flash luminances for the scotopic ERG filters were measured on the scotopic luminous efficiency curve. The results of these measurements for the five intensity settings on the PS 22 are listed in Tables 5 and 6, respectively.

Photodiode

Compared to the Pritchard 1980 PL photometer, a sensitive photodiode is a relatively inexpensive and much more portable device which can be used to measure the single flash energy output of the ERG photostimulus. For direct detection of stimulus energy by a photodiode, the signal current (iDD) is equal to the signal power (Ps) times a constant factor $(\frac{nq}{nv})$ for a given wavelength, where n = quantum efficiency, hv = quantum energy, and q = electronic charge (Compton, 1975). Therefore, the photodiode current will be directly proportional to the stimulus power, and the amplitude of the photodiode response displayed on the oscilloscope will be directly proportional to the radiant intensity of the photostimulus. The photodiode response can then be calibrated to the photometric measurement of the stimulus.

We used an SGD-100A photodiode for measurements of our photo-stimulus because its ability to respond to an extremely short flash of light (Figure 3). The photodiode apparatus (Figure 4) was temporarily mounted on the Pritchard photometer so that simultaneous measurements could be made on our ERG photostimulus. The front surface of the photodiode was positioned one meter away from the posterior, inner surface of the ganzfeld. The output was connected by a cable with 550 ohms rated resistance to a Tektronix 7313 storage oscilloscope. These measurements are also listed in Tables 3, 4, 5 and 6.

These data were then plotted on graphs so that any future measurements made with the photodiode apparatus can be easily converted to photometric units (Figures 5, 6, and 7). Since the SGD-100A photodiode response to different wavelengths does not coincide with that of the Pritchard photo-meter, we must use a separate graph for each wavelength filter.

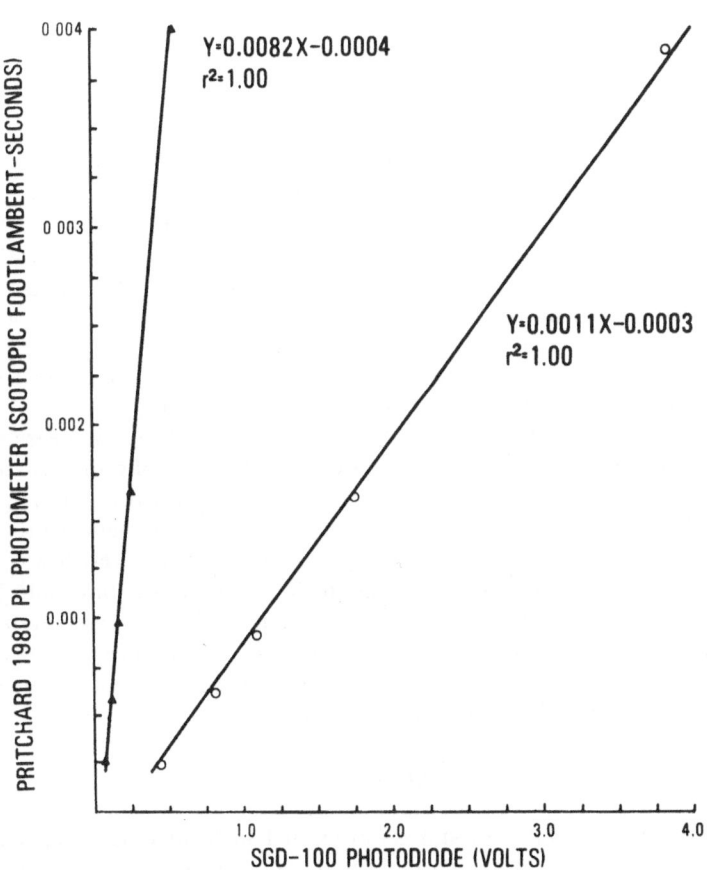

Fig. 7. SGD-100A photodiode vs. Pritchard photometer, o Wratten #26; ▲ Wratten #47, 47A, 47B, ND 1.0

401

Table VI. Integrated light values and photodiode output for each of the PS 22 intensity settings using long and short wavelength scotopic ERG filters. #26, long wavelength. #47, 47A, 47B, ND 1.0, short wavelength, scotopically balanced

PS 22 Intensity Settings	Integrated Light Value (Footlambert-Seconds)	Photodiode (Volts)
Wratten #26		
1	0.00023	0.44
2	0.00055	0.82
4	0.00090	1.10
8	0.00161	1.75
16	0.00390	3.80
Wratten #47, 47A, 47B, ND 1.0		
1	0.00024	0.07
2	0.00056	0.13
4	0.00093	0.17
8	0.00166	0.26
16	0.00400	0.54

CONCLUSION

The calculated integrated light values for the ERG photostimulus using the Tektronix J-16 digital photometer correspond relatively well with the actual values as measured with the Prichard 1980 PL photometer. The variations between these values are probably not highly significant since the visual system generally responds according to logarithmic changes in stimulus intensity. However, the necessary calculations are based on a number of assumptions that we would rather not have to make.

The Pritchard 1980 PL photometer enables us to directly measure the single flash luminance of the ERG stimulus in convenient, photometric terms. But it is a rather expensive instrument to be used only for this purpose.

The SGD-100A photodiode apparatus is well suited for calibration of the ERG stimulus because of its accuracy, portability, and relatively low cost. It is capable of measuring the photostimulus in photometric units, and these measurements appear to be more precise than the human visual response. With the aid of this calibration device, the ERG can more accurately assess retinal function in the clinic and the data obtained in one clinic can be more confidently compared to data from other clinics.

SUMMARY

The ERG photostimulus should be calibrated in footlambert-seconds, i.e. integrated light value. A standard photometer can be used to form a reasonable estimate of the integrated light value. The Pritchard 1980 PL photometer enables us to accurately measure the integrated light value. The